HIKE

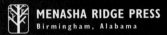
MENASHA RIDGE PRESS
Birmingham, Alabama

60 HIKES WITHIN 60 MILES

SACRAMENTO

INCLUDING
AUBURN, FOLSOM, AND DAVIS

SECOND EDITION

JORDAN SUMMERS

60 HIKES WITHIN 60 MILES: SACRAMENTO

Copyright © 2012 Jordan Summers
All rights reserved
Printed in the United States of America
Published by Menasha Ridge Press
Distributed by Publishers Group West
Second edition, first printing

Library of Congress Cataloging-in-Publication Data

Summers, Jordan, 1951–
    60 hikes within 60 miles, Sacramento : including Auburn, Folsom, and Davis / Jordan Summers.
        p. cm. — (60 hikes within 60 miles)

    Summary: "Hiking enthusiast Jordan Summers introduces area residents and visitors to an array of the best day hikes from casual riverside nature hikes to rugged foothill treks within roughly an hour's drive of Sacramento. Carefully researched on foot and filled with detailed descriptions of firsthand trail notes, this newly updated edition of *60 Hikes within 60 Miles: Sacramento* helps hikers discover their choices with concise at-a-glance information highlighting details such as location, access, directions, distances, scenery, and preparation details that help hikers get the most from each outing. Precise maps, descriptive text, photos, and trailhead coordinates guide you on your way quickly and keep you on route reliably. Discover the varied geology, the cultural history, and the natural beauty of the Foothills, Mother Lode, and Delta Regions in *60 Hikes within 60 Miles: Sacramento*." —Provided by publisher.

    ISBN-13: 978-0-89732-604-9 (pbk.)
    ISBN-10: 0-89732-604-0 ()
    1. Hiking—California—Sacramento Region—Guidebooks. 2. Sacramento Region (Calif.)—Guidebooks. I. Title. II. Title: Sixty hikes within sixty miles, Sacramento.
    GV199.42.C22S239 2012
    796.5109794'5—dc23

                        2012008680

Editor: Ritchey Halphen
Cover design: Scott McGrew
Cartography and elevation profiles: Steve Jones, Scott McGrew, and Jordan Summers
Text design: Steveco International
Cover and interior photos: Jordan Summers
Author photo: Karin Connolly
Photo editor–proofreader: Donna Poehner
Indexer: Rich Carlson

Menasha Ridge Press
P.O. Box 43673
Birmingham, AL 35243
menasharidge.com

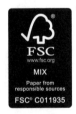 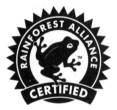

DISCLAIMER

TO MY GRANDCHILDREN—TAYLOR, DEACON, AND FINN—HIKING AS FAR AS THEY CAN, WHENEVER THEY WANT.

— JORDAN SUMMERS

TABLE of CONTENTS

ACKNOWLEDGMENTS

SHARING THE OUTDOORS—helping hikers of all abilities get out there, have fun out there, and return safely from there—is one of my passions, one that I could realize only with the guidance, knowledge, and support of many people, a considerable number of whom are unaware of their important contributions.

I am so grateful to Molly Merkle at Menasha Ridge Press for giving me the opportunity to write this second edition of *60 Hikes within 60 Miles: Sacramento.* And I am especially grateful to Ritchey Halphen for his patience, coaching, and project expertise, without which there would be no guidebook for you to follow. I also owe thanks to fellow outdoor activist Rachel Freytag for her help in getting this book into hikers' hands.

A sincere recognition is due to the many volunteers and trail crews who have worked so hard to create or maintain the trails described in this book. We would be unable to visit such beautiful wild places without these folks' valuable contributions.

I'm grateful as well to the many rangers, park volunteers, and fellow hikers who gladly answered my questions, helped me pinpoint features, or told me about interesting hikes, trailheads, conditions, scenery, or natural history.

In particular, I owe thanks to the overnight crew of the Cool Fire Department, for their help with temporary parking situations; to miners Mike and Ken, who filled me in on their friend Dan—the lost miner of Euchre Bar; to Kathy Brown at the Cosumnes River Preserve, for explaining riparian-area trail closures; to Jennifer Reed with the Yolo County Flood Control and Water Conservation District, for schooling me in seasonal water releases and flow rates; to our friend Deb Young, for her reality checks regarding my difficulty-rating system; and especially to Tami Rakstad-Schaner of the Calaveras Big Trees Association and Wendy Harrison of California State Parks, for their knowledge of trails, natural history, and local information at Calaveras Big Trees and Indian Grinding Rock state parks.

Additional thanks are due to Jim Ricker and Ron Gould and volunteers of the North Fork American River Alliance, who are continuing the efforts of Russell Towle to preserve historic trails, or access to them, in the North Fork region. I am grateful for their efforts and their advice on hiking the Green Valley Trail from the Alta trailhead.

I truly appreciate the efforts of Erin Harrington at REI, Sara and Michael Barlow at Trailmix.net, and Sandra and Steve Felderstein, along with their fellow supporters of the Sacramento Library Foundation, in helping popularize this guidebook.

And as steps go, hiking with friends is the best way to do it. Trey Ish and his daughter, Katie, brought along "Cookie Dave" for a great day on Ruck-A-Chucky Rapids Trail. My friend Trig Rosenblatt joined me in hiking River of Skulls and Lodi Lake trails and dished out words of support whenever I needed them.

My daughter, Ashley, and her three children joined my partner, Karin, and me in hiking the Independence Trail's West Branch. My grandson Deacon shouldered a pack and hiked with me on the East Branch. Ashley met me early for hikes on American Canyon–Dead Truck, Diggins Loop, and Humbug trails. Karin handled several urban and Delta hikes as well.

I am deeply grateful to Karin—who wanted to be with me on every hike but waited patiently for me at home for most; who kept me supplied with trail bars and hydrating mix; who made breakfast for every predawn departure; who viewed pictures of every feather, cone, leaf, rock, and flower; who approved of each of my new gear requirements; and who cheerfully encouraged me with her excitement to hear of each new hike.

—*Jordan Summers*
Elk Grove, California, 2012

FOREWORD

WELCOME TO MENASHA RIDGE PRESS'S *60 Hikes within 60 Miles.* Our strategy was simple: First, find a hiker who knows the area and loves to hike. Second, ask that person to spend a year researching the most popular and very best trails around. And third, have that person describe each trail in terms of difficulty, scenery, condition, elevation change, and all other categories of information that are important to hikers. "Pretend you've just completed a hike and met up with other hikers at the trailhead," we told each author. "Imagine their questions, and be clear in your answers." An experienced hiker and writer, author Jordan Summers has selected 60 of the best hikes in and around the Sacramento metropolitan area. From the greenways and urban hikes that make use of parklands to flora- and fauna-rich treks along the cliffs and hills in the Foothills, he provides hikers (and walkers) with a great variety of hikes—and all within roughly 60 miles of Sacramento.

You'll get more out of this book if you take a moment to read the Introduction, which explains how to read the trail listings. The "Topographic Maps" section will help you understand how useful topos will be on a hike, and will also tell you where to get them. And though this is a where-to rather than a how-to guide, those of you who have not hiked extensively will find the Introduction of particular value. As much for the opportunity to free the spirit as well as to free the body, let these hikes elevate you above the urban hurry.

All the best,
The Editors at Menasha Ridge Press

ABOUT THE AUTHOR

JORDAN SUMMERS has had more fun sleeping on rock, snow, and dirt than any one person should be allowed.

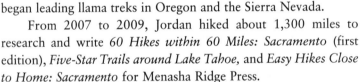

As a boy in Virginia, he would camp in the woods behind his house. Since then, he's spent absurd amounts of time in the three major ranges and many minor ones, and in forests, canyons, and deserts in every season and weather condition.

Quite naturally, Jordan's children were both veteran hikers by the age of 5. They became llama-wranglers and guides a few years later, when their dad said goodbye to Santa Monica, California, and began leading llama treks in Oregon and the Sierra Nevada.

From 2007 to 2009, Jordan hiked about 1,300 miles to research and write *60 Hikes within 60 Miles: Sacramento* (first edition), *Five-Star Trails around Lake Tahoe,* and *Easy Hikes Close to Home: Sacramento* for Menasha Ridge Press.

In 2009, Jordan solo-hiked 1,100 miles of the Pacific Crest Trail from the California–Mexico border to Echo Lake Dam. Dedicated to a young family friend, his hike raised significant contributions for RP Fighting Blindness's genetic research to cure retinitis pigmentosa, an inherited eye disease that causes sudden-onset blindness in young adults. The hike's theme: . . . *to see what I can see.*

Jordan is an alumnus of the National Outdoor Leadership School (NOLS) Wilderness Outdoor Educator program, a Leave No Trace trainer, and an NOLS/Wilderness Medicine Institute–certified Wilderness First Responder. All of these affiliations help him pursue his passion: to help hikers of all abilities get out there, have a great time there, leave no trace there, and come home safely from there.

A volunteer for the Tahoe Rim Trail Association, Jordan lives in the Sacramento suburb of Elk Grove, California, with his partner, Karin Connolly. Most importantly, he and Karin frequently get to hike with his children and grandchildren.

PREFACE

MY FIRST HIKES as a 6-year-old were wonderful experiences among the frogs and snakes, the turtles and crayfish, the poison ivy and mosquitoes. I would drag my army-surplus pup tent to a clear spot in the big trees near the creek at my home in Virginia. A sandwich was dinner. The stars were my night-light. And I was always home by breakfast. Honestly, the first song I ever learned was "The Bear Went over the Mountain."

So it's no exaggeration to say that I truly have a passion for hiking. I've had the good fortune to have lived on both coasts, in both the North and South, and in between. And I can sincerely say that hiking has never been better than it is here now in the Sacramento region.

Sacramento is considered the gateway to the central Sierra Nevada. Interstate 80 and US 50 lead from Sacramento to the crystal-clear waters of Lake Tahoe and the snowcapped ridges of the Pacific Crest. Millions of avid outdoor enthusiasts pass through the Sacramento Valley and the Foothills annually on their way to these natural treasures.

In the days before European settlement, this area served as an important gateway for Native Americans. The Maidu, Nisenan, Miwok, and others capitalized on this lush riparian land for trading opportunities, valuable food crops, and plentiful game migrations.

Then the Gold Rush opened up Sacramento as the gateway for the miners, ranchers, farmers, anglers, loggers, and engineers who followed them. And the Sacramento region continues today as a gateway for outdoor recreation.

From strolls down a riverside promenade in the city to near-vertical monster slopes in a remote river canyon, there's something here for all types of hikers. Broad tidal marshlands, verdant riparian woodlands, crystal-clear creeks, cascading streams, plummeting waterfalls, ice-cold swimming holes, wild rushing rivers, old-growth forests, historic mining towns, colorful profusions of

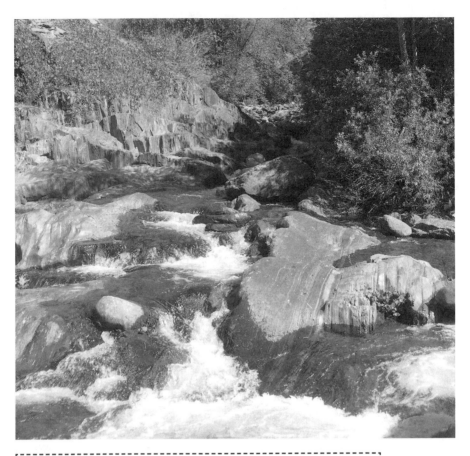

The North Fork of the Middle Fork of the American River displays its geologic treats at El Dorado Canyon.

wildflowers, and a dozen other wonderful things can be found within a 60-mile radius of Sacramento.

Of course, there are the expected attractions: wildflowers, rivers, trees, and photo opportunities on every hike. However, this book touches on the special things, the hidden gems that make each hike memorable in its way. Stand on the porch of a forty-niner's cabin and behold his view of the river. Walk through a grove of valley oaks more than half a millennium old whose acorns the Miwok women turned into flour on the ancient grinding rock. Walk across the windswept grasses atop a levee, where you might see, in a single day, endangered, threatened, and migrating bird species nesting or feeding there.

Whether you're new to the area or a resident trail vet, you'll discover something new in this book. The websites I've included should lead you to further investigation about hikes and history in this region. *Did you know that Yankee Jim was hanged for attempting to steal a schooner in San Diego?*

If you're an experienced hiker but you want to learn more natural history, a number of the hikes I've profiled have excellent interpretive displays. You may rediscover a trail that you haven't thought about for years, or you could learn about a new one just around the corner.

Preparing for the hikes is just part of the fun. Check the details and, with the information in this book, some maps, and pleasant weather, you're off—as that song from my childhood says—*to see what you can see.*

ABOUT THE HIKES

With the help of Google Earth, we can visualize the Sacramento region: the Sacramento Valley, the Delta, and the Foothills. No single word can characterize the diverse geography of this area.

The Sacramento Valley, almost featureless except for the Sutter Buttes, is surrounded by rugged and interesting terrain. The Yuba River joins the Feather and then adds the Bear before becoming the Sacramento River in the north. To the west are the Coast Ranges, which trend northwest–southeast from the coast right up to the valley. The southern border is broken by slough and levee, holding the fresh- and salt water in a delicate balance at the confluence of the Sacramento and San Joaquin rivers above San Pablo Bay. The east is filled with the tortured geology of continents in collision. Its river canyons claw their way from their source in the snows of the Sierra Nevada: the North, Middle, and South forks of the American River and the Rubicon, Cosumnes, Mokelumne, and Calaveras rivers all make their mark and add to the physical and historic makeup of the Foothills.

SACRAMENTO AND VICINITY

Sacramento is known as the City of Trees, and its dozens of neighborhood parks are notable for their majestic arbors. Sacramento's Capitol Park, William Land Park, and the University of California, Davis, Arboretum have excellent trails that wind through magnificent tree displays.

WEST SACRAMENTO VALLEY

Tule elk, bald eagles, and a host of mammals and birds make the dry hills to the west of the Sacramento Valley their home. The hills run northwest–southeast and edge right up to the valley about 10 miles west of Interstate 5. The lands that are open to the public here are often administered jointly by the U.S. Bureau of Land Management (BLM) and the California Department of Fish and Game. Hunting is regulated in the Cache Creek Natural Area. Summers are brutally dry in these hills, making hydration a real challenge. However, Cache Creek flows year-round. It not only has excellent whitewater recreation but also attracts migratory birds. The spring and fall migrations offer spectacular wildlife-viewing opportunities.

DELTA AREA

The Sacramento–San Joaquin River Delta drains virtually the entire western slope of the Sierra Nevada. This inverted delta, one of only a few worldwide, creates a tidal marshland that is an important resting spot for migrating waterfowl. The recovery of the Delta region is a fascinating story, and you can learn about it while visiting Grizzly Island Wildlife Area or the Cosumnes River Preserve. The California Department of Fish and Game and The Nature Conservancy, along with other contributing organizations, have allied to preserve several remaining examples of the once-vast riparian forest in this area.

FOOTHILLS SOUTH

Bounded only by an arbitrary line approximately along US 50 to Tahoe, the southern Foothills area has gems that beg to be explored. There are no straight lines here, so driving times would be outlandish if the roads weren't in such beautiful country. It is a stretch to see the Big Trees, but a stretch that's worthwhile, and one not to be found any closer. The dams and reservoirs on the Calaveras and Mokelumne rivers protect against floods, provide reliable drinking water, and offer excellent hiking and other recreational opportunities.

FOOTHILLS CENTRAL

In an ideal world, great hikes would be equally distributed for easy access by all. The area from US 50 along the South Fork of the American River to Interstate 80, including the Middle and North forks, is truly outdoors central. The natural features here offer hiking enthusiasts of all persuasions something exciting and memorable. Home of the Mother Lode, birthplace of the Gold Rush, and route of the Emigrant Trail and Pony Express, the Foothills between Placerville and Auburn are as exciting a place for day hikes as any in the country. Six sites hiked here are listed on the National Register of Historic Places. You can discover even more historic sites by taking the route less traveled to explore on your own.

Access is arranged largely along the canyons of the American's three forks and the Yuba's south fork. The North Fork of the American is reachable from both I-80 and Foresthill Road, which also provides access to its Middle Fork. The South Fork is reached via CA 49 through either Auburn or Placerville. The confluence of the North and Middle forks is a focal point of activity in the Auburn State Recreation Area, where I hiked many fine routes for this book. The North and South forks are united at the upper end of Folsom Lake State Recreation Area, accessible from both I-80 and US 50.

FOOTHILLS NORTH

On the north side of I-80, the hikes lead to geologically interesting features and Gold Rush–era sites. The South Yuba River trailheads can be accessed from Marysville or Nevada City. They lead to such historic locations as the longest single-span wood-covered bridge in the United States, the richest hardrock gold mine and largest hydraulic gold mine of the era, and the first wheelchair-accessible wilderness trail in the nation.

RECOMMENDED HIKES

HIKE CATEGORIES

> ✓ configuration
> ✓ difficulty
> ✓ length (mi.)
>
> ✓ bird-watching
> ✓ dogs permitted
>
> ✓ easiest
> ✓ flat

REGION / Hike #/Hike name	page	configuration	difficulty	length (mi.)	bird-watching	dogs permitted	easiest	flat
SACRAMENTO AND VICINITY								
1 Capitol Park Loop	22	Loop	Cakewalk	2	✓	✓	✓	✓
2 Old Sacramento State Historic Park	26	Loops	Cakewalk	1.75		✓	✓	✓
3 Riverwalk Park	30	Out-and-back	Cakewalk	1.5	✓	✓	✓	✓
4 William Land Park Trail	34	Out-and-back	Cakewalk	3	✓	✓	✓	✓
5 Effie Yeaw Nature Center Trails	37	Loops	Easy	2.5	✓		✓	✓
6 UC Davis Arboretum Trail	42	Loop	Cakewalk	3.5	✓		✓	✓
7 Davis–Covell Greenbelt	46	Loop	Cakewalk	2.7		✓	✓	✓
WEST SACRAMENTO VALLEY								
8 Homestead– Blue Ridge Trail	52	Loop	Challenging	5.1	✓			
9 Blue Ridge– Fiske Peak Trail	59	Out-and-back	Challenging	8.6	✓	✓		
10 High Bridge Trail	64	Out-and-back	Moderate	5.6	✓	✓		
11 Judge Davis Trail	68	Out-and-back	Challenging	11.5	✓	✓		
12 Redbud Trail	72	Out-and-back	Hard	15.5	✓	✓		
13 Perkins Creek Ridge Trail	77	Out-and-back	Hard	12.4	✓	✓		
14 Johnson Ridge– Gunsight Rock Trail	81	Out-and-back	Challenging	9.2	✓	✓		

REGION Hike #/Hike name	page	configuration	difficulty	length (mi.)	bird-watching	dogs permitted	easiest	flat
DELTA AREA								
15 Grizzly Island Wildlife Area Trail	88	Loop	Easy	4.5	✓		✓	✓
16 River Bend–Majestic Oaks Loop Trail	92	Loop	Easy	3	✓		✓	✓
17 Lodi Lake Nature Trail	97	Loops	Cakewalk	2.5	✓		✓	✓
18 Cosumnes River Preserve Trails	101	Loops	Cakewalk	4.1	✓		✓	✓
FOOTHILLS SOUTH								
19 China Gulch Trail	108	Out-and-back	Challenging	11	✓			
20 River of Skulls Trail	113	Loop	Cakewalk	1		✓		
21 Big Trees North Grove Trails	117	Loops	Cakewalk	3			✓	✓
22 Big Trees South Grove Trail	122	Out-and-back	Moderate	5.4				
23 Indian Grinding Rock Loop Trails	128	Loops	Cakewalk	1.8			✓	✓
24 Jenkinson Lake Trail	133	Loop	Moderate	9		✓		✓
FOOTHILLS CENTRAL								
25 Pioneer Express Trail	140	Out-and-back	Moderate	9.5				
26 Avery's Pond Trail	144	Out-and-back	Easy	4.1			✓	✓
27 Rattlesnake Bar–Horseshoe Bar Trail	149	Out-and-back	Easy	4.7		✓	✓	
28 Sweetwater Trail	153	Out-and-back	Moderate	5.4		✓		✓
29 Monroe Ridge Trail	157	Loop	Moderate	2.9				
30 Dave Moore Nature Area Trail	161	Loop	Cakewalk	1.1	✓	✓	✓	✓
31 South Fork American River–Gerle Loop Trail	165	Loop	Easy	2.6		✓		✓

HIKE CATEGORIES

✓ configuration	✓ bird-watching	✓ easiest
✓ difficulty	✓ dogs permitted	✓ flat
✓ length (mi.)		

REGION Hike #/Hike name	page	configuration	difficulty	length (mi.)	bird-watching	dogs permitted	easiest	flat
32 South Fork American River Trail	169	Point-to-point	Challenging	11.6		✓		
33 Cronan Ranch Trails	174	Loops	Moderate	4.5		✓		
34 Olmstead Loop Trail	178	Loop	Moderate	9	✓			
35 Robie Point Firebreak Trail	183	Out-and-back	Moderate	6		✓		
36 Lake Clementine Trail	187	Out-and-back	Moderate	4.4		✓		
37 Confluence Trail	192	Out-and-back	Easy	3.5		✓		
38 Quarry Road Trail to American Canyon Falls	195	Out-and-back	Challenging	14.5		✓		
39 American Canyon–Dead Truck Trail	200	Loop	Moderate	5.3		✓		
40 Wendell T. Robie Trail	204	Out-and-back	Challenging	8.5		✓		
41 Ruck-A-Chucky Rapids Trail	208	Out-and-back	Moderate	6.4		✓		
42 Foresthill Divide Loop Trail	213	Loop	Moderate	10		✓		
43 Codfish Falls Trail	218	Out-and-back	Easy	3			✓	
44 North Fork Middle Fork American Trail	223	Out-and-back	Moderate	2.2		✓		
45 Yankee Jim's–Indian Creek Trail	229	Out-and-back	Moderate	3		✓		
46 Windy Point Trail	234	Out-and-back	Moderate	3				
47 Stevens Trail West	238	Out-and-back	Moderate	7.4		✓		
48 Stevens Trail East	244	Out-and-back	Moderate	7		✓		
49 Green Valley Trail	249	Out-and-back	Hard	6	✓	✓		
50 Euchre Bar Trail to Humbug Canyon	254	Out-and-back	Challenging	8.8				
51 American Eagle Mine Trail	259	Out-and-back	Moderate	1.8				
FOOTHILLS NORTH								
52 Hidden Falls Trails	266	Connected loops	Moderate	5.5		✓		
53 Fairy Falls Trail	271	Out-and-back	Moderate	5.1		✓		
54 Hardrock Trail	276	Loops	Moderate	4.4			✓	
55 Independence Trail: East Branch	280	Out-and-back	Easy	4.5			✓	✓

REGION Hike #/Hike name		page	configuration	difficulty	length (mi.)	bird-watching	dogs permitted	easiest	flat
FOOTHILLS NORTH (continued)									
56	Independence Trail: West Branch	284	Out-and-back	Easy	4.8			✓	✓
57	Buttermilk Bend Trail	288	Out-and-back	Easy	2.5			✓	
58	Point Defiance Trail	292	Out-and-back	Moderate	2				
59	Humbug Trail	296	Out-and-back	Moderate	5.6				
60	Diggins Loop Trail	300	Loops	Moderate	5.4				

HIKE CATEGORIES

✓ configuration
✓ difficulty
✓ length (mi.)

✓ bird-watching
✓ dogs permitted

✓ easiest
✓ flat

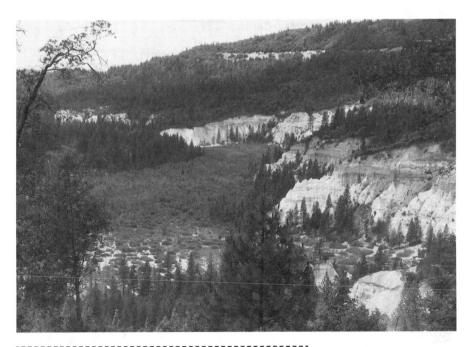

The scars left behind after the Gold Rush, such as the ones here at Malakoff Diggins State Historic Park, are slowly fading.

MORE RECOMMENDED HIKES

HIKE CATEGORIES

- ✓ handicapped access
- ✓ historical sites/ruins
- ✓ jogging
- ✓ kids
- ✓ most difficult
- ✓ streams/rivers
- ✓ steep
- ✓ waterfalls/cascades
- ✓ wildflowers
- ✓ wildlife-viewing

REGION / Hike #/Hike name	handicapped access	historical sites/ruins	jogging	kids	most difficult	streams and rivers	steep	waterfalls/cascades	wildflowers	wildlife-viewing
SACRAMENTO AND VICINITY										
1 Capitol Park Loop	✓		✓	✓					✓	
2 Old Sacramento State Historic Park	✓	✓	✓	✓		✓				
3 Riverwalk Park	✓		✓	✓		✓				
4 William Land Park Trail	✓		✓	✓					✓	
5 Effie Yeaw Nature Center Trails	✓		✓	✓		✓			✓	✓
6 UC Davis Arboretum Trail	✓		✓	✓					✓	
7 Davis–Covell Greenbelt	✓		✓	✓						
WEST SACRAMENTO VALLEY										
8 Homestead–Blue Ridge Trail		✓			✓	✓	✓	✓	✓	✓
9 Blue Ridge–Fiske Peak Trail					✓				✓	✓
10 High Bridge Trail				✓		✓			✓	✓
11 Judge Davis Trail					✓	✓			✓	✓
12 Redbud Trail					✓	✓			✓	
13 Perkins Creek Ridge Trail					✓		✓		✓	✓
14 Johnson Ridge–Gunsight Rock Trail					✓				✓	

REGION Hike #/Hike name	handicapped access	historical sites/ruins	jogging	kids	most difficult	streams and rivers	steep	waterfalls/cascades	wildflowers	wildlife-viewing
DELTA AREA										
15 Grizzly Island Wildlife Area Trail			✓			✓			✓	✓
16 River Bend–Majestic Oaks Loop Trail	✓			✓		✓			✓	✓
17 Lodi Lake Nature Trail	✓			✓		✓			✓	✓
18 Cosumnes River Preserve Trails	✓			✓		✓			✓	✓
FOOTHILLS SOUTH										
19 China Gulch Trail			✓						✓	
20 River of Skulls Trail				✓		✓			✓	
21 Big Trees North Grove Trails	✓			✓					✓	
22 Big Trees South Grove Trail				✓		✓			✓	
23 Indian Grinding Rock Loop Trails	✓	✓		✓					✓	
24 Jenkinson Lake Trail			✓	✓		✓		✓	✓	
FOOTHILLS CENTRAL										
25 Pioneer Express Trail	✓		✓	✓		✓				
26 Avery's Pond Trail		✓		✓					✓	
27 Rattlesnake Bar–Horseshoe Bar Trail			✓	✓						
28 Sweetwater Trail				✓						
29 Monroe Ridge Trail		✓		✓		✓				✓
30 Dave Moore Nature Area Trail	✓	✓		✓		✓			✓	✓
31 South Fork American River–Gerle Loop Trail			✓	✓		✓			✓	✓
32 South Fork American River Trail					✓	✓			✓	✓
33 Cronan Ranch Trails		✓	✓	✓		✓			✓	✓
34 Olmstead Loop Trail			✓			✓			✓	✓
35 Robie Point Firebreak Trail			✓	✓		✓			✓	
36 Lake Clementine Trail		✓	✓	✓		✓			✓	

REGION / Hike #/Hike name	handicapped access	historical sites/ruins	jogging	kids	most difficult	streams and rivers	steep	waterfalls/cascades	wildflowers	wildlife-viewing
37 Confluence Trail			✓	✓		✓			✓	
38 Quarry Road Trail to American Canyon Falls		✓	✓	✓		✓		✓		
39 American Canyon–Dead Truck Trail						✓	✓	✓		
40 Wendell T. Robie Trail						✓		✓	✓	
41 Ruck-A-Chucky Rapids Trail		✓	✓	✓		✓		✓		
42 Foresthill Divide Loop Trail			✓			✓			✓	✓
43 Codfish Falls Trail				✓		✓		✓	✓	
44 North Fork Middle Fork American Trail		✓				✓			✓	
45 Yankee Jim's–Indian Creek Trail		✓				✓		✓	✓	
46 Windy Point Trail						✓	✓	✓	✓	
47 Stevens Trail West		✓	✓	✓		✓		✓	✓	
48 Stevens Trail East		✓		✓		✓			✓	✓
49 Green Valley Trail		✓			✓	✓	✓		✓	✓
50 Euchre Bar Trail to Humbug Canyon		✓		✓	✓	✓	✓		✓	✓
51 American Eagle Mine Trail		✓			✓	✓			✓	✓
FOOTHILLS NORTH										
52 Hidden Falls Trails	✓		✓	✓		✓		✓	✓	✓
53 Fairy Falls Trail		✓		✓		✓		✓	✓	
54 Hardrock Trail		✓	✓	✓						
55 Independence Trail: East Branch		✓		✓		✓			✓	
56 Independence Trail: West Branch	✓	✓	✓	✓		✓		✓	✓	
57 Buttermilk Bend Trail				✓		✓			✓	
58 Point Defiance Trail				✓		✓			✓	
59 Humbug Trail		✓				✓		✓	✓	
60 Diggins Loop Trail		✓		✓						

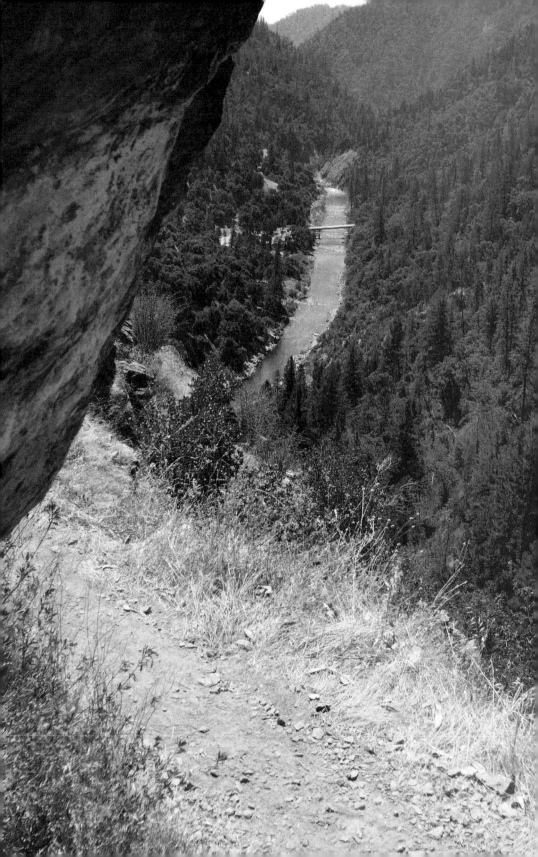

INTRODUCTION

Welcome to *60 Hikes within 60 Miles: Sacramento*. If you're new to hiking or even if you're a seasoned trailsmith, take a few minutes to read the following introduction. It explains how this book is organized and how to use it.

HOW TO USE THIS GUIDEBOOK

THE OVERVIEW MAP AND OVERVIEW-MAP KEY

Use the overview map on the inside front cover to assess the exact locations of each hike's primary trailhead. Each hike's number appears on the overview map, on the map key facing the overview map, and in the table of contents. As you flip through the book, a hike's full profile is easy to locate by watching for the hike number at the top of each right-hand page.

REGIONAL MAPS

The book is divided into regions, and prefacing each regional section is an overview map. The regional maps provide more detail than the overview map, bringing you closer to the hike.

TRAIL MAPS

Each hike contains a detailed map that shows the trailhead, the route, significant features, facilities, and topographic landmarks such as creeks, overlooks, and peaks. The author gathered map data by carrying a Garmin GPSMAP 60CSx unit while hiking. This data was downloaded into DeLorme's digital-mapping program Topo USA and then processed by expert cartographers to produce the highly accurate maps in this book. Each trailhead's GPS coordinates are included with each profile (see discussion following).

LEGEND

A map legend that details the symbols found on trail maps appears on the inside back cover.

ELEVATION PROFILES

Corresponding directly to the trail map, each hike contains a detailed elevation profile. The elevation profile provides a quick look at the trail from the side, enabling you to visualize how the trail rises and falls. Key points along the way are labeled. Note the number of feet between each tick mark on the vertical axis (the height scale). To avoid making flat hikes look steep and steep hikes appear flat, height scales are used throughout the book to accurately depict the hike's climbing difficulty.

GPS TRAILHEAD COORDINATES

This book includes the GPS coordinates for each trailhead in latitude–longitude format. These numbers tell you where you are by locating a point west (latitude) of the 0° meridian line that passes through Greenwich, England, and north or south of the 0° longitude line that belts the Earth, a.k.a. the equator.

For readers who own a GPS unit, whether handheld or aboard a vehicle, the latitude–longitude coordinates provided on the first page of each hike may be entered into the unit. Just make sure yours is set to navigate using WGS84 datum. Now you can navigate directly to the trailhead.

Many trailheads, which begin in parking areas, can be reached by car, but other hikes still require a short walk to reach the trailhead from a parking area. In those cases, a handheld GPS unit is necessary to continue the navigation process. Still, readers can easily access all trailheads in this book by using the directions given, the overview map, and the trail map, which shows at least one major road leading into the area. But for those who enjoy using the latest GPS technology to navigate, the necessary data has been provided.

In this book, latitude–longitude coordinates are expressed in degrees and decimal minutes. For example, the coordinates for Hike 1, Capitol Park Loop (page 22), are as follows: N38° 34.634′; W121° 29.599′. To convert GPS coordinates given in degrees, minutes, and seconds to the format shown above, divide the seconds by 60. For more on GPS technology, visit **usgs.gov.**

HIKE PROFILES

Each hike contains seven key items: an In Brief description of the trail, a Key At-a-Glance Information box, directions to the trail, trailhead coordinates, a trail map, an elevation profile, and a trail description. Many hike profiles also include notes on nearby activities. Combined, the maps and information provide a clear method to assess each trail from the comfort of your favorite reading chair.

IN BRIEF

A "taste of the trail." Think of this section as a snapshot focused on the historical landmarks, beautiful vistas, and other sights you may encounter on the hike.

KEY AT-A-GLANCE INFORMATION

The following information gives you a quick idea of the statistics and specifics of each hike:

LENGTH How long the trail is from start to finish. There may be options to shorten or extend the hikes, but the mileage corresponds to the described hike. Use the Description as a guide to customizing the hike for your ability or time constraints.

CONFIGURATION A description of what the trail might look like from overhead. Trails can be loops, out-and-backs (trails on which one enters and leaves along the same path), point-to-points, figure-eights, or a combination of shapes.

DIFFICULTY This is a highly subjective matter, and I was tempted to stick with the tried-and-true 1–5 scale and let the reader guess what it means. But based on conversations with other hikers, equipment manufacturers, guides, clients, and my children, I've been able to successfully employ common terminology in describing trail effort:

> *Cakewalk:* Level ground; effortless, short, shaded; almost a catered affair.
>
> *Easy:* Like an A-ticket ride. No real sweat. Just fun.
>
> *Moderate:* Now you sweat some. Uphill, downhill, navigate.
>
> *Challenging:* Long; uphill, downhill, navigate. A workout.
>
> *Hard:* Vertical exposure; elevation gain/loss; scrambling; route-finding; long or remote.

WATER required How much hydration (in liters) you'll need to bring along.

SCENERY A short summary of the hike's attractions and what to expect in terms of plant life, wildlife, natural wonders, and historic features.

EXPOSURE A quick check of how much sun you can expect on your shoulders during the hike.

TRAFFIC Indicates how busy the trail might be on an average day. Trail traffic, of course, varies from day to day and season to season. Weekend days typically see the most visitors. Other trail users whom you may encounter are also noted.

TRAIL SURFACE Indicates whether the trail surface is paved, rocky, gravel, dirt, boardwalk, or a mixture of surfaces.

HIKING TIME How long it takes to hike the trail. A slow but steady hiker will average 2–3 miles an hour, depending on the terrain.

SEASON Time(s) of year when the hike is accessible.

ACCESS A notation of any necessary fees or permits to access the trail or park at the trailhead. For a list of California state parks and recreation areas that charge fees, visit **parks.ca.gov/?page_id=23294**. You can obtain an annual day-use pass at park offices (when they're staffed) or online at **store.parks.ca.gov/park-passes**. City and county parks typically require no permits or fees.

MAPS Here, you'll find a list of maps that show the trail topography, including U.S. Geological Survey (USGS) topo maps and local trail maps. The Auburn State Recreation Area has a map that clearly identifies each of its 50 trails. In addition, the Tahoe National Forest map shows a number of trails and trailhead access points.

WHEELCHAIR ACCESS Indicates whether all or part of the hike can be enjoyed by persons with disabilities.

FACILITIES What you can expect in terms of restrooms and water at the trailhead or nearby.

DRIVING DISTANCE How far away the hike is by car from a starting point given in the Directions—for example, the junction of I-80 and the Capital City Freeway.

SPECIAL COMMENTS Any extra details that don't fit into the categories above.

DIRECTIONS

Used in conjunction with the overview map, the driving directions will help you locate each trailhead. Once there, park only in designated areas.

GPS TRAILHEAD COORDINATES

The trailhead coordinates can be used in addition to the driving directions if you enter the coordinates into your GPS unit before you set out. See page 2 for more information.

DESCRIPTION

This is the heart of each hike. Here, the author summarizes the trail's essence and highlights any special traits the hike has to offer. The route is clearly outlined, including any landmarks, side trips, and possible alternate routes along the way. Ultimately, the Description will help you choose which hikes are best for you.

NEARBY ACTIVITIES

Look here for information on nearby activities or points of interest. These include parks, museums, restaurants, or even a brew pub where you can get a well-deserved beer after a long hike. (Note that not every hike has a listing.)

WEATHER

Sacramento sits in the middle of the Central Valley, almost midway between the Sierra Nevada and Coast Ranges. Its Mediterranean climate brings warm days and cool nights in the spring and summer along with cool, wet winters, as shown in the table opposite. In short, Sacramento has a climate that's very hiker-friendly.

The Sacramento Valley, however, has more than one face when it comes to the weather you may encounter on a given day. Near sea level, in the middle of a geologic bathtub, Sacramento itself endures very hot summer days when temperatures exceed 90°F for more than 60 days from June through September. In winter, the rain and fog return the moisture lost in the valley, while the snowstorms that coat the sierra sometimes dip into the Foothills.

Spring and autumn are the colorful seasons in the Sacramento Valley and the Foothills. Spring is an explosion of color, with wildflowers and trees blooming and budding everywhere that water soaks the soil. Trails that cross creeks and streams should be approached with some planning and caution during the spring runoff. Wet rocks are slippery, and running water is often stronger than hikers realize before it's too late. Hike with a partner or use trekking poles at creek crossings at this time of year.

SACRAMENTO MONTHLY TEMPERATURE AND PRECIPITATION AVERAGES						
	JAN	FEB	MAR	APR	MAY	JUN
HIGH	53.8°F	60.5°F	64.7°F	71.4°F	80.0°F	87.4°F
LOW	38.8°F	41.9°F	44.2°F	46.3°F	50.9°F	55.5°F
PRECIPITATION	3.84"	3.5"	2.8"	2.8"	2.8"	2.8"
	JUL	AUG	SEP	OCT	NOV	DEC
HIGH	92.4°F	91.4°F	87.5°F	78.2°F	63.7°F	53.9°F
LOW	58.3°F	58.1°F	55.8°F	50.6°F	42.8°F	37.7°F
PRECIPITATION	0.0"	0.0"	0.3"	0.8"	2.1"	2.4"

These hot days in the valley that are so important for crops mellow somewhat as one climbs into the foothills of the Sierra Nevada. However, as the sun ascends and extends its rays into these foothill canyons and drainages, they too become ovenlike as the summer days grow. Temperatures exceeding 100°F are not uncommon either in the valley or in the foothill canyons. This seasonal heat wave can really temper your choice of trails to hike. The slow-moving pools on the forks of the American River are excellent destination points on a summer hike.

Looking at the temperature and precipitation chart, you can see that these same four months enjoy as little moisture as they do cool days. This makes summer hiking a bit more demanding and forces hikers to think carefully about their water needs for the day. Hydrate yourself thoroughly before your hike, and be sure to carry enough water to replenish lost body fluids.

Your hiking experience will change with the seasons. In midsummer, streams that flowed with gusto in the spring may be completely dry, and the picturesque falls you want to hike to may not be much more than a trickle. Nevertheless, wildlife still abounds. Deer are in velvet, and the remaining water sources can be great places to observe in the early morning and evening.

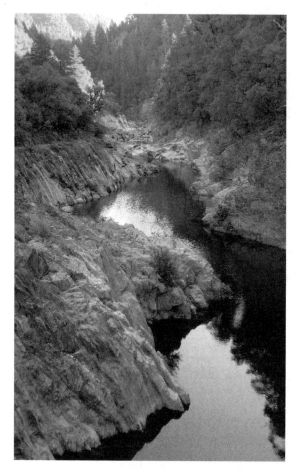

The North Fork of the American River, as viewed from the last upriver footbridge to cross it

Autumn is, of course, a multicolored extravaganza in the Foothills, where the native trees and plants—oak, ash, sycamore, redbud, maple, toyon, willow, cottonwood, and others—change from green to red and gold. Not to be outdone, the Sacramento Valley is awash in colors of both native and ornamental trees and plants. With moderate temperatures and infrequent rainfall, autumn is a very popular time of year to hike.

You can expect mild temperatures in the winter, when this area realizes the majority of its rainfall. Winter months, when the highs are generally in the 50s and 60s and the lows are rarely under 40, may be ideal for difficult hikes that might otherwise sap your strength in the summer. In this season, the Sacramento region receives the majority of its rainfall—that is, almost 75 percent of its annual precipitation—in just four months. The positive side is that this water charges all the drainages, creeks, and rivers with the raw material for real hiking wonders: cascades, waterfalls, wildflowers, and wildlife. The only downside is that some Foothills trails turn rather sticky after a soaking rain.

Every hike in this book but two is walkable at any time of year. Both exceptions are in Calaveras Big Trees State Park. The South Grove Trail at this park is closed when snows block the road leading to the grove. However, the North Grove Trail is converted to a cross-country-skiing trail when snowfall conditions permit. No other trails described in this book are closed unless the trailhead is temporarily inaccessible. On occasion, Foresthill Road closes at China Wall after a snowstorm in the Foothills region. A few of the unpaved and unimproved trailhead-access roads, such as Drivers Flat Road, Ponderosa Way, and Yankee Jim's Road, are extremely difficult to navigate after it rains.

WATER

How much is enough? Well, one simple physiological fact should persuade you to err on the side of excess when deciding how much water to pack: a hiker working hard in 90°F heat needs about 10 quarts of fluid per day. That's 2.5 gallons—12 large water bottles or 16 small ones. In other words, pack one or two bottles even for short hikes.

While it's no problem to carry adequate supplies of water on these day hikes, some hikers and backpackers hit the trail prepared to purify water found along the route. This method, while less dangerous than drinking untreated water, comes with risks if not properly performed. Purifiers with ceramic filters are the safest. Many hikers pack the slightly distasteful tetraglycine–hydroperiodide tablets to debug water (sold under the names Potable Aqua, Coughlan's, and others). Aquamira chlorine dioxide drops are nearly tasteless and almost weightless; gravity filters and hydration systems with inline filters are convenient and effective as well. SteriPEN is an ultraviolet-light treatment device that weighs about 10 ounces. If none of these methods is available, bringing the water to a boil is enough to kill the pathogens.

Probably the most common waterborne bug that hikers face is giardia, which may not hit until one to four weeks after ingestion. It will have you living in the bathroom, passing noxious rotten-egg gas, vomiting, and shivering with chills. Other parasites to worry about include E. coli and cryptosporidium, both of which are nastier and harder to kill than giardia.

For most people, the pleasures of hiking make carrying water a relatively minor price to pay to remain healthy. If you're tempted to drink "found water," do so only if you understand the risks involved. Better yet, hydrate before your hike, carry (and drink) 6 ounces of water for every mile you plan to hike, and hydrate after the hike. If in an emergency situation you find yourself having to choose between drinking untreated water and getting dehydrated, by all means drink it—if you get sick, see a doctor after your rescue.

ESSENTIAL EQUIPMENT

One of the first rules of hiking is to be prepared for anything. The simplest way to be prepared is to carry the essentials. In addition to carrying the items that follow, you need to know how to use them, especially navigation items. Always consider worst-case scenarios such as getting lost, hiking back in the dark, broken gear (for example, a broken hip strap on your pack or a water filter getting plugged), twisting an ankle, or a brutal thunderstorm. The items listed here don't cost a lot of money, don't take up much room in a pack, and don't weigh much, but they might just save your life.

EMERGENCY TOOLS: Signal whistle, signal mirror, knife, multitool, cord

EXTRA CLOTHING: Insulation layer, gloves, rain gear, socks, soft-shell jacket

FOOD: Nutrition bars, snacks, or meals for the day, plus extra; always try to return with some food.

FIRE: Matches, lighter, fire starter, or stove with full fuel bottle/canister

FIRST-AID KIT: With fresh supplies, instructions, and the knowledge to use them

LIGHT: Headlamp with fresh batteries

MAP AND COMPASS: Trail or topographic map, simple compass, the route description, and the knowledge to use them

SUN PROTECTION: Hat, sunglasses, sunscreen, lip balm

SHELTER: A space blanket or Siltarp can provide immediate sun or rain protection for accident victims.

TREKKING POLES: In addition to keeping your footing steady, they can act as a third leg, monopod, shelter pole, cougar and bear defense, poison-oak deflector, or handy implement for poking and irritating creatures while dawdling.

WATER: Full bottles, plus extra or water-treatment tablets/purifying filter

WHISTLE: More effective in signaling rescuers than your voice

This list is fully weather- and trip-dependent. If you hike in Capitol Park in the spring, you will require virtually none of this gear. If, however, you hike on the Stevens Trail in the fall, you might need and use every bit of it. The list will help you structure and plan for the requirements of each trip. The only item I haven't yet used is the whistle.

No matter where you hike, though, it's a good idea to consider other, *nonessential* gear that could add to your experience, comfort, or general pleasure.

GEAR AND CLOTHING RECOMMENDATIONS

It should be as easy as throwing on a pair of cutoffs and T-shirt, but it simply isn't. Depending on a hike's difficulty, length, location, and season, your individual clothing and equipment needs will change.

Here's a list of the gear and clothing I've worn or carried on these hikes, in addition to the items listed previously as essential equipment:

BANDANNA: Great mosquito-swatter, brow-wiper, impromptu hat

BINOCULARS: 8x21, compact size

CAMERA

DAY PACK: 20–30 liters (depending on how many books you carry)

FOOTWEAR: Lightweight hiking boots, trail runners, or hiking shoes are all made to stand up to the hikes in this book.

FIELD GUIDES: Paper and pencil

GAITERS: Almost a must, they keep dirt, sticks, seeds, and other crud from getting inside boots; good protection against poison oak.

GPS DEVICE and extra batteries

LIGHTWEIGHT LONG-SLEEVED SHIRT: To protect your arms when the sun is blistering down at lunchtime

SHORTS: Cargo pockets are a fashion plus for holding far too many gadgets, snacks, and paper scraps.

SIT PAD: Insulation for the keister; great for kneeling while getting that macro shot

SOCKS AND LINERS: Two pairs of socks are a sure way to protect against blisters.

TRIPOD: Compact and flexible for a variety of surfaces

WICKING T-SHIRT: A good base layer or outerwear in summer

WICKING UNDERWEAR: Cotton feels great until it gets sweaty. Cotton clothing should be avoided when hiking.

FIRST-AID KIT

A typical kit may contain more items than you think necessary. The following are just the basics. If you carry nothing else for first aid, a blister-treatment kit should be it. That will cover 90 percent of the on-trail owies you'll ever have.

Prepackaged kits in waterproof bags (Atwater Carey and Adventure Medical make a variety of kits) are available. Even though there are quite a few items listed here, they pack down into a small space:

Ace bandages or Spenco joint wraps

Antibiotic ointment (Neosporin or the generic equivalent)

Aspirin or acetaminophen

Band-Aids

Benadryl or the generic equivalent, diphenhydramine (in case of allergic reactions)

Butterfly-closure bandages

Epinephrine in a prefilled syringe (for people known to have severe allergic reactions to such things as bee stings)

Gauze (one roll)

Gauze compress pads (a half-dozen 4 by 4–inch pads)

Hydrogen peroxide or iodine

Insect repellent

Matches or pocket lighter

Moleskin/Spenco Second Skin

Sunscreen

Your personal daily medications

HIKING WITH CHILDREN

No one is too young for a hike in the outdoors. Be mindful, though. Flat, short, and shaded trails are best with an infant. Toddlers who haven't quite mastered walking can still tag along, riding on an adult's back in a child carrier. Use common sense to judge a child's capacity to hike a particular trail, and always assume that the child will tire quickly and need to be carried.

When packing for the hike, remember the child's needs as well as your own. Make sure children are adequately clothed for the weather, have proper shoes, and are protected from the sun with sunscreen. Kids dehydrate quickly, so make sure you have plenty of fluid for everyone. Hikes suitable for children are included in the chart on pages xix–xxi.

GENERAL SAFETY

To some potential mountain enthusiasts, the steep slopes and deep canyons seem perilous. No doubt, dangerous situations can occur outdoors, but as long as you use sound judgment and prepare yourself before hitting the trail, you'll be much safer in the woods or mountains than in most urban areas of the country. It's better to look at a backcountry hike as a fascinating chance to discover the unknown rather than a setting for potential disaster. These tips will help make your trip safer and easier.

- **Always carry food and water, whether you're planning to go overnight or not. Food will give you energy, help keep you warm, and sustain you in an emergency until help arrives. You never know if you'll have a stream nearby when you become thirsty. Bring potable water, or treat water before drinking it from a stream or other source.**

- **Stay on designated trails. Most hikers get lost when they leave the path. Even on the most clearly marked trails, you usually reach a point where you have to stop and consider the direction in which to head. If you become disoriented, don't panic. As soon as you think you may be off-track, stop, assess your current direction, and then retrace your steps back to the point where you went awry. Using map, compass, and this book—and keeping in mind what you've passed thus far—reorient yourself and trust your judgment about which way to continue. If you become absolutely unsure of that, return to your vehicle the way you came in. Should you become completely lost and have no idea how to return to the trailhead, remaining in place along the trail and waiting for help is most often the best option for adults and always the best option for children.**

- **Be especially careful when crossing streams. Whether you're fording the stream or crossing on a log, make every step count. If you're not sure you can maintain your balance on a foot log, go ahead and ford the stream instead. When fording a stream, use a trekking pole or stout stick for balance and face upstream as you cross. If a stream seems too deep to ford, turn back. Whatever is on the other side isn't worth risking your life for.**

- **Be careful at overlooks. While these areas may provide spectacular views, they are potentially hazardous. Stay back from the edge of outcrops and be absolutely sure of your footing.**

- **Standing dead trees and storm-damaged living trees pose a real hazard to hikers and tent campers. These trees may have loose or broken limbs that**

could fall at any time. When choosing a spot to rest or a backcountry
campsite, look up.

- Know the symptoms of heat exhaustion. Excessive sweating, faintness or
dizziness, clammy skin, vomiting, and paleness are all common symptoms. If
symptoms arise, remove extra clothing, move to the shade, and drink plenty
of water.

- Likewise, know the symptoms of hypothermia. Shivering and forgetfulness
are the two most common indicators of this insidious killer. Hypothermia
can occur at any elevation, even in the summer, especially when the hiker is
wearing lightweight cotton clothing. Get the victim shelter, hot liquids, and
dry clothes or a dry sleeping bag.

- Bring your brain. A cool, calculating mind is the single most important piece
of equipment you'll ever need on the trail. Think before you act. Watch your
step. Plan ahead. Avoiding accidents before they happen is the best recipe
for a rewarding and relaxing hike.

- Ask questions. Forest and park employees are there to help. It's a lot easier
to gain advice beforehand and avoid a mishap away from civilization when
it's too late to amend an error. Use your head out there, and treat the place as
if it were your own backyard.

ANIMAL AND PLANT HAZARDS

MOUNTAIN LIONS

MOUNTAIN LIONS MAY BE FOUND IN THIS AREA. ALTHOUGH SELDOM SEEN, THEY
CAN BE UNPREDICTABLE AND HAVE BEEN KNOWN TO ATTACK HUMANS WITHOUT
WARNING. These words, or words to their effect, are often seen at trailheads or
recreation-area entrances throughout the Sacramento region. Mountain lions are a
real and potential danger on many hiking trails, especially in the Foothills. In 1994,
a lone runner was killed by a mountain lion as she jogged on a trail near Auburn.

Also known as cougars or pumas, mountain lions are everywhere in California and are most abundant where there is a supply of deer and groundcover.
They are tan-coated, have black-tipped ears and tail, weigh between 75 and 150
pounds, and are about 7 feet long from nose to tail.

Never approach a mountain lion. If confronted, do anything to make yourself appear larger: raise your outspread arms, wave trekking poles or tree limbs,
and gather other hikers (especially children) next to you. Act threatening, but give
the mountain lion an escape path. Avoid bending over or turning your back on it.
Do not run. Make noise, yell, and throw rocks or anything you can grab without
bending over.

If you're attacked, try to remain standing, as mountain lions will try to bite
the neck or head. Always try to fight back. In 2007, a 65-year-old woman successfully used a ballpoint pen to fight off the mountain lion that was attacking her

husband in Prairie Creek Redwoods State Park. The couple survived their ordeal thanks to her quick action.

CALIFORNIA BLACK BEARS

With the possible exception of mountain lions, most animals will be scared of you and won't pose a threat as long as you respect their space. California has a large population of black bears, which are actually cinnamon to dark brown in color. The threat from black bears is that they are very intelligent and they are always searching for large quantities of food. Despite weighing between 200 and 500 pounds, black bears can run up to 30 miles an hour.

Again, bears want your food. Take every precaution to keep it under your control. Do not leave food out and unattended. If a bear is already eating your food or shredding your pack in search of snacks, let him have it. Perhaps you can walk away with just a great story. Do not try to retrieve your food from a bear.

If you do encounter a black bear on the trail, do not run. Make eye contact, but don't stare. Pick up small children to keep them from running. If a bear approaches, make yourself appear larger by spreading your arms or holding your jacket open. Make as much threatening noise as you can by yelling or banging gear together. If a bear is after you and not your food, throw rocks or sticks and make every attempt to fight back.

TICKS

Ticks like to hang out in the brush that grows along trails. In the summer their numbers seem to explode, but you should be tick-aware during all months of the year. Ticks, which are arachnids and not insects, need a host to feast on in order to reproduce.

The ticks that alight on you while you hike will be very small, sometimes so tiny that you won't be able to spot them. Primarily of two types, deer ticks and dog ticks, both need a few hours of actual attachment before they can transmit any disease they may harbor. Note that Lyme disease has been reported in every county covered by this book, and the threat of contracting it is real.

Deer ticks are the size of a pencil point, dog ticks the size of the pencil's eraser. Both may settle in shoes, socks, and hats, and they may take several hours to actually latch on. The best strategy is to visually check every half-hour or so while hiking, do a thorough check before you get in your car, and then, when you take a posthike shower, do an even more thorough check of your entire body. Ticks that haven't attached are easily removed but not easily killed. If you pick off a tick in the woods, just toss it aside. If you find one on your body at home, dispatch it and then send it down the toilet. For ticks that have become embedded, removal with tweezers is best.

SNAKES

Rattlesnakes, as well as other species of snakes, are important members of the natural community. They will not attack, but they will defend themselves if disturbed or cornered. Rattlesnakes will usually warn you with the buzz of their rattle.

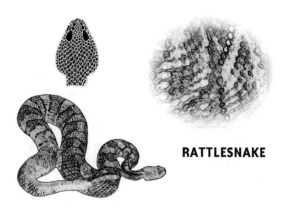

The Northern Pacific rattlesnake—the only pit viper that is native to Northern California—makes its home in the Foothills around Sacramento, so some caution is required when you travel in its habitat. Rattlesnakes like to rest on warm rocks and in small spaces,

RATTLESNAKE

often moving in and out of warmth to maintain body temperature. Be careful when you step over logs or boulders. Don't place your foot in a spot you can't see. Watch where you place your hands when scrambling. Snakebites occur most often you inadvertently touch the snake.

Rattlesnakes eat rodents, lizards, squirrels, rabbits, and sometimes birds, but not humans. The Northern Pacific rattlesnake is most active in the spring and hunts at dawn, dusk, or night. Mating occurs in the spring, and young are born in the fall. Rattlers are rather shy and will usually move out of your way before you are aware of them.

If you encounter a rattlesnake, consider how lucky you are to see this beautiful creature. It can't hurl itself at you to strike, but if you get within the distance of its body length—about 5 feet—you're within the strike zone. Do not try to touch or move the snake. Give it distance and respect. Step back. Take a picture. Walk away with another great story.

It is unlawful to kill or harm rattlesnakes or any other wildlife in California state parks.

POISON OAK

Recognizing this plant and avoiding contact with it is the most effective way to prevent the painful, itchy rashes associated with it. Poison oak occurs as either a vine or a shrub, with three shiny identical leaflets. Urushiol, the oil in the plant's sap, is responsible for the rash. Usually within 12–14 hours of exposure (but sometimes

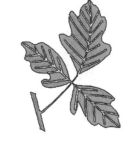

much later), raised lines and/or blisters will appear, accompanied by a terrible itch. Refrain from scratching, because bacteria under your fingernails can cause infection and spread the rash to other parts of your body. Wash and dry the rash thoroughly, applying calamine lotion or other product to help dry the rash. If itching or blistering is severe, seek medical attention. Remember that oil-contaminated clothes, pets, or hiking gear can easily spread the rash to you or someone else, so wash not only any exposed parts of your body but also clothes, gear, and pets.

MOSQUITOES

You will encounter mosquitoes on most of the hikes in this book. Although it's not a common occurrence, individuals can become infected with the West Nile virus after being bitten by an infected mosquito. Culex mosquitoes, the primary varieties that can transmit West Nile virus to humans, thrive in urban rather than natural areas. They lay their eggs in stagnant water and can breed in water that's been standing for more than five days. Most people infected with West Nile virus have no symptoms of illness, but some may become ill, usually 3–15 days after being bitten.

In the Sacramento area, spring and summer are the highest risk periods for West Nile virus. At this time of year—and anytime you expect mosquitoes to be buzzing around—you may want to wear long sleeves, long pants, and socks. Loose-fitting, light-colored clothing is best. Spray clothing with insect repellent. Follow the instructions on the repellent, and take extra care with children.

TIPS FOR ENJOYING THE SACRAMENTO REGION

Before you go, visit the various websites in this book. This will help you get oriented to the region's roads, features, and attractions. Detailed maps of specific parks or recreation areas are available online, at stores, or from the agencies themselves (see "Managing Agencies" at the end of this book). They will really help you get around the forest's backcountry. In addition, the following tips will make your visit enjoyable and more rewarding:

- Investigate different areas of the region. The Delta offers flat hikes with huge wildlife populations. The Western Sacramento Valley cloaks its dry hills with golden fields splattered with oak. The southern Foothills' broad and rolling hills conceal reservoirs and lakes for Bay Area residents. The northern Foothills are a wild, steep jumble of geologic catastrophes displaying the remnants of the region's mining legacy

- Take your time along the trails. Pace yourself. The Foothills are filled with wonders both big and small. Don't rush past a tiny salamander to get to that overlook. Stop and smell the wildflowers. Peer into the clear rivers for trout. Don't miss the trees for the forest. Shorter hikes allow you to stop and linger more than long hikes. Something about staring at the front end of a 10-mile trek naturally pushes you to speed up. That said, take close notice of the elevation profiles that accompany each hike: if you see many ups and downs over large elevation changes, you'll obviously need more time. Inevitably you'll finish some of the hikes long before or after the times suggested. Nevertheless, leave yourself plenty of time for those moments when you simply feel like stopping and taking it all in.

- We can't always schedule our free time when we want, but try to hike during the week and avoid the traditional holidays if possible. Trails that are packed in the spring and fall are often clear during the hottest months of

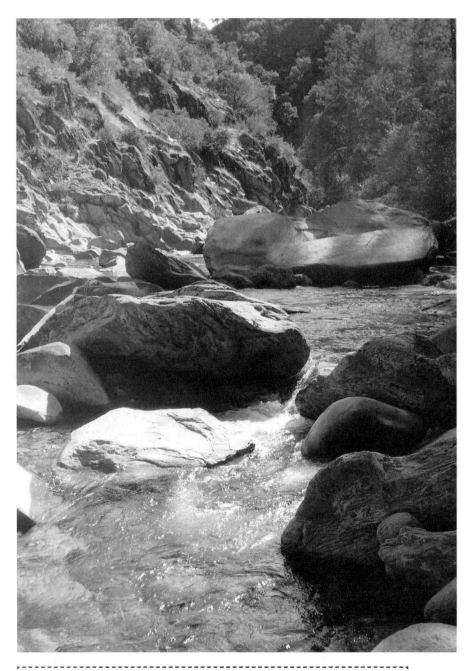

Steep canyon walls tighten around the upper reaches of the North Fork of the Middle Fork of the American River.

summer. If you're hiking on a busy day, go early in the morning; it'll enhance your chances of seeing wildlife. The trails really clear out during rainy times; don't hike during a thunderstorm, though.

TOPO MAPS

The maps in this book have been produced with great care and, used with the hiking directions, will direct you to the trails and help you stay on course. However, you will find superior detail and valuable information in the USGS's 7.5-minute series topographic maps. One well-known free topo service on the Web is **Microsoft Research Maps** (msrmaps.com). Online services such as **Trails.com** charge annual fees for additional features such as shaded relief, which makes the topography stand out more. If you expect to print out many topo maps each year, it might be worth paying for such extras. The downside to USGS topos is that most are outdated, having been created more than 30 years ago. But they still provide excellent topographic detail.

Digital topographic-map programs such as DeLorme's Topo USA enable you to review topo maps of the entire United States on your computer. Data gathered while hiking with a GPS unit can be downloaded into the software, letting you plot your own hikes. Of course, Google Earth (**earth.google.com**) does away with topo maps and their inaccuracies, replacing them with satellite imagery and its inaccuracies. Regardless, what one lacks the other augments. Google Earth is an excellent tool whether or not you have difficulty with topos. Getting a quick set of eyes on the ground can be invaluable when you're planning your hike.

If you're new to hiking, you might be wondering, "What's a topographic map?" In short, a topo indicates not only linear distance but elevation as well, using contour lines. These lines spread across the map like dozens of intricate spiderwebs. Each line represents a particular elevation, and at the base of each topo, a contour's interval designation is given. If the contour interval is 20 feet, then the distance between each contour line is 20 feet. Follow five contour lines up on the same map, and the elevation has increased by 100 feet.

Let's assume that the 7.5-minute-series topo reads "contour interval 40 feet," that the short trail we'll be hiking is 2 inches in length on the map, and that it crosses five contour lines from beginning to end. What do we know? Well, because the linear scale of this series is 2,000 feet to the inch (roughly 2.75 inches representing 1 mile), we know that our trail is about four-fifths of a mile long (2 inches equals 4,000 feet). But we also know we'll be climbing or descending 200 vertical feet (five contour lines are 40 feet each) over that distance. And the elevation designations written on occasional contour lines will tell us if we're heading up or down.

In addition to the sources listed in Appendix B, topos are available at major universities and some public libraries. If you want your own and can't find them locally, visit The USGS Store (**store.usgs.gov**).

BACKCOUNTRY ADVICE

Some hikes in this book on BLM land and in national forests let you camp along the way or at the destination. No permit is required before you enter the backcountry to camp. However, you should practice low-impact camping. Adhere to the adages "Pack it in, pack it out," and "Take only pictures, leave only footprints." Practice Leave No Trace camping ethics while in the backcountry; for basic information on how to do so, visit **lnt.org.**

Open fires are permitted except during dry times, when the U.S. Forest Service may issue a fire ban. Backpacking stoves are strongly encouraged and fires are discouraged.

You must protect your food from bears and other animals to keep them from becoming dependent on humans for their sustenance. Wildlife can learn to associate backpacks and backpackers with easy food sources, thereby influencing their behavior. Bear-proof canisters or odor-sealing bags will help prevent advertising your food's location. Bear-bag hanging has been improved and simplified with a technique called the PCT bear-bag method (check YouTube for video demonstrations). It can be used quickly and effectively in areas that do not require the use of bear-proof food containers. You can also help ensure that no bears visit your camp for food by maintaining a clean camp environment, cooking 100 feet away from your campsite, hanging all food and scented articles 100 feet from your campsite, and sleeping with no food or scented items in your tent.

Solid human waste must be buried in a hole at least 3 inches deep and at least 200 feet away from trails and water sources; a trowel is basic backpacking equipment.

Following the previous guidelines will increase your chances of a pleasant, safe, and low-impact interaction between humans and nature. Forest and park regulations can change over time, so contact the appropriate managing agency to confirm the status of any regulations before you enter the backcountry.

TRAIL ETIQUETTE

Whether you're on a city, county, state, or national-park trail, always remember that great care and resources (from nature as well as from your tax dollars) have gone into creating these trails. Treat trails, wildlife, and fellow hikers with respect.

- **HIKE ON OPEN TRAILS ONLY. Respect trail and road closures (ask if you're not sure), avoid possible trespassing on private land, and obtain all permits and authorization as required. Also, leave gates as you found them or as marked.**

- **LEAVE ONLY FOOTPRINTS. Be sensitive to the ground beneath you. This also means staying on the existing trail and not blazing any new trails. Pack out what you pack in. No one likes to see the trash someone else has left behind.**

- **NEVER SPOOK ANIMALS. An unannounced approach, a sudden movement, or a loud noise can startle them. A surprised animal can be dangerous to you, others, and itself. Give animals plenty of space.**

- **PLAN AHEAD. Know your equipment, your ability, and the area in which you are hiking—and prepare accordingly. Be self-sufficient at all times; carry** necessary supplies for changes in weather or other conditions. A well-executed trip is a satisfaction to you and to others.

- **BE COURTEOUS TO OTHER HIKERS,** bikers, equestrians, and others you encounter on the trails.

- **MOST OF THE TRAILS DESCRIBED HERE** welcome hikers, bikers, and equestrians. There are also runners, hunters, anglers, and critters galore who use them. Many of the trailheads sport triangular signs suggesting that hikers and bikers should yield to equestrians, bikers should yield to hikers, and, whenever it's safe, everyone should yield to uphill hikers, bikers, or equestrians.

- **WHEN YOU ENCOUNTER EQUESTRIANS,** it's very helpful to move off-trail to the downhill side and greet the rider. This helps the horse understand that you are not a predator that wants to eat it.

- **IF POSSIBLE, TAKE BREAKS IN LOCATIONS** where you can move off the trail onto a nonvegetated area.

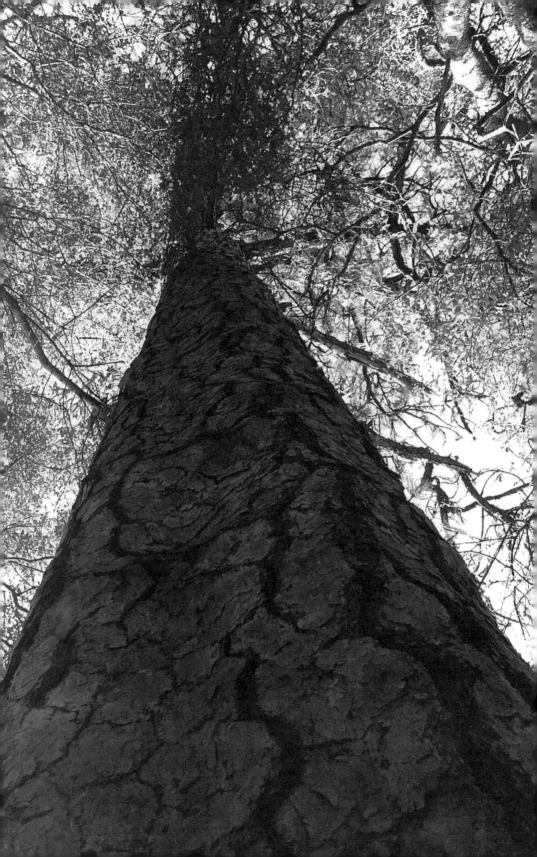

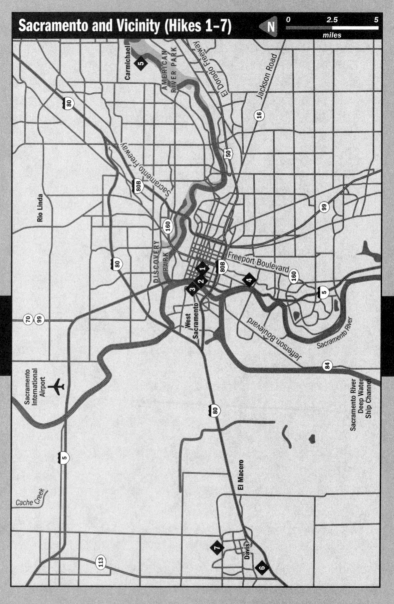

Sacramento and Vicinity (Hikes 1–7)

N

0   2.5   5
miles

Carmichael

AMERICAN RIVER PARK

El Dorado Freeway

Jackson Road

80

16

50

Sacramento Freeway

808

Rio Linda

99

160

DISCOVERY PARK

Freeport Boulevard

80

808

160

4

5

70   99

West Sacramento

Jefferson Boulevard

Sacramento River

Sacramento International Airport

84

Sacramento River Deep Water Ship Channel

80

El Macero

Cache Creek

5

113

Davis

7

6

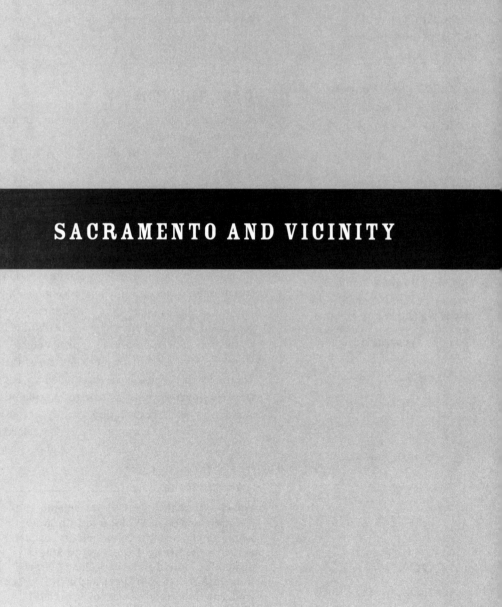

SACRAMENTO AND VICINITY

1 CAPITOL PARK LOOP

KEY AT-A-GLANCE INFORMATION

LENGTH: 1.5 miles

CONFIGURATION: Loop

DIFFICULTY: Cakewalk

WATER REQUIRED: 1 liter

SCENERY: Arboretum, statuary, monuments, memorials

EXPOSURE: Some sun, some shade

TRAIL TRAFFIC: Moderate

TRAIL SURFACE: Paved walkways

HIKING TIME: 2 hours

SEASON: Year-round

ACCESS: No fees or permits

MAPS: USGS Sacramento East; park-brochure map

WHEELCHAIR ACCESS: Yes

FACILITIES: On- and off-street parking; water fountains; benches

DRIVING DISTANCE: 1 mile

SPECIAL COMMENTS: This route can be walked in any direction, depending on your interests or the location of your parking space.

GPS TRAILHEAD COORDINATES

Latitude   N38° 34.634´
Longitude   W121° 29.599´

IN BRIEF

The California State Capitol Park is one of the most outstanding capitol grounds in any state. You can meander aimlessly through the dozen or so memorials, which are spread among hundreds of trees, bushes, and flowers from around the world in this 40-acre Victorian-style garden.

DESCRIPTION

Capitol Park can be accessed from any point along its 12-city-block length, so it seems natural to start closest to where you park. The starting point of this hike is on the north side steps at 11th Street. You can get a pamphlet at the State Capitol Museum, which offers a good map and an informative description of the park's many features.

Several major plantings, or "beautifications," were undertaken between the park's inception in 1869 and the most recent beautification in 1951, when the capitol annex was built. Rather than plantings having been added to the park, only memorials have been erected since the 1950s. Some of the oldest trees, the "heritage" plantings, have succumbed to age or storms over the years and are to be replaced during the next beautification.

The sidewalks encircling the park are lined with palms, and the walkways throughout the

----

Directions ─────────────────────────────➤

From I-5 North in downtown Sacramento, exit at J Street and drive 12 blocks to 15th Street, where you'll turn right. Drive 2 blocks to L Street and take another right. On-street parking is available around Capitol Park along L Street from 9th Street to 15th Street, and on N Street as well. Pay stations take cash, coins, or credit. There are also several covered garages nearby.

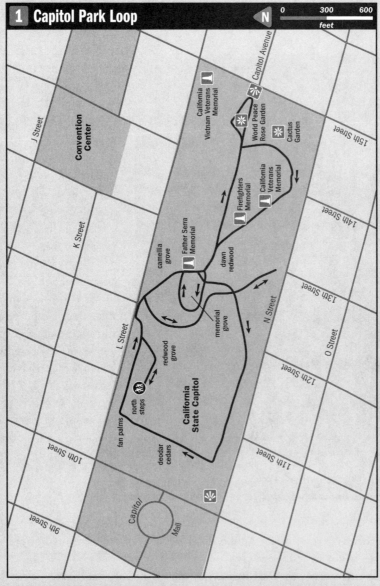

1 Capitol Park Loop

N — 0 · 300 · 600 feet

J Street

Convention Center

K Street

California Vietnam Veterans Memorial

Capitol Avenue

World Peace Rose Garden

Cactus Garden

15th Street

California Veterans Memorial

Firefighters Memorial

14th Street

camellia grove

Father Serra Memorial

dawn redwood

L Street

memorial grove

N Street

13th Street

O Street

redwood grove

north steps

California State Capitol

12th Street

fan palms

deodar cedars

10th Street

11th Street

9th Street

Capitol Mall

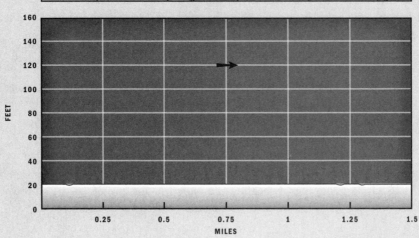

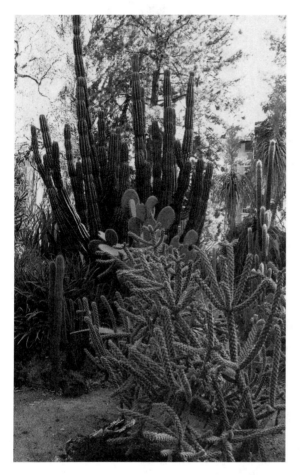

The Cactus Garden features plants donated by schoolchildren in 1914.

park are lined with trees; both sets of paths have been designed for the easiest and most complete access to the park's features. Paths are not always at right angles, so the park has a very natural appearance.

There is no one specific direction for visitors to travel through this park. If you turn right from the starting point, you will see a line of coast redwoods, which were original plantings from the 1872 beautification. A grove of coast redwood and giant sequoia is planted on the north side of the capitol, just to the east of the security entrance. One of the trees in this grove is called the "moon tree" by park staff because the seed was carried on an Apollo lunar mission and then planted on its return. The tree is not signed, however.

As you angle toward L Street, you will see the sole Italian stone pine remaining from the original planting in 1872. Turn right at 12th Street and head to the east entrance of the capitol, where you have some excellent photo opportunities. From here, walk east on the central promenade, where memorials and commemorative gardens lie on either side of you.

Next, walk to the 15th Street end of the park, where you will have more excellent photo opportunities of the capitol. The World Peace Rose Garden features a fragrant and colorful garden with benches dedicated by notable women who are themselves dedicated to peace.

The California Vietnam Veterans Memorial is adjacent to the rose garden. Its striking theme features stylized ammunition and starkly contrasting white limestone that holds black-granite panels bearing the names of missing or dead California veterans of that war. The inside of the circular monument features reliefs and sculptures representing various aspects of armed service in Southeast Asia. The centerpiece of the memorial is a life-size bronze statue of a 19-year-old soldier.

The Firefighters Memorial, also made of granite and bronze, dramatically depicts the dangers facing firefighters in action. These two sculptures were added in 2002. Out toward N Street is the California Veterans Memorial, which is dedicated to all Californians who have served in the armed forces. Its use of photography and stone is unique.

An Indian grinding rock is to the west before you reach another coast redwood–giant sequoia grove with a comfortable bench, encouraging rest and contemplation. Make your way north again, where the Spanish-American War Memorial, the Civil War Memorial, and the Liberty Bell Memorial are grouped among flowers and trees. An example of the dawn redwood, the only deciduous redwood species, is here. From the interior of China, it was long thought to be extinct.

The life-size monument featuring Father Junipero Serra is prominently featured in front of the colorful camellia grove. Standing beneath a lamppost shaped like a shepherd's crook, Father Serra's bronze statue looks down on a bronze relief map of California mounted on a black marble pedestal.

You can wander around the inside perimeter sidewalk on the west side of the capitol, where a row of deodar cedars flanks the walkway for two city blocks. The corner is yet another good spot from which to take some pictures.

Walking along these pathways on a weekend morning is a real pleasure at Capitol Park, where you can find both natural and man-made art. The architecture is classic and unimposing. The gardens and groves, with their thousands of flowers, bushes, and trees, are just waiting for you to view, smell, touch, photograph, and wander among them.

NEARBY ACTIVITIES

Old Sacramento features original buildings and excellent restorations, along with dining and entertainment. Hike 2 (see next profile) guides you through the streets of Old Sacramento State Historic Park.

OLD SACRAMENTO STATE HISTORIC PARK

2

KEY AT-A-GLANCE INFORMATION

LENGTH: 1.75 miles

CONFIGURATION: Loops

DIFFICULTY: Cakewalk

WATER REQUIRED: None

SCENERY: Restored 19th-century buildings

EXPOSURE: Shade inside every door

TRAIL TRAFFIC: Busy

TRAIL SURFACE: Cobblestone pavement, wooden sidewalk

HIKING TIME: 1–2 hours

SEASON: Year-round

ACCESS: Always open, no fees or permits

MAPS: USGS Sacramento West

WHEELCHAIR ACCESS: Yes

FACILITIES: All amenities are available here.

DRIVING DISTANCE: 1 mile

SPECIAL COMMENTS: Brochure with street map at oldsacramento.com

GPS TRAILHEAD COORDINATES

Latitude   N38° 37.863´

Longitude   W121° 30.395´

IN BRIEF

In the middle of the 19th century, Old Sacramento was a pioneer post, a glint-in-the-eye trading town with decent growth prospects. When the discovery of gold was announced, the nonnative population of California rose from fewer than 15,000 in 1848 to more than 100,000 by 1850, then exceeded 250,000 by 1852. Old Sacramento bore the brunt of that growth explosion and, surviving repeated floods and fires, quickly became a noted transportation terminus and communication hub, as well as the enduring center of California's government.

DESCRIPTION

The golden glimmer of the sun-drenched Tower Bridge almost forces you to turn in to Old Sacramento to escape the glare. Once you find yourself on Front Street, a quick look around tells you that you are in another era.

The cobblestone streets and wooden sidewalks of Old Sacramento are as appealing as you might expect, inviting its 5 million annual visitors to stroll . . . and stroll some more. With more than 50 reconstructed 19th-century buildings, the entire 1850s business district lies within the park's limits and was designated a National Historic Landmark in 1965.

Directions

Old Sacramento is downtown and can be reached via I-5's J Street exit. Follow the signs for covered, street, or open-lot parking. Enter Old Sacramento at Third and I streets or at Capitol Mall and Front Street.

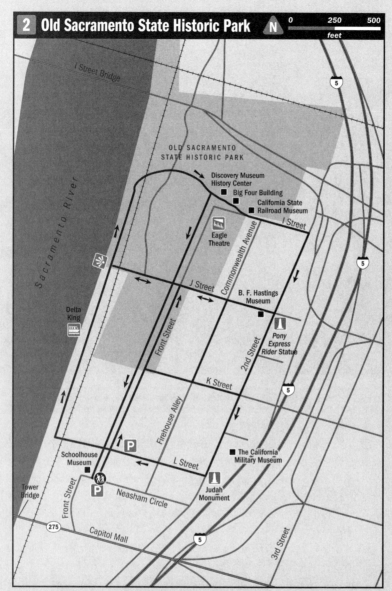

2 Old Sacramento State Historic Park

N

0   250   500
feet

I Street Bridge

5

OLD SACRAMENTO
STATE HISTORIC PARK

Discovery Museum
History Center
■ Big Four Building
■ California State
■ Railroad Museum

Sacramento River

Eagle
Theatre

I Street

Commonwealth Avenue

5

Delta
King

J Street

B. F. Hastings
Museum

■

2nd Street

Front Street

Pony
Express
Rider Statue

5

K Street

Firehouse Alley

P

L Street

■ The California
Military Museum

Schoolhouse
Museum
■

P

Judah
Monument

Tower
Bridge

Front Street

Neasham Circle

275

Capitol Mall

5

3rd Street

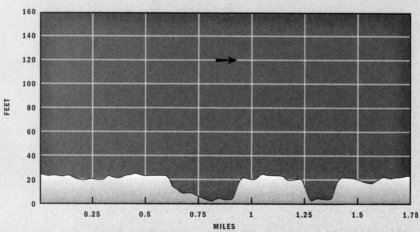

FEET

160
140
120
100
80
60
40
20
0

0.25   0.5   0.75   1   1.25   1.5   1.75

MILES

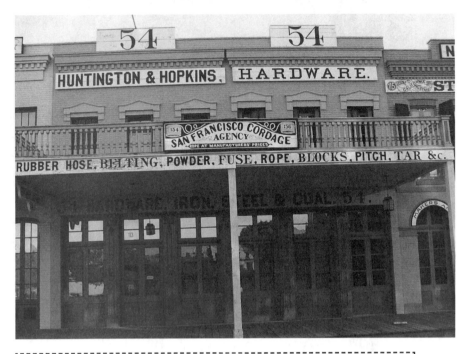

The Big Four Building, named for Mssrs. Huntington, Hopkins, Stanford, and Crocker, who organized the Central Pacific Railroad and founded the Southern Pacific Railroad here

The Sacramento Schoolhouse Museum is a natural starting point for your walk among these restored historic buildings. Stroll through the Waterfront Park on your way to the market, where the activity of vendors recalls that of the original waterfront. While John Sutter was going about setting up an agricultural empire, Sam Brannan was doing business with a steady tide of businesspeople arriving by riverboat.

The waterfront was the center of activity in Sacramento. Riverboat fans will enjoy the close-up views of the *Delta King*, which can be seen between the market and the railroad station. Look across the street from the passenger station to see the historic Eagle Theatre. It was the first theater to be opened in California, in 1849, and it was the first theater in California to be closed by flooding, in 1850.

Across the street from the freight station is the Booth Building, which housed wholesale dry goods and groceries. It appears that in the 20 years since John Sutter settled here, pioneers had made the transition from hunting rabbits for dinner to buying groceries at the store.

You will probably see or hear old steam trains traveling back and forth along the spur tracks heading past the station platforms and the Discovery Museum into the California State Railroad Museum. Trains operate on a 6-mile round-trip route for a 40-minute excursion on the Sacramento River levees. Volunteers from around Sacramento maintain and operate the trains, which run on weekends from April through September. They will gladly interrupt their tasks to answer questions.

Pass a cluster of picnic tables huddled under the massive sycamore tree shading the front of the Discovery Museum. The entrance is just beyond the branches' reach. If you are walking between the two museums on I Street, notice the historic Big Four Building, which housed the offices of the Central Pacific Railroad and the Huntington and Hopkins Store. The entrance to the California State Railroad Museum is just past the Big Four Building. When you exit there, look across the street at the patio-dining area below the street. You are looking down on what was once the ground or street level before the city was raised 12 feet in 1862 to thwart further destruction caused by flooding.

On the left is the famous *Pony Express Rider* statue by Thomas Holland, one of the most popular items on display. This 15-foot-tall, 3,800-pound bronze casting accurately portrays the rider and horse, according to contemporary accounts, which include Mark Twain's commentary on the rider's clothing. However, riders wore skullcaps more often than the hat depicted.

The western terminus of the Pony Express was across the street in the historic B. F. Hastings Building, which has housed a number of illustrious tenants. Built immediately after the Great Fire of 1852, it once contained the Wells Fargo office and the California Supreme Court. It was also the western terminus for the transcontinental telegraph. Today it houses the Old Sacramento State Historic Park Visitor Center and the Wells Fargo Museum.

Pass the tall, narrow, brightly painted Sacramento Engine Company No. 3 (unless you're ready for an excellent meal), and look for the sculpture on the left. Theodore Judah's remembrance, detailed here in this intricately carved rock, can scarcely reflect the monumentality of his great achievement—engineering the Central Pacific Railroad's route across the Sierra Nevada Mountains.

Wander up and down the streets and sidewalks of Old Sacramento to see more historic buildings. The Lady Adams Building, the oldest in the city, houses a popular costume and variety shop. The Union Hotel, rebuilt with brick after the 1852 fire, was a fine hostelry in its day.

Sidewalk vendors ply their trade in front of the saloons, hotels, restaurants, and an assortment of shops that occupy the rest of the buildings composing Old Sacramento. Regardless of its occupant, the building itself is sure to have a story or secret for you to discover.

NEARBY ACTIVITIES

Walk across the river on the Tower Bridge to West Sacramento's Riverwalk, which is described in Hike 3 (see next profile). Head east down the Capitol Mall to Capitol Park, also described in Hike 1 (see previous profile).

3 RIVERWALK PARK

KEY AT-A-GLANCE INFORMATION

LENGTH: 1.5 miles

CONFIGURATION: Out-and-back

DIFFICULTY: Easy

WATER REQUIRED: 1 liter

SCENERY: Sacramento riverfront

EXPOSURE: Completely exposed

TRAIL TRAFFIC: Moderate

TRAIL SURFACE: Paved sidewalks and pathways

HIKING TIME: 30 minutes

SEASON: Year-round

ACCESS: No fees or permits

MAPS: USGS Sacramento West

WHEELCHAIR ACCESS: Yes

FACILITIES: Picnic areas, pit toilets

DRIVING DISTANCE: 1 mile

SPECIAL COMMENTS: Both garage and on-street metered parking are available in Old Sacramento and West Sacramento. Work is under way to extend Riverwalk to the south, past Raley Field, adding 0.6 mile to the walkway.

GPS TRAILHEAD COORDINATES

Latitude   N38° 34.874´

Longitude   W121° 30.586´

IN BRIEF

West Sacramento's Riverwalk Park offers a fresh perspective on the Sacramento River at the embarcadero. Shade trees line the riverbank, where you can picnic and watch boat traffic. The promenade will ultimately reach from the Lighthouse Marina to the locks at the Port of Sacramento. The walk currently runs from the Tower Bridge to a block south of the I Street Bridge. Pass the Grand Staircase and the renowned Ziggurat Building on your way to crossing the railroad bridge as you return to Old Sacramento.

DESCRIPTION

The most convenient, and most interesting, place to park is on the cobbled streets of Old Sacramento. Whether you use the garage or metered parking on the street, walk out to the Tower Bridge, which you will cross to reach the Riverwalk arch. Alternatively, there is a pedestrian access point to Riverwalk in the cul-de-sac at the end of Second Avenue on the north side of the Ziggurat Building.

Look east and you will be met with an excellent view of the white dome of the capitol, sitting handsomely above its surrounding trees. A right turn places you squarely in front of the Tower Bridge—gleaming gold at any time of day but shining brightest at sunrise.

Directions _____

From I-5 North in downtown Sacramento, take the Old Sacramento exit onto J Street, then head toward the Tower Bridge. Turn right into Old Town Sacramento and park. Walk across the Tower Bridge and turn right beneath the Riverwalk archway, which is your trailhead.

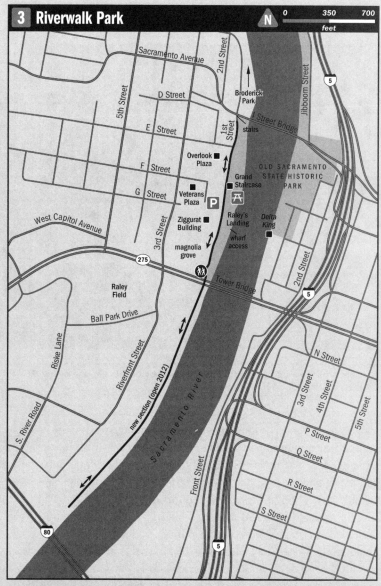

3 Riverwalk Park

N

0   350   700
feet

Sacramento Avenue

2nd Street

5th Street

D Street

Broderick Park

Jibboom Street

5

E Street

1st Street

I Street Bridge

stairs

Overlook Plaza

F Street

OLD SACRAMENTO STATE HISTORIC PARK

Grand Staircase

G Street

Veterans Plaza

P

Ziggurat Building

Raley's Landing

Delta King

West Capitol Avenue

3rd Street

magnolia grove

wharf access

2nd Street

5

275

Tower Bridge

Raley Field

Ball Park Drive

N Street

Riske Lane

Riverfront Street

3rd Street

4th Street

5th Street

S. River Road

new section (open 2012)

Sacramento River

P Street

Q Street

Front Street

R Street

80

S Street

5

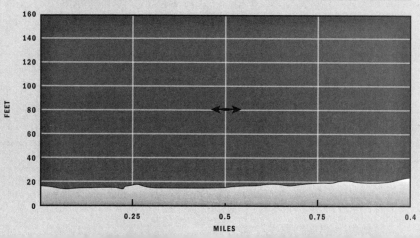

160
140
120
100
80
60
40
20
0

FEET

0.25   0.5   0.75   0.4

MILES

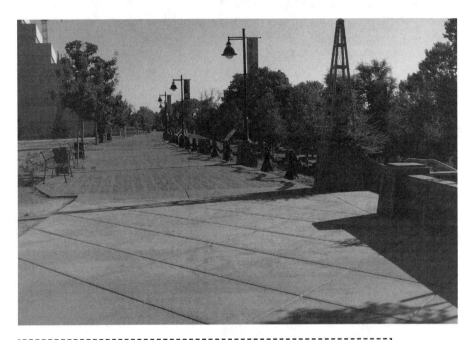

As you amble north toward the Ziggurat Building, Union Plaza (to the right) and similar small plazas line the scenic riverfront promenade.

The bridge's gold paint pays homage to the mineral that made the boat landing at Sacramento a turning point in the lives of so many following the spring of 1848.

Built in 1935 for less than $1 million, the Tower Bridge originally accommodated trolleys in the middle of four traffic lanes. Pedestrians have always been able to walk across the 737-foot bridge on its outside walkways. Walk to the west and look up under the arched trusses. The 200-foot center span and the equipment used to lift it weigh more than 5 million pounds.

Once on the West Sacramento side of the river, turn right at the brick-paved entry to the Riverwalk. The Flemish settler known as John Schwartz settled West Sacramento in the 1840s. He and his brother founded salmon fisheries, along with drying, pickling, and other seafood operations along the river's shores. They later sold land to the McDowell family; when Mr. McDowell was killed in a bar fight, his widow subdivided her land, which became known as the Town of Washington and was later renamed Broderick.

At about the same time, a hopeful but unlucky gold miner named Mike Bryte retreated from the Foothills and took up dairy farming on the west banks of the Sacramento. The community known as Bryte was established after his farm was subdivided. The communities of Broderick and Bryte, also called East Yolo, eventually became incorporated as the town of West Sacramento.

From the arched entrance, walk toward the river. The first set of steps, decorated with a derrick, is Union Square, which is dedicated to the port laborers who had worked here and at the Port of Sacramento in the early days. An iron anchor chain borders the promenade to the north. Below you, just past the picnic area and the trees along the shore, are a water-taxi stop and a fishing pier.

Through a break in the sycamore, you can see the *Delta King* moored on the opposite bank, below the train depot in Old Sacramento. Bird's-eye-view drawings from 1849 show a river port active with ships of all types on both shores. Most maritime commerce today is handled in the deep-water Port of Sacramento. Now a local landmark, the Ziggurat Building is the largest office building in West Sacramento and is known not only for its unique terraced design but also for its use of seismic dampers. The Ziggurat Building overlooks the Raley's Landing boat wharf. A wooden boardwalk provides access to the wharf through the giant cottonwoods; there are picnic tables on the lawn on either side of the boardwalk.

Pass the simple Veterans Plaza just before the Grand Staircase, which fans out down to the picnic areas. From this vantage, the views are dramatic in all directions. Before you stand the waterfront buildings of Old Sacramento, sandwiched between the transportation system of centuries past and the architecture of a modern city. Before continuing north, turn around for an image of ancient and modern architecture juxtaposed here in West Sacramento.

Just opposite E Street are another overlook and a plaza that offer great vistas of Sacramento's skyline and the Sacramento River, along with views of waterfowl and shorebirds.

The path continues north from this plaza, past the restrooms and water fountains, and appears to end just ahead. Actually, here you have three choices: you can turn around and walk past the Tower Bridge to the new section, which opened in the fall of 2011; you can walk down the stairs to the dirt path and walk under the I Street Bridge for about 0.35 mile to Broderick Park; or you can walk straight ahead and climb the stairs of the I Street Bridge and walk across it to Old Sacramento. This double-decker bridge is one of two built in 1911. The original 1911 bridge at M Street no longer exists, but the one at I Street remains. Stroll across the Sacramento River for an excellent view. When the Amtrak Capitol Corridor rumbles beneath you, you'll swear the whole bridge is going to shake apart. The sidewalk exits onto the circular ramp leading into Old Sacramento. Wind along Second Street and turn up J Street.

NEARBY ACTIVITIES

The California State Railroad Museum is on I Street, next to the Big Four Building in Old Sacramento. It's open daily (except Thanksgiving, Christmas, and New Year's Day) from 10 a.m. to 5 p.m. Admission: $9 adults, $4 youths ages 6–17, children age 5 and under free. For more information, visit **csrmf.org**.

For information regarding Old Sacramento, a brochure is available online at **oldsacramento.com**.

4   WILLIAM LAND PARK TRAIL

KEY AT-A-GLANCE INFORMATION

LENGTH: 3 miles

CONFIGURATION: Out-and-back

DIFFICULTY: Cakewalk

WATER REQUIRED: 1 liter

SCENERY: Tree-filled city park

EXPOSURE: Shaded

TRAIL TRAFFIC: Moderate

TRAIL SURFACE: Sand and gravel

HIKING TIME: 1 hour

SEASON: Year-round, sunrise–sunset

ACCESS: No fees or permits

MAPS: USGS Sacramento East, Sacramento West; park map at tinyurl.com/landparkmap

WHEELCHAIR ACCESS: Yes

FACILITIES: Restrooms, parking, phone, water

DRIVING DISTANCE: 2 miles

SPECIAL COMMENTS: Land Park, with its varied features, has an active, family-oriented atmosphere.

GPS TRAILHEAD COORDINATES

Latitude   N38° 32.386´

Longitude   W121° 30.130´

IN BRIEF

Leading through a grand old city park, this biking and jogging track is a wonderful place to hike among the native and ornamental trees, which border some wonderfully architected homes. Parking is near Fairytale Town. The route begins in front of the zoo, winds along the fishing pond and the golf course, and then leads on to circumnavigate the ball fields.

DESCRIPTION

When you need a place to hike that's close to home yet still has a natural look and feel to it, William Land Park is the place to visit. Most people think of children's attractions when they think of Land Park. While the zoo and Fairytale Town are worth visiting, this 146-acre park offers a host of other attractions, such as a nine-hole golf course; fields for soccer, baseball, and softball; fishing ponds; and basketball courts. The clean, broad jogging and walking track winds among all of these.

William Land Park was added to Sacramento's park system with the purchase of this land in 1918. William Land, a former Sacramento mayor and hotel owner, willed the city of Sacramento $250,000 for "recreation sport for children and a pleasure ground for the poor." Although the city had decided on this

----

Directions ⟶

From J Street and I-5 in downtown Sacramento, drive 1.6 miles on I-5 South to the Sutterville Road exit. Take Sutterville Road east 0.4 mile and turn left on Land Park Drive. Take the first right turn to park next to Fairytale Town. The sand-and-gravel trail begins across from the zoo entrance at 15th Avenue and Land Park Drive.

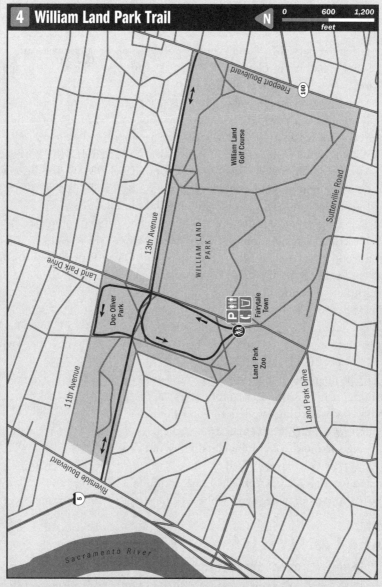

Freeport Boulevard

160

William Land
Golf Course

Sutterville Road

13th Avenue

Land Park Drive

WILLIAM LAND
PARK

Doc Oliver
Park

Fairytale
Town

Land Park
Zoo

11th Avenue

Land Park Drive

Riverside Boulevard

5

Sacramento River

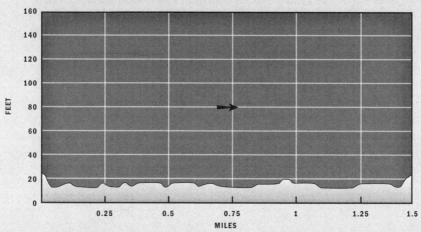

160

140

120

100

80

60

40

20

0

FEET

0.25   0.5   0.75   1   1.25   1.5

MILES

property for the park, Mr. Land's niece opposed the site's purchase and declared that her uncle had never liked the location. Despite that, the zoo was opened in 1927 and Fairytale Town was opened in 1959.

At the sign declaring BEGIN BIKE LANE, just across from the zoo entrance, you will usually see a few daily athletes stretching and warming up as they ready themselves for a workout. This is where your 3-mile route begins as well.

Walk under the Douglas firs, foothill pines, and coast redwoods as you head north past the amphitheater. Pass the fishing pond, where you will hear whoops and cries of delight as youngsters reel in their first perch. You may hear other sorts of shouts as you pass golfers critiquing their latest shot.

There is a great deal of flexibility in how each individual completes this route, but the described track continues straight north across 13th Avenue on the way to looping around the baseball field at the top of Doc Oliver Park. Take a left on 11th Avenue and walk under the shade of the valley oaks and sycamores along there.

Turn left to continue south on sycamore-lined 13th Street as it rounds the ball fields before you bear right onto 13th Avenue. This street section, 0.3 mile long, takes you to Riverside Boulevard, where you will make a U-turn. Backtrack past the south end of the Doc Oliver fields, and continue along 13th Avenue 0.5 mile to Freeport Boulevard and back.

The promenade along 13th Avenue is made to seem so much larger by the towering cottonwood and sycamore trees in the park. Valley oaks, with their spreading limbs inviting strollers to enter their shade, dot the margin of the golf course. Houses lining the avenues around the park have added to the natural tone here, being surrounded by ornamental trees and shrubs.

Now that you have walked the two "arms" of the hike, cross Land Park Drive and walk to 13th Street. Then turn south on 13th Street and walk the 0.25 mile to 15th Avenue, where you will cross the street to your starting point.

NEARBY ACTIVITIES

Nine holes of golf can be arranged here by contacting the pro at William Land Park Golf Course, 1701 Sutterville Road, Sacramento, CA 95822; 916-277-1207.

EFFIE YEAW NATURE CENTER TRAILS

5

IN BRIEF

This 77-acre nature preserve offers a glimpse of the once-vast riparian and oak woodlands, shrub lands, meadows, and aquatic habitats along the American River. Deer, coyotes, wild turkeys, rabbits, snakes, hawks, owls, woodpeckers, songbirds, and waterfowl add to the adventure of three self-guided walking trails.

DESCRIPTION

The Effie Yeaw Nature Center captures a time when Maidu Nisenan people camped along this area each summer, enjoying the plentiful food in this riparian habitat that once extended 5 miles on either side of the American River. Deer, rabbit, squirrel, fox, turkey, fowl, crayfish, and salmon, and plentiful valley oaks, willows, sedges, and reeds—all essential ingredients of life to Native Americans—could be found where you now walk.

In the 1950s and 1960s, Effie Yeaw, a teacher, conservationist, and environmental educator, began leading natural- and cultural-history walks in this area formerly known as Deterding Woods.

- -

Directions ───────────────────➤

From downtown Sacramento, take US 50 East 5 miles to the Watt Avenue North exit. Follow Watt Avenue north 0.8 mile to Fair Oaks Avenue. Turn right on Fair Oaks and drive 4 miles to Van Alstine (El Camino to the left). Turn right on Van Alstine and, in 0.3 mile, turn left on California. Go 0.2 mile to Tarshes Drive, where you will turn right at the Ancil Hoffman Park sign. Drive 0.4 mile along Tarshes Drive to the entrance kiosk and then 0.2 mile to San Lorenzo Way; then turn left and head 0.1 mile to the nature-center parking lot. The trailheads are on either side of the nature center.

KEY AT-A-GLANCE INFORMATION

LENGTH: 0.75–2.5 miles

CONFIGURATION: 3 loop trails

DIFFICULTY: Cakewalk

WATER REQUIRED: 1 liter

SCENERY: Riparian zone

EXPOSURE: Mostly shaded

TRAIL TRAFFIC: Varies

TRAIL SURFACE: Pebble and duff, river cobble and sand

HIKING TIME: 0.5–2 hours

SEASON: The trails are open daily, from dawn to dusk. The nature-center building is open November–January, 9 a.m.–4 p.m.; February–October, 9 a.m.–5 p.m.; closed Thanksgiving, Christmas Day, and New Year's Day; closed Mondays and Tuesdays.

ACCESS: No fees or permits

MAPS: USGS Carmichael; trail maps available online and at nature center

WHEELCHAIR ACCESS: Possible, but note that the trails can be bumpy, slippery, and muddy in spots.

FACILITIES: Restrooms, picnic tables, outdoor theater, gift shop

DRIVING DISTANCE: 7 miles

SPECIAL COMMENTS: Dogs, horses, bicycles, and smoking are prohibited on these trails.

GPS TRAILHEAD COORDINATES

Latitude   N38° 37.044´
Longitude   W121° 18.702´

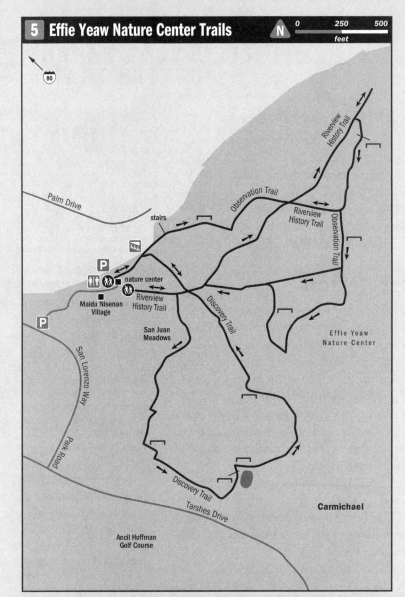

N

0   250   500
feet

Palm Drive

80

Observation Trail

Riverview History Trail

Riverview History Trail

Observation Trail

stairs

P

nature center

Riverview History Trail

Maidu Nisenan Village

P

San Juan Meadows

Discovery Trail

Effie Yeaw Nature Center

San Lorenzo Way

Park road

Discovery Trail

Tarshes Drive

Carmichael

Ancil Hoffman Golf Course

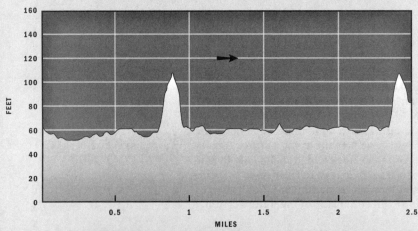

160
140
120
100
80
60
40
20
0

FEET

0.5   1   1.5   2   2.5

MILES

Yeaw raised interest in preserving the lands along the river and worked with the Sacramento County Parks Department to develop the concept of a parkway along the river that would include these grounds. Most importantly, her vision helped stimulate the formation of the Save the American River Association (SARA) and establishment of the American River Parkway.

As you walk from the parking lot to the nature center, pause and read the interpretive signs for the native California species displayed here. Look to your right at the Maidu Nisenan summer village, where you will see authentic examples of a tule shelter, grinding rock, acorn granary, and fire pit, plus a shade shelter.

Pick up a free map of the nature-preserve trails inside the center. You have a choice of three trails, which start in two different spots: The Observation Trail and Discovery Trail begin at a trailhead behind the center. The Riverview History Trail begins (and the Discovery Trail ends) near the huge walnut tree to the left of the picnic tables next to the Maidu village.

The interpretive signs on these trails are among the best in any park system. Each consecutively numbered sign has a symbol that indicates the trail, drawings or pictures, and complete descriptions—all etched into a durable metal sign.

The Discovery Trail, the Observation Trail, and the Riverview History Trail have common starting points, common ending points, and parts of the trail in common—but not all in the same way. If it sounds confusing, relax. These trails are delightful and well signed. So while you might easily get off one route and onto another, there is no danger of becoming "temporarily mislocated."

Step back out of the nature center, turn left, and walk around the building. Pass the Himalayan blackberries on your right, then pass the small outdoor theater, and your trailhead is another 10 feet.

This is a dual trailhead—straight ahead for the Observation Trail and right for the Discovery Trail. The Observation Trail both starts and ends here. The Discovery Trail starts here but ends at the start of the Riverview History Trail.

Ahead, on the Observation Trail, you will start with a winding, nicely shaded, duff-covered trail that leads to a bench atop the only stairs on the trails. Look at the moss covering the north side of the trees in this damp valley-oak grove. Momentarily, the trail will open up and join the Riverview History Trail for a brief bit of full sunshine. In this open area, the native grasses and sedges proliferated after floods.

Pay close attention as you approach the river. The Observation Trail turns right, and the Riverview History Trail turns left 10 feet farther along. Take the Observation Trail, heading south on this duff trail and ignoring the first trail that comes in from the right. Although that trail from the right will reconnect with this trail and lead back to the center, the Observation Trail continues ahead. Look to the left at the moonscape of large river cobble and boulders. This spectacular scene is just part of the original land granted to John Sutter.

Make a right onto the next trail and plunge into a thick copse of live oak, where you can feel the air temperature drop. Sample more blackberries if there

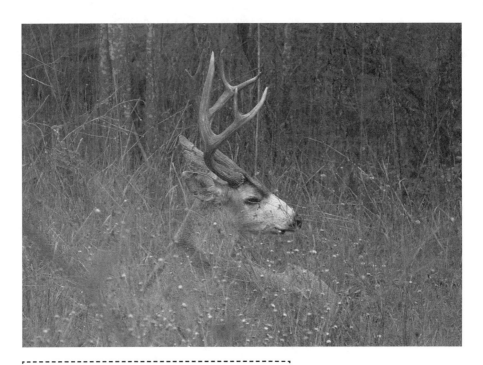

Protected wildlife thrives in the nature center's sanctuary.

are any left. The undergrowth is so lush and the foliage so thick that it's difficult to hear or see others, which affords a nice sense of solitude. Take a break at the bench, where the trail turns briefly north.

A small meadow ringed by live oak offers a nice spot for deer to browse. The trail crosses Riverview History Trail but soon turns toward the nature center, so don't let the deer capture your attention at this junction. A short uphill section returns you to the trailhead and the start of Discovery Trail.

On Discovery Trail, you will descend gently alongside Himalayan blackberries, past giant—fallen and decomposing—valley oak, alongside Dutchman's pipevine, all of which provide habitat for beetles, ground squirrels, hummingbirds, and woodpeckers.

As you look to your right, you will see deer lounging near the trail and around the margin of San Juan Meadows. The meadow is defined by huge valley oaks. Found only in California, these prototypically spreading oaks are the largest species of oak in North America. Deer and rabbit are plentiful here, and opportunities for outstanding wildlife photos abound. But stay on the trails—particularly in this area. As in most parks, this one also posts cautions about poison oak and even has interpretive signs pointing it out along this section of the trail.

Turkeys are abundant in this area, and you will notice their signs everywhere if you don't slip on or trip over them first. And they roost in trees! Enjoy the sandy, winding trail as you read the signs on the way to the nature pond. A clean bench there makes a great perch to observe bugs, reptiles, and birds.

After winding through sedge-filled groves of live oak and western redbud, the trail begins to turn to sand and river cobble. At the junction with the River-view History Trail, turn left. Walk past your initial crossing with this trail and head west along the San Juan Meadows. The Discovery Trail ends where the Riverview History Trail begins—at the huge two-toned walnut tree.

Now at the beginning of the Riverview History Trail, you've seen and crossed several parts of it. The trail, made of river cobble and sand, is partly service road and is therefore potholed in spots. On this, the most openly exposed of all the trails, walk straight; the trails you walked earlier cross your path. You will angle toward the American River. Beautiful modern homes on the cliffs above you stand in stark contrast to the quiet as you approach the river. You will take a much smaller footpath off to the right, angling another 50 feet toward the river. If you happen to miss this turn, you'll find a bench about 100 feet ahead. Turn there and come back to this trail alongside the river.

Head south along the trail and try to imagine the view without the remains of gold dredging. A bench ahead on your right is a great spot for that and for bird-watching.

At the next signed junction to the right, you will turn and retrace your steps from the Observation Trail as the Riverview History Trail now joins with it for the return to the nature center.

NEARBY ACTIVITIES

The Effie Yeaw Nature Center (inside Ancil Hoffman County Park, 2850 San Lorenzo Way, Carmichael, California; 916-489-4918) offers programs for all ages every Saturday and Sunday at 1:30 p.m. Visit **sacnaturecenter.net** for details, a calendar, and maps.

Folsom State Recreation Area has a 90-mile network of multiuse trails that includes the Pioneer Express Trail (Hike 25, page 140) as well as a 21-mile segment of the American Discovery Trail, the nation's first coast-to-coast nonmotorized recreation trail.

6 UC DAVIS ARBORETUM TRAIL

KEY AT-A-GLANCE INFORMATION

LENGTH: 3.5 miles

CONFIGURATION: Loop

DIFFICULTY: Cakewalk

WATER REQUIRED: 1 liter

SCENERY: Flora from around the world

EXPOSURE: Mostly shaded

TRAIL TRAFFIC: Light

TRAIL SURFACE: Asphalt, pebble, and sand

HIKING TIME: 2 hours, plus lingering time

SEASON: Year-round

ACCESS: No fees or permits

MAPS: USGS Merritt, Davis; interactive map at arboretum .ucdavis.edu/visitor_map.aspx

WHEELCHAIR ACCESS: Yes

FACILITIES: Water fountains and restrooms in various locations near the trail. See UC Davis Arboretum map for exact locations.

DRIVING DISTANCE: 14 miles

SPECIAL COMMENTS: This hike is not only beautiful and enjoyable but accessible and educational, too.

GPS TRAILHEAD COORDINATES

Latitude   N38° 31.898′

Longitude   W121° 45.545′

IN BRIEF

More than 4,000 plants and flowers are on display at the University of California, Davis, Arboretum in 18 collections and gardens. If you want to learn about the flora in California's biozones, a few hours among these magnificent gardens and collections will satisfy your interest.

DESCRIPTION

The UC Davis Arboretum Trail winds peacefully along an interstate highway and city streets. You start this hike by walking southwest through fragrant lavender, rosemary, and other herbs growing on both sides of the Mediterranean Collection along Putah Creek Lagoon.

When Putah Creek's channel was diverted in the 1870s, what remained was this abandoned oxbow—the old north channel—which dried up over the years and became the sole depression among otherwise flat farmland. From its beginnings as an actual farm for

----

Directions

From I-5 South in downtown Sacramento, drive 13 miles on I-80 West to Davis. Take Exit 71/UC Davis and turn right on Old Davis Road. Turn at the first left onto California Avenue, then take the next left onto La Rue Road. Turn left on Putah Creek Lodge Road, then right into the parking area. Parking is also available in Lots 47 and 48 on La Rue Road and costs $6; you can use a credit card or $1 bills. Parking is limited on weekdays, but on weekends it's free and more broadly available. The trail described here starts at the Putah Creek Lodge footbridge. You can begin your hike from any point along the path, but this hike begins at the Mediterranean collection, at the footbridge on the side of the creek opposite the Putah Creek Lodge.

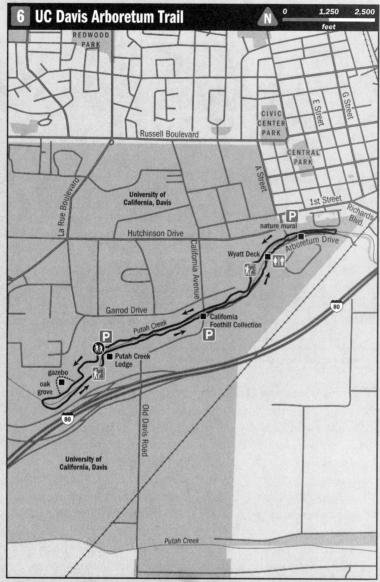

N

0   1,250   2,500

feet

REDWOOD PARK

Russell Boulevard

CIVIC CENTER PARK

CENTRAL PARK

E Street

G Street

University of California, Davis

A Street

1st Street

La Rue Boulevard

Richards Blvd.

Hutchinson Drive

nature mural

P

California Avenue

Wyatt Deck

Arboretum Drive

Garrod Drive

Putah Creek

California Foothill Collection

P

80

P

gazebo

Putah Creek Lodge

oak grove

80

Old Davis Road

University of California, Davis

Putah Creek

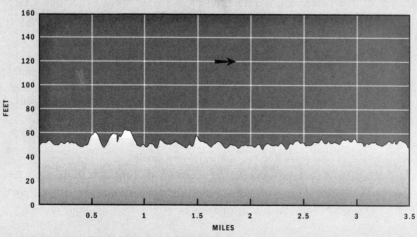

FEET

160

140

120

100

80

60

40

20

0

0.5   1   1.5   2   2.5   3   3.5

MILES

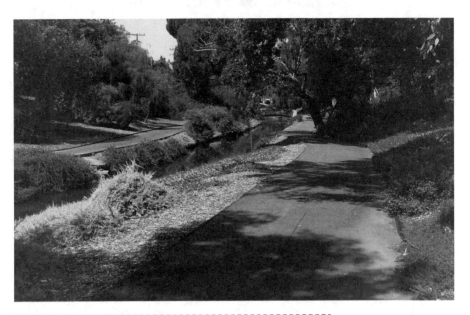

Beautiful sights and pungent scents surround the pathway through the
Mediterranean collections of aromatic trees and plants.

horticultural instruction in World War I until 1936, the arboretum area became
the collection point for an abundance of unwanted materials. The arboretum was
founded February 29 of that same year, when students, faculty, and administra-
tors joined in their traditional "leap day campus-improvement project." This
included the arboretum's "first planting," which comprised many of the trees seen
along the south shore from Wyatt Deck to the California Avenue Bridge.

The design and placement of the arboretum included plants native to California that have low water requirements, and protected the magnificent 400-year-
old valley oaks (*Quercus lobata*) growing in the California Foothill Collection.
Caretakers of the arboretum have adhered to the principle of using the natural
landform whenever possible. The larger ponds at the south end of the arboretum
were sculpted, but you may not notice this as you walk around the vine-covered
gazebo and its fragrant white-flower garden. The oak grove to the far right is
popular for catching shade on hot summer days.

The plants lining the trail represent those specifically native to the various
regions of California and, more generally, to the regions of the world where a
Mediterranean climate predominates. You will find gardens and collections in this
100-acre arboretum that represent areas such as South Africa, Australia, or South
America; specific plants are also grouped by type, as in the oak groves, the redwood grove, and the acacia collection, and there are demonstration gardens and
horticultural theme gardens, like the white-flower garden.

As you might expect, you're never far from shade on this trail, but a broad-
brimmed hat will help keep you cool as you browse around at the boathouse,
where an early-California garden displays plants found in the state before the

Gold Rush. There really are no empty spaces—understory trees and bushes, grasses, and flowers seem to occupy the terrain and line the creekside path.

Pass to the right of Putah Creek Lodge with its inviting fire pit and seating area, through the South American Collection with its lush Cuyamaca cypress, and then into the dense, cool shade of the acacia grove. As you walk around the little side trails and groves, notice the soil underfoot on these bordered trails. The silt and plant debris deposited alongside this former channel were the ingredients that created the rich sandy loam that is so beneficial to all of the plants here. Towering Torrey pines and spreading California sycamore suddenly dwarf any understory plants, but California poppies can be counted on for color.

There are very few surprising turns on this trail, and all are clearly marked. Aleppo pine, buckeye, and California box elder lead into the valley-oak grove as you head toward the Mondavi Center for the Performing Arts. The California Foothill Collection features live oak, toyon, mesa oak, gray pine, and a streamside covered with wild grapes, in addition to a 5-foot-diameter valley oak.

Flowers and shrubs accompany you past Mrak Hall Drive, and native California plants fill the side gardens just ahead of Wyatt Deck and the redwood grove. California fuchsia, dwarf coyote bush, Torrey pine and Santa Cruz ironwood, Catalina Island mountain mahogany, Canary Island pine and sand mesa manzanita, shooting star, and penstemon are all part of this impressively colorful display.

Leap Day 1941 saw the planting of the redwood trees in this grove. Because they are not native to the valley, these coast redwoods were hand-watered by energetic students, who were responsible for the trees' maturing into the grove you see today. This is the spot to stop and take notes and pictures and have a drink or a snack. The picnic tables offer solitude within these giant trees.

Art and nature are as important as the gardens to the arboretum. The huge, colorful, and oversized nature lesson that is found in the tunnel-wall mural is an example of that partnership. Take the left fork after this tunnel and enter the Australian collection. Your turnaround takes you to the other side of the creek, onto a dirt path just opposite the mural tunnel. Meander through the North Coast Collection opposite the redwood grove. Your dirt path will return to asphalt at the next footbridge. Formosan redwood, Soquel coast redwood, and egg-shaped sculptures precede the desert collection, with its sunny patch of blossoming prickly-pear cactus and looming agave plant.

Gray pine, Oaxaca pine, Chinese juniper, and a long line of redbud lead into the South American Collection and back to the trailhead.

NEARBY ACTIVITIES

Group tours can be arranged with 30 days' notice by calling 530-752-4880.

7 DAVIS-COVELL GREENBELT

KEY AT-A-GLANCE INFORMATION

LENGTH: 2.7 miles

CONFIGURATION: Loop

DIFFICULTY: Cakewalk

WATER REQUIRED: 1 liter

SCENERY: Urban green space with wildlife-viewing platforms

EXPOSURE: Plenty of sun and shade

TRAIL TRAFFIC: Moderate but not crowded

TRAIL SURFACE: Asphalt pavement

HIKING TIME: 1.5 hours

SEASON: Year-round

ACCESS: No fees or permits

MAPS: USGS Davis, Merritt

WHEELCHAIR ACCESS: Yes

FACILITIES: Restrooms at trailhead and at Northstar Park

DRIVING DISTANCE: 15 miles

SPECIAL COMMENTS: This hike features playgrounds, lawn sculptures, and a nature walk.

GPS TRAILHEAD COORDINATES

Latitude   N38° 33.615´
Longitude W121° 44.861´

IN BRIEF

The Davis–Covell Greenbelt links the Davis Community Park and Northstar Park while it weaves through neighborhoods and their playgrounds. The well-lit asphalt path has location signs and easy access to all the adjacent communities.

DESCRIPTION

The Davis–Covell Greenbelt is a wonderful path to walk and includes a surprising diversity of interesting sights. The described hike begins at the pedestrian overpass at the north end of the Davis Community Park. An alternative starting point, also with parking and restrooms, is at Northstar Park, at the north end of the greenbelt. If you're arriving on foot, almost every side street along the path accesses the greenbelt, which winds through the surrounding communities.

Once across the bridge, the trail splits at the first playground. You will be returning along the path to the left. Walk straight, generally north-northwest, along the greenbelt as it meanders through Covell Park. The names of the streets you pass all have a Spanish theme, and nearly every street has an entrance to the greenbelt. Within the first 0.5 mile, you will

---

Directions ⟶

From I-5 South in downtown Sacramento, take I-80 West 9.5 miles to Exit 72B/Richards Boulevard in Davis. Turn right at First Street and then left on F Street, one block later. Continue north on F Street 1.3 miles to West Covell Boulevard. Turn left on West Covell Boulevard, then left again into the parking lot just before the pedestrian overpass. Your trailhead is at the end of the overpass.

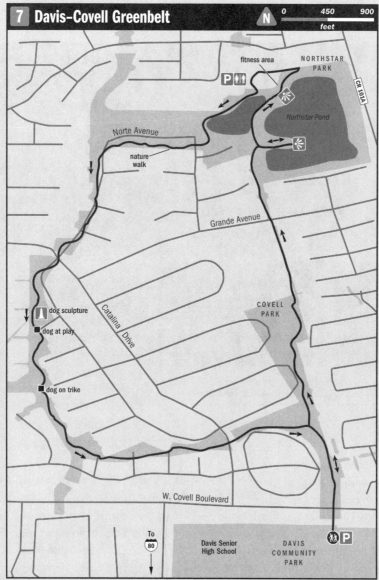

NORTHSTAR PARK

fitness area

Northstar Pond

CR 101A

Norte Avenue

nature walk

Grande Avenue

Catalina Drive

dog sculpture

dog at play

dog on trike

COVELL PARK

W. Covell Boulevard

To 80

Davis Senior High School

DAVIS COMMUNITY PARK

0   450   900

feet

N

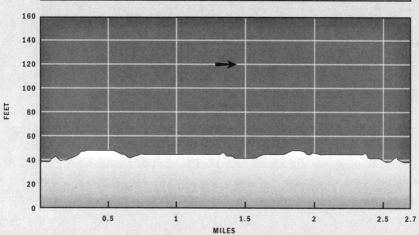

FEET

160
140
120
100
80
60
40
20
0

0.5   1   1.5   2   2.5   2.7

MILES

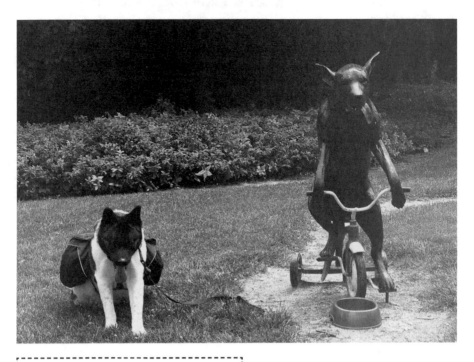

The Hugest Tongue in Davis contest was a draw.

see tennis courts, benches, barbecue grills, swings, slides, merry-go-rounds, and other leisure amenities.

Continue past the empty field to your left and cross Grande Avenue. A fence to your right marks the border of the Northstar Park wetland area. A variety of waterfowl inhabits this small pond and, from the sounds of it, so does a bevy of frogs. A nicely architected viewing platform extends into the wetland, allowing you to observe the wildlife. Egrets, herons, Canada geese, mallards, and coots compose just a partial list of birds that live or visit here. An identically designed but much smaller viewpoint is just 500 feet down the path on these tiny wooded islands.

Pass the aerating pond to the left of the path and walk toward Anderson Road, where you will turn left. A fitness and warm-up area sits on the path's left, just 100 feet past the smaller viewpoint. This is a good reason for beginning an exercise run at the Northstar Park and using the parking lot on the west side of the Tandem Properties building.

Continuing on the described path takes you through the parking lot, past the restrooms on the left, southward toward your trailhead. You will once again pass the aerating pond, with the playing fields of Northstar Park to your right.

You'll come to a nature walk on your right just after the playing fields. An information kiosk lists a huge variety of trees, shrubs, and flowers found here and also along the path. Walk west along the gravel path through the shady nature area, and make sure to look up as you pass under the welded arbors for an important message.

Exit the nature walk and turn to the south again. Within a few minutes, you'll cross Catalina Drive and reach another of the small parks along the walk. Eucalyptus trees tower over the path as you enter Greenbelt Area #10. You may not have expected artwork to be among the interesting things you'd be seeing on this walk. Rendered in bronze and natural stone, several clever installations liven the pathway. Keep a lookout for a turkey-chasing dog along here. As you pass Ecuador Place, you may notice another friendly dog ready to share his water with your pup. And as you watch out for bicycles along the path, be on the alert for happy tricycle riders around Estrella Place.

The route described here continues straight south. But if you want to wander farther to the west, turn right and walk through the tunnel under Anderson Road; when the trail ends, just one block farther west, you can pick up an alternate trail back to the north. Your path continues through signed greenbelt areas with playgrounds, Frisbee fields, picnic tables, and benches before crossing Catalina Drive and reentering Covell Park to the east. At the playground, take the path to the right and head toward the pedestrian overpass where you began your walk.

NEARBY ACTIVITIES

If you have children with you on this walk, you may want to visit the Davis Art Center, which is in the same parking lot as your trailhead. They offer a host of excellent programs for young artists of all interests.

If you don't have children with you, stop in for a bite at Redrum Burgers, at the intersection of Olive Drive and Richards Boulevard. When Murder Burger, a straightforward burger-and-beer joint, expanded to Rocklin, residents objected to the violent nature of the name, and so a renaming contest was held wherein Redrum was conceived. It continues to be known for its wide variety of beers and low-fat-beef burgers (ask about the Zoom).

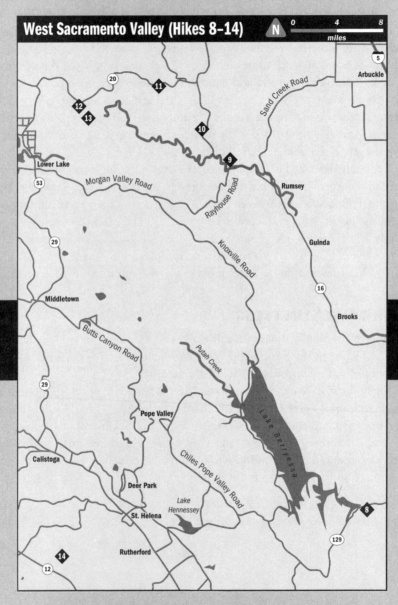

West Sacramento Valley (Hikes 8–14)

N

0   4   8
miles

Arbuckle

5

20

11

12

13

10

9

Sand Creek Road

Lower Lake

53

Morgan Valley Road

Rayhouse Road

Rumsey

Knoxville Road

Guinda

29

16

Middletown

Brooks

Butts Canyon Road

Putah Creek

29

Pope Valley

Lake Berryessa

Calistoga

Chiles Pope Valley Road

Deer Park

Lake Hennessey

St. Helena

8

Rutherford

129

14

12

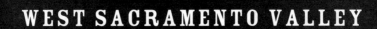

WEST SACRAMENTO VALLEY

8 HOMESTEAD-BLUE RIDGE TRAIL

KEY AT-A-GLANCE INFORMATION

LENGTH: 5.1 miles

CONFIGURATION: Loop

DIFFICULTY: Challenging

WATER REQUIRED: 3 liters

SCENERY: Ranges from idyllic canyon streams to spectacular views of Lake Berryessa

EXPOSURE: Mostly shaded trail with some brief exposure

TRAIL TRAFFIC: Light, with only 5,000 visitors annually

TRAIL SURFACE: Sand and rock, dirt and duff

HIKING TIME: 4–5 hours

SEASON: Year-round, sunrise–sunset

ACCESS: No fees or permits

MAPS: USGS Monticello Dam, Mount Vaca

WHEELCHAIR ACCESS: None

FACILITIES: None

DRIVING DISTANCE: 36 miles

SPECIAL COMMENTS: Dogs and bikes are prohibited on these trails.

GPS TRAILHEAD COORDINATES

Latitude   N38° 30.529´

Longitude W122 05.819´

IN BRIEF

Offering adventurous day hikers spectacular views of Lake Berryessa from the solitude of a ridgeline trail, this informative and physically demanding hike is hard to surpass. Start the morning walking along a seasonal canyon stream on a self-guided interpretive trail, which culminates at an abandoned homestead site. Then tighten your laces as you ascend the "monster stairs" to a ridgeline trail where what was once ocean floor now stands on its side. This loop takes hikers through seven habitat zones, or biozones, which support a vast array of fauna and flora.

DESCRIPTION

Every hiker has yearned for the trail that seems like an all-you-can-eat buffet for the naturalist. Set in the Stebbins Cold Canyon Reserve, the Homestead–Blue Ridge Trail serves it up. The Homestead Trail is an easy hike along an interpretive trail. In a short time, you'll learn about trees, shrubs, flowers, reptiles, amphibians,

----

Directions ⟶

From the junction of I-80 West and the Capital City Freeway, drive 10 miles on I-80 West to CR 113 North. Take CR 113 North 2.1 miles to the Russell Road exit. Turn left and drive another 12 miles to Winters.

Continue straight on CR 128 toward Lake Berryessa. Pass Pleasants Valley Road after 4.5 miles and drive another 4.5 miles to a bridge across Putah Creek, just past Canyon Creek Resort, with a vista upstream to Monticello Dam. Cross the bridge and park in the second, smaller parking area on the right 0.2 mile after the bridge. The trailhead is directly across the road. The trail finishes just 100 yards up the road from your trailhead.

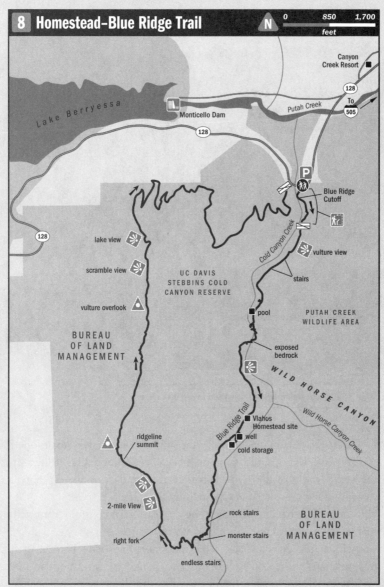

8 Homestead–Blue Ridge Trail

N

0   850   1,700
feet

Canyon Creek Resort

128

To 505

Putah Creek

Monticello Dam

128

Lake Berryessa

P

Blue Ridge Cutoff

Cold Canyon Creek

lake view

vulture view

scramble view

stairs

vulture overlook

UC DAVIS STEBBINS COLD CANYON RESERVE

pool

PUTAH CREEK WILDLIFE AREA

exposed bedrock

BUREAU OF LAND MANAGEMENT

WILD HORSE CANYON

Blue Ridge Trail

Wild Horse Canyon Creek

Vlahos Homestead site

well

ridgeline summit

cold storage

2-mile View

rock stairs

right fork

monster stairs

BUREAU OF LAND MANAGEMENT

endless stairs

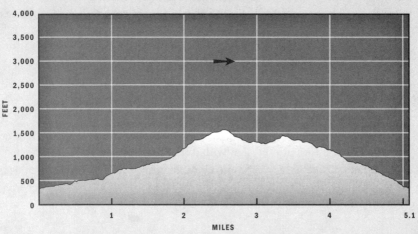

FEET

4,000
3,500
3,000
2,500
2,000
1,500
1,000
500
0

1   2   3   4   5.1
MILES

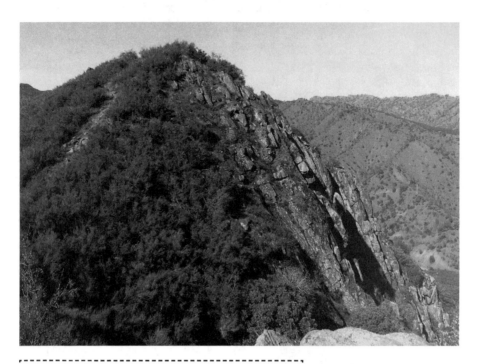

The Coast Ranges consist mostly of upended ancient seafloor.

insects, and rocks. At about 1 mile, you will encounter the abandoned Vlahos Homestead overlooking Cold Canyon Creek. Ascending Blue Ridge Trail after the homestead site will take you through grassland, woodland, chaparral, and lower montane zones up to a newly maintained ridgetop trail.

The Coast Range was formed by the deposition of coastal sediment falling to the ocean floor more than 160 million years ago; these layers of sand, clay, and silt eventually solidified into rock. That metamorphic rock—with layers still visible—was uplifted by the collision of the Pacific and North American plates. And those uplifted rocks have been further eroded and their sediments sent out to sea again. At present, they are highly visible in the middle of your trail, near the apex of the hike.

The Stebbins Cold Canyon Reserve is part of the University of California Natural Reserve System and is managed by UC Davis. This means that naturalists—amateur and professional alike—have wonderful resources available at the UCD NRS website (nrs.ucdavis.edu/stebbins.html). In-depth species lists and geologic information are provided to enhance your hike.

Step through the opening in the gate across the road from the parking area, and you will see an informational sign with a trail map immediately on your left. Distance markers posted every 0.25 mile along the trail help you track your location. This combination of trails is a long, narrow loop of about 2 miles per long leg, generally running south–north with the canyons.

Follow my cautions in the Introduction regarding poison oak, rattlesnakes, and mountain lions, because all are prevalent throughout the reserve. Watch your footing on the rock-speckled trails—they're both slippery when wet and easy to stumble over.

Immediately the trail forks, the left fork heading uphill on Pleasants Ridge Trail. The Homestead Trail begins down the right fork, across some landslide debris, and then past the right-turn cutoff over to the Blue Ridge Trail. You continue to the left, stepping over rocks that do not appear to be normal river cobble; in fact, they are debris from a 1995 mudslide. As you hike this trail, you can see signs of slumping in the surrounding hills.

Another green gate signals the area boundaries and provides another permanent trail map to study. A sign-in register bordered by toyon stands ready for you to log your visit. The sand-and-rock trail diverges left at some coyote brush, with the creek on the right.

As you gain a bit of elevation along this manzanita-shaded trail, look up to the right to view the distinctive V of turkey vultures as they circle in front of the rocky ridge (which you will later hike). The trail continues south, gaining about 20 feet above the creek; a series of stairs will help you across a 1982 land slump. You can't help but notice the energetic croaking of frogs along this section, which is shaded by bay laurel, manzanita, and live oak.

Get used to the word *stairs,* because they are the preferred (for sound soil-management practices) elevation assist in the reserve. When you reach more stairs, turn and take in the view of the Coast Range as it disappears into the Central Valley. Now climb 18 steps, and in 10 yards descend 15 steps. After 0.5 mile, as you continue to ascend the drainage, you can see the scar made by seasonal runoff.

Pause next to gentle cascades and pools among the spicebush plant after taking any one of the short side trails over to the creek. Some of the pools have been created by rock and cobble dams. These pools support a diverse community of aquatic insects, amphibians, and mammals.

Boulder-hop across the stream at the trail, but be careful not to get tangled in the brush on the opposite side. In another 250 feet, you will have a rare opportunity to see some exposed bedrock along the stream to your left. Your trail alternates from rocky to sandy now, as foothill pine becomes the predominant large tree. Just after you cross a little bridge, around 0.75 mile along, a large cottonwood stands in the middle of the creek.

Stairs will help you through some steep spots along here; the live oak and foothill pine provide nice shade, and the dense mat of moss and ferns helps keep you cool. The trail narrows and slithers uphill, but the sunlight never makes it through this tunnel of brush. Emerging at about 1 mile, you are greeted with a wonderful view up the canyon and the sight of an exemplar foothill pine, whose needles shimmer green and silver in the sunlight.

Walk through the space in the fence that says NO ENTRY and head toward the large clearing in front of you. Slightly ahead and to the right are the remains of the Vlahos Homestead. From atop the stone foundations, you can look out at Cold Canyon Creek and its confluence with Wild Horse Canyon Creek. Can you imagine a house sited here with goats corralled in the flat area in front of you? Just down the path are the remains of a well and a retaining wall or building foundation. Past the well, down the path to the left and across the drainage, is the cold-storage shed. Built of cemented stone into a hillside and covered with limbs and dirt, this room would have stayed quite cool. If you cross for a closer look, be aware that there is a beehive in the fork of the tree on the left, immediately next to the cold storage.

Retreating back to the well site, ascend the right-hand trail as it crosses the drainage farther uphill. You are now on the Blue Ridge Trail. As you approach 1.25 miles along the shaded trail, try to spot the witch's butter—the bright-orange fungus on downed pine limbs. You may also try to keep an eye open for signs on the ground of roosting turkeys. With so many species in this reserve, you are sure to see signs of many, but some are more obvious than others. On or next to the trail, look for signs of weasels and coyote in addition to raccoon and skunk.

Toyon will continue providing shade as you approach about six steps in the rock. After clambering over these giant steps, notice the moss-covered boulders surrounded by white alder. In another few paces, you'll come upon—you can hardly avoid—a huge, impressive madrone that is actually two individual trees, each with trunks about 16 inches in diameter. A few more monster stairs will warm you up for the 200 more to come over the next 0.5 mile. (But who's counting?)

As you approach the ridge, the trail will be squeezed by chaparral, but after your last ten steps, you will level out among scrub oak and ceanothus. At the junction with the Tuleyome Trail, take the right fork, climbing somewhat steeply, and as you near a high spot around the 2-mile point, turn to the northwest for a wonderful view of Lake Berryessa through the clearing.

Brush closes in against the rocky trail on the way to the next high clearing. Some rocks on the left side of the trail can provide a nice off-the-trail viewpoint to cool your feet. Or you may want to continue on this easy dirt trail section to the next summit, at around 1,460 feet. Watch along here for surprising displays of larkspur and Indian paintbrush.

Ahead, toward a beautiful overlook, you will be stopped by what appears to be a dead end. The brush is close in, and there appears to be no way forward, only retreat. Turn left and clamber over the boulder you're facing. Now you'll see your clear trail continuing. Before you leave this spot, take a look below to your right. Do you see that distinctive V again? The turkey vultures will circle above and below you, their heads always down, their eyes always scanning, their wings almost motionless. Listen quietly as one passes just overhead, and hear its nearly silent glide.

A great spot for pictures and snacks lies just ahead, as boulders provide an overlook for you to dangle your legs from while you lean back against the rocks. Leaving this beautiful overlook, your rock-and-dirt trail descends slightly to the

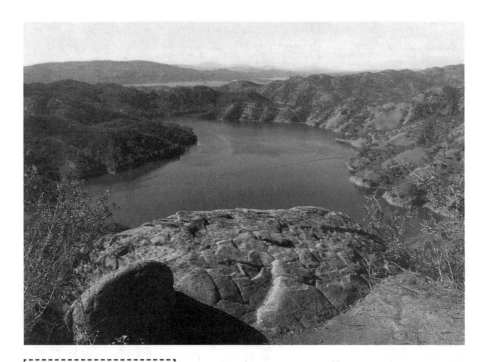

Vista point over Lake Berryessa

east side of the ridge. The trail continues to be easily distinguished, but a short stretch does wander along the ridgeline atop boulders.

Rocky and slightly steep as it exits the ridge's north end, your trail will level out at about the time you are shaded and cooled by some large manzanita. The hills to your east will momentarily come into view, and the manzanita will continue to crowd your northward trail. Just before the trail emerges from the brush, tread cautiously across the left side of a rock jumble. After a bit of exposure, you're back in the shade.

When you cross the next boulder patch, the trail will exit ahead to the right. Initially, walk around to the left of the rocks and cross the boulders; the trail will seem obvious as you look to the north. The next summit point along the dirt trail is at 2.75 miles. Right after this spot, you'll run into some leg-stretching boulder stairs. It's a bit tight along here, so don't let your pack catch on the brush.

Looking ahead, your trail becomes wide and obvious, and it climbs slightly but steadily. Look down at the line in the center of the trail: on closer inspection, that line is not one but hundreds of alternating light and dark strata of the ancient (160-million-year-old) sediments compressed to just inches thick over millennia. The sediments—silt, sand, and clay—fell to the ocean floor and have been altered by heat and pressure, tilted up by the collision of the Pacific and North American plates, and eroded again by the power of water . . . and your boots.

There is a bit of a scramble on the south side of this next summit. As you skirt the summit and exit the north end, go around the big boulder, using it as a handhold. Once around the boulder, turn left, not straight. A freshly maintained trail picks up here, where you will head downhill. Watch the first three steps—they are tall.

The 3.25-mile point, marked with an impressive rock outcrop, offers hikers an impressive vista over Lake Berryessa. The pictures here are well worth carrying a camera for. Your trail continues north, trending gently downhill. It levels out just before a trail-restoration zone. This newly constructed portion of the trail enters a copse of trees that breaks briefly, giving you a view of the uplifted rock that anchors the Monticello Dam across Putah Creek.

This trail was reconstructed by crews from the California Department of Forestry and Fire Protection Delta Conservation Camp and staff members from the University of California, Davis, Natural Reserve System. In 2000, to make the trail safer and more accessible, some 200 of the wooden steps were carried in and set in place by hand.

Just as you pass the manzanita that seems to grow out of a boulder in the newly dug trail, look ahead to the right to see your destination—just in time, as the shadow of another vulture crosses your path. As you descend to the gate at the end of the trail, you can enjoy the butterflies on the larkspur. The gate, another informational sign, and a register are at the 4.75-mile mark. Walk ahead to the road, then go about 100 yards right, to the parking lot across the road.

BLUE RIDGE-FISKE PEAK TRAIL 9

IN BRIEF

Tighten your bootlaces and clean the camera lens for the hike to Fiske Peak. This well-maintained trail ascends steadily through a lush foothill-woodland forest to the peak of vertically uplifted ocean floor—revealing views from the Coast Range to the Central Valley.

DESCRIPTION

If any entirely uphill hike can be enjoyed, it's this one. Your hike begins at the white gate on CR 40, where you'll see a notification that the bridge is out (it isn't), along with several other important but not-very-useful signs. Descend and cross the low-water bridge that straddles Cache Creek. River rafters are required to portage here, so they take the opportunity for a lunch break right near the trailhead. After crossing the creek, walk uphill and watch for a sign about 50 paces to the left, indicating the trailhead's location. Turn left and walk to the yellow gate; step through on the left and follow the doubletrack over toward the rafters' picnic grounds.

Directions ⟶

From Sacramento near Arco Arena, take I-5 North 55 miles to Williams and take Exit 577/ CA 20 West. Drive 18 miles on CA 20 West to the junction with CA 16 South in Wilbur Springs. Take CA 16 South 8.9 miles to old CR 40. Your landmark is the campground 0.7 mile before the turnout on the right. You may use Cache Creek Canyon Regional Park for a fee; otherwise, you may park under the trees along old CR 40 for free. After situating your car at the parking area, walk 375 feet to your trailhead at the white gate and barricade that stand across the old CR 40.

---

i **KEY AT-A-GLANCE INFORMATION**

LENGTH: 8.6 miles

CONFIGURATION: Out-and-back, up-and-down

DIFFICULTY: Hard

WATER REQUIRED: 3–4 liters

SCENERY: Coast mountains and valleys, foothill woodland, huge wooded vista from several vantage points along trail and summit

EXPOSURE: Surprisingly shaded on most of the trail

TRAIL TRAFFIC: You leave the river crowds behind at the trailhead.

TRAIL SURFACE: Dirt and duff

HIKING TIME: 4–5 hours

SEASON: Year-round, sunrise–sunset

ACCESS: $6 day-use fee at Cache Creek Canyon Regional Park; free parking under trees next to highway

MAPS: USGS Glascock Mountain; area-specific maps at blm.gov/ca/ st/en/fo/ukiah/cachecreek

FACILITIES: Cache Creek Canyon Regional Park offers about 40 parking spaces, picnic tables, recycling containers, and pit toilets.

WHEELCHAIR ACCESS: None

DRIVING DISTANCE: 91 miles

SPECIAL COMMENTS: Hydrate before hiking, and carry water in your pack. Streams are seasonal.

GPS TRAILHEAD COORDINATES

Latitude   N38° 54.595´

Longitude   W122° 18.415´

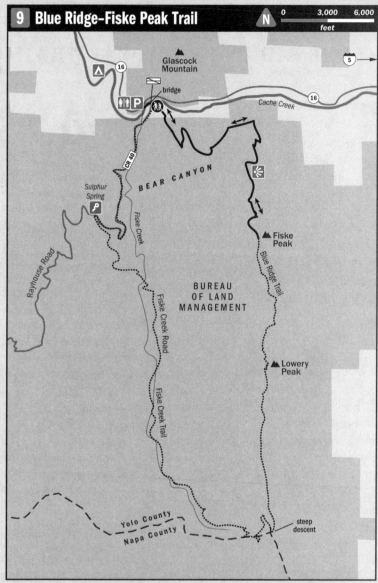

N

0   3,000   6,000
feet

Glascock
Mountain

16

5

bridge

16

Cache Creek

P

CR 40

BEAR CANYON

Sulphur
Spring

Fiske Creek

Fiske Peak

Blue Ridge Trail

Rayhouse Road

BUREAU
OF LAND
MANAGEMENT

Fiske Creek Road

Fiske Creek Trail

Lowery
Peak

Yolo County

Napa County

steep
descent

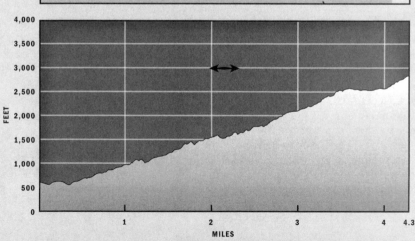

4,000
3,500
3,000
2,500
2,000
1,500
1,000
500
0

FEET

1   2   3   4   4.3

MILES

A sign on your right marks the trailhead and advises you of the distances to several points: Blue Ridge (3 miles), Fiske Peak (4 miles), and Fiske Creek Road (8.5 miles). Check your packs for loose fasteners and turn uphill (right) into a foothill-pine and live-oak forest that surrounds the singletrack. You will ascend steadily on the dirt-and-duff trail as the creek veers left.

This splendid trail winds through a manzanita grove where foothill pines loom overhead and young grasses beneath. Unfairly, this well-groomed trail is filthy with poison oak. In an ironic twist, the poisonous plant is decorated with beautiful Indian pink, Indian warrior, and Indian paintbrush. But resist the temptation to wade in for a closer look: on this hike, there will be few, if any, water sources to wash off the itch-inducing oils.

You'll next encounter a few minutes of gentle contouring, some gentle ascents, some monster uphills, and finally a stream to cross as you head into another uphill covered with fiddlenecks and blue dicks.

In a few minutes you'll reach the 1-mile mark, just about at the point where you can look back down Still Gulch—the canyon you've just ascended. If you're here in the spring, you'll see redbud trees highlighting the hillside whenever you emerge from cover to glimpse them.

The geological features of this area are primarily sedimentary and metamorphic rock. At this moment you are walking on flat sandstone and mudstone, alluvial deposits that long ago slumped to the seafloor and then were scraped up again as plates collided. Some deposits were deeper, older, and more dramatically inclined, as in the case of the metamorphic rock vertically oriented and exposed at Cache Creek. Notice that the plates here are horizontal. At other points in the hike, these strata will be oriented at various angles.

As you survey the surrounding hills, you may pick up on other ways the hills have been formed. As the incline becomes steeper, material on top loses its grip and slumps to a lower elevation. Look at the hillsides above the highway directly below you, and you can see evidence of hill formation due to slumping.

If you're here early enough in the season, you can linger around the next stream crossing, captivated by the sound of the water cascading gently above and below your crossing point. Shooting stars have been added to the displays of Indian pink, Indian warrior, and Indian paintbrush. You never have to wait long to hear the sound of hummingbirds as they take long draughts from each plant.

After 1.5 miles, the vista of the creek below and of the surrounding hillsides is matched only by the much-closer splash of yellow poppy and rabbitbrush. Turn your back on the creek below and continue ascending. The trail makes no unexpected direction changes other than to enter and exit ravines. When boulders in the trail block your path 2.2 miles along, climb over them. You may notice that the cool areas along the trail support a variety of mosses and ferns, including California maidenhair fern and bracken fern. The views are plentiful as you walk in and out of the shade of huge, spreading manzanitas.

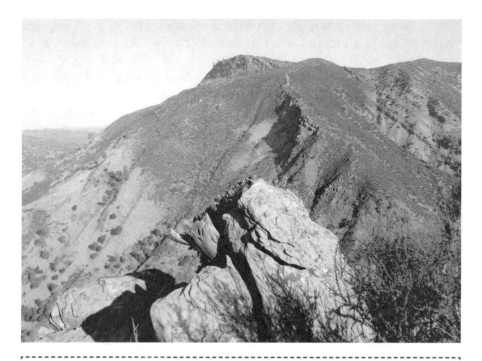

These gigantic slabs of former ocean floor rose from fantastic depths to add acreage to California—and form the Coastal Ranges.

Shortly after some switchbacks at 2.5 miles, you will see a signpost on the right indicating that you're now at the 2,000-foot elevation point. This is a welcome sign on a hike that is more up than out. You will be impressed by the maintenance crews' handiwork as the trail widens through the next set of switchbacks. Now you can be a bit less worried about being crowded by poison oak.

Look for an outcropping on the right with a hollow beneath it. You've hiked about 3 miles at this point. In another 0.25 mile, use caution as you cross the trail reroute around a ravine. The shade of a large foothill pine at the 3.25-mile point provides a nice rest spot before you ascend another 150 feet to the ridge. Continue across the outcroppings and the fire-scorched manzanita. Fence lizards skitter out of your way as you approach an intersection with a sharp peak visible to your right and more uphill trail to your left.

Continue on the trail to your left, but first gaze out from the peak ahead of you on the right. A use-trail and some hunters' campsites are hidden in the brush as you make your way uphill to the peak at 2,631 feet. This is a great spot for lunch; the warmth of the sun and rocks balances the steady chill winds that support a squadron of turkey vultures purposefully gliding by, eye-to-eye with you for a momentous instant.

Your trail to Fiske Peak—easily seen from this high vantage point—heads south and continues gaining elevation along a series of short uphill efforts until you reach a flat area at 2,850 feet. In front of you is a rectangular patch of grass about 10 feet by 15 feet. Before you enter that grassy area, the trail turns left and, 10 feet later, turns left again for the final steps up to the USGS marker on 2,868-foot Fiske Peak. An ammo can holds the peak-baggers' log, which you should sign and read: you've earned it.

From this peak you can visually grasp the earth-building process by observing the arrangement of the mountains in this coastal range: a series of north–south ridgelines interrupted by valleys that lie along earthquake fault lines. A look over the east side of the ridgeline reveals the Cache Creek Valley and the town of Rumsey.

If this hike has satisfied your sense of adventure and properly tired you, then make a U-turn to retrace your steps downhill.

NEARBY ACTIVITIES

The Cache Creek Natural Area has several excellent trails developed by the BLM. One of these is the High Bridge Trail (see next profile), which begins at the turnout on the west side of CA 16, 4.5 miles south of CA 20.

Cache Creek Regional Park Campground is on CA 16, 0.7 mile north of CR 40. RV and tent sites are available for a fee.

10 HIGH BRIDGE TRAIL

KEY AT-A-GLANCE INFORMATION

LENGTH: 5.6 miles

CONFIGURATION: Out-and-back

DIFFICULTY: Moderate

WATER REQUIRED: 2 liters

SCENERY: Hillsides of blue oak and wildflowers

EXPOSURE: Shade is all around, but the trail is often quite sunny.

TRAIL TRAFFIC: Light

TRAIL SURFACE: Dirt

HIKING TIME: 3 hours

SEASON: Year-round

ACCESS: No fees or permits

MAPS: USGS Glascock Mountain; trail map at blm.gov/ca/st/en/fo/ukiah/cachecreek

WHEELCHAIR ACCESS: None

FACILITIES: Parking area, pit toilet, picnic tables

DRIVING DISTANCE: 77.5 miles

SPECIAL COMMENTS: This trail is for hikers and equestrians, but not for bikers. Binoculars are a super accessory for this hike.

GPS TRAILHEAD COORDINATES

Latitude   N38° 57.396´

Longitude   W122° 20.618´

IN BRIEF

You will see magnificent groves of blue oaks, vistas of distant hills, and fields full of grasses and wildflowers, but you *won't* see a bridge on this trail. This hike climbs 700 feet in about 3 miles on a dirt trail that is graded for a practically effortless ascent. If you climb to the ridge early enough, you'll have a great perch from which to focus your binoculars on the wildlife at Bear Creek.

DESCRIPTION

Your trailhead is to the left of the steel-cable gate marked TRAIL. It winds down to cross Bear Creek on the mineral-encrusted boulders lining its banks. Turn sharply left at the bottom of the hill around the old fire rings, and follow the sandy path about 75 feet through the willows to the rocky cobble at the creek. Choose the path across that keeps you driest. Once across the creek, step up onto the conglomerate of rocks and turn again to the southwest. You will see the path ahead leading up the spur of a ridge. Rejoin the path, and you will gain some elevation over the creek as you walk around this

----

Directions _____➤

From Sacramento near Arco Arena, take I-5 North 55 miles to Williams and take Exit 577/CA 20 West. Drive 18 miles on CA 20 West to the junction with CA 16 South in Wilbur Springs. Take CA 16 South 4.3 miles to the trailhead parking lot, on the right. The unmarked turn-in, immediately after the second bridge over Bear Creek, has ample parking, a pit toilet, and two picnic tables. The trailhead is in the southwest corner of the parking area.

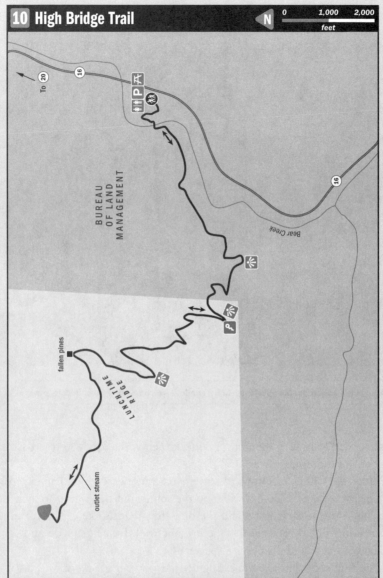

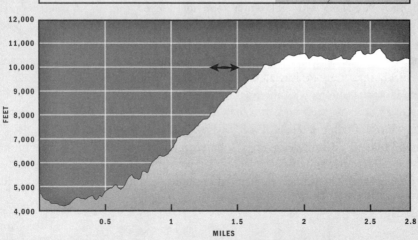

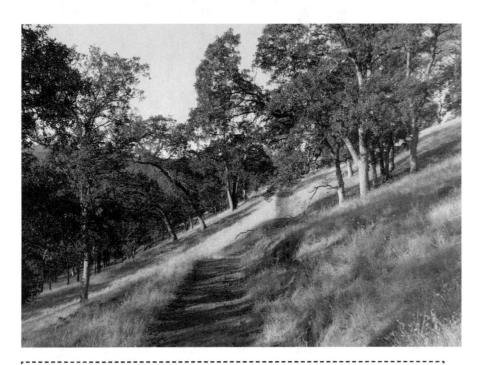

Trailside blue oaks cover hikers with pleasant shade, a welcome relief from the late-summer sun.

sparsely treed hillside and enter a ravine, which will allow you to cross the confluence of two drainages.

After just 100 feet of upward travel, you are rewarded with an exceptionally striking view of the creek and valley to the south. But this is not, in fact, the best view. Climb to the next vista, and the one after that. Make certain to take your camera along when you hike this picturesque trail. In fact, sunrise and sunset on the blue-oak-studded hillsides are spectacular.

The trail sometimes becomes slightly narrow, but for the most part it's wide enough to walk along with children at your side. Indeed, there is no point on this trail that would prove difficult for kids over age 4. The pond at the end of the hike has a sufficient stock of frogs, turtles, and birds to interest everyone. Look for signs of mammalian visitors along the margins of the pond. Tree frogs and pond turtles slip quickly into the muddy water when you approach. You will see raccoon and coyote footprints, along with the tracks of deer and birds of all types.

On the way to the pond, you may find yourself thinking only of the sound of the wind through the trees. In fact, this trail will lull you into actually enjoying an uphill hike. BLM trail designers and builders deserve kudos for this easy route into the wilderness. Your first and only barrier along the trail is a rusty-hinged white gate, which should present itself after about 45 minutes of hiking. You will have traveled 1.5 miles and will be about 500 feet above the trailhead.

A quartet of stout manzanita presents a rare change in the tree foliage as the trail meanders through the grasses. After about 2 miles of hiking, you will have reached roughly 1,500 feet elevation. If you look uphill and around you, the blue oaks seem to have flowed downhill from the ridge summit, almost blanketing the slope down to the creek. However scarce the foothill pines are on this slope, they are just as prolific on the facing slope as the oaks are on this one.

Now descend slightly toward a switchback in the crux of a ravine marked by two decaying foothill pines lying in its streambed. From this last switchback, which heads southwest, the trail will slowly resume a northwest heading for slightly less than 0.5 mile up to your destination.

The trail crosses an outlet stream just 0.1 mile before the pond. Climb to the left and around to the ranch road. While this is a stock pond, it's easy to see the footprints of several other mammals: coyote, fox, muskrat, and raccoon; you can also watch fish, turtles, and frogs as they all take a swipe at some of the thousands of grasshoppers that hatch here. A lone oak at the far end of the pond on the east side may provide a shady vantage point for your pondside picnic. Another rest spot with a great view is atop the rocks to the right, just after you climb out of the first ravine on your return—a place this explorer named Lunchtime Ridge.

11 JUDGE DAVIS TRAIL

 KEY AT-A-GLANCE INFORMATION

LENGTH: 11.5 miles

CONFIGURATION: Out-and-back

DIFFICULTY: Challenging

WATER REQUIRED: 3–4 liters

SCENERY: Panoramic views of Wilson Valley and Cache Creek

EXPOSURE: Some welcome shade from blue-oak groves; trail is 75% exposed.

TRAIL TRAFFIC: Enjoy your solitude.

TRAIL SURFACE: Dirt and duff, dirt and rock, grass

HIKING TIME: 4–5 hours

SEASON: Year-round, sunrise–sunset

ACCESS: No permits required, but check dfg.ca.gov/lands/wa/region2 for hunting dates.

MAPS: USGS Wilson Valley, Wilbur Springs; local maps at blm.gov/ca/st/en/fo/ukiah/cachecreek.html

FACILITIES: Pit toilets and parking at trailhead

WHEELCHAIR ACCESS: None

DRIVING DISTANCE: 75 miles

SPECIAL COMMENTS: This is an easy route into Cache Creek. The wildlife-viewing is superb above Wilson Valley. Bikes are prohibited on the wilderness trails. Check water-flow rate at ycfcwcd.org/waterinfo.html.

GPS TRAILHEAD COORDINATES

Latitude   N39° 00.515´
Longitude   W122° 24.955´

IN BRIEF

As a Yolo County judge from 1851 to 1862, Isaac Davis had questionable legal credentials—what with no legal training at all—but this trail is anything but crooked. As a matter of fact, it used to be way too straight. This route to the creek has been modified to make it more knee-friendly and environmentally sound. The views from above Wilson Valley are spectacular, more so through binoculars.

DESCRIPTION

Cache Creek Natural Area covers more than 70,000 acres of public lands open to mixed use. A variety of wildlife is supported in this area, which includes lush riparian forest along the creeks, hillside blue-oak woodlands, foothill-woodland forest, and dense chaparral.

In particular, the Wilson Valley on Cache Creek—your destination—is a haven for both wildlife and plant life. Bald eagle, tule elk, wild turkey, coyote, mountain lion, bear, black-tailed deer, and jackrabbit all thrive on the wide variety of grasses, berries, and aquatic life in this secluded area.

From your trail you can overlook the entire habitat and its inhabitants all at once. Early morning and evening are prime viewing

- -

Directions ─────────────────────→

From Sacramento near Arco Arena, take I-5 North 55 miles to Williams and take Exit 577/CA 20 West. Take CA 20 West 22.6 miles, watching for the Colusa–Lake county line. The parking lot for the trailhead is exactly 0.1 mile ahead on the left, below the road grade. Park in the lot to the right of the pit toilet. Your trailhead starts between the two large posts here. *Note:* Do not confuse this with the gated trail that starts to the left of the pit toilet.

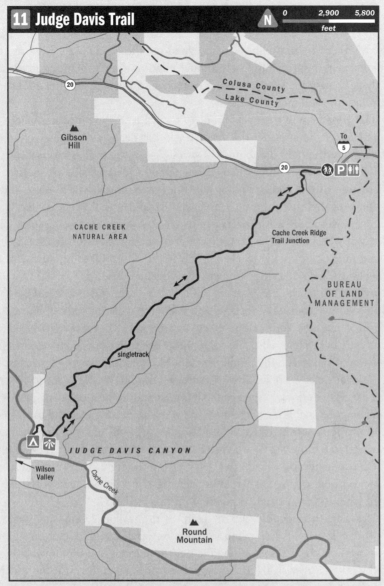

N

| 0 | 2,900 | 5,800 |

feet

20

Colusa County
Lake County

Gibson
Hill

To
5

CACHE CREEK
NATURAL AREA

Cache Creek Ridge
Trail Junction

BUREAU
OF LAND
MANAGEMENT

singletrack

JUDGE DAVIS CANYON

Wilson
Valley

Cache Creek

Round
Mountain

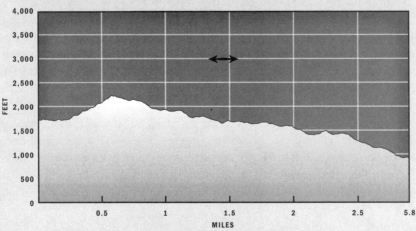

4,000										
3,500										
3,000										
2,500										
2,000										
1,500										
1,000										
500										
0										

FEET

0.5   1   1.5   2   2.5   5.8

MILES

hours, whether you're up above or down along the creek. Waterfowl use this as an important rest spot along their annual migration. Free-roaming herds of tule elk, which browse the grasslands and chaparral, often seek out the cool shade of the creek in the summer.

Start your hike in the parking lot to the right of the pit toilet, where a pair of stout posts stand astride a dirt singletrack that heads west, somewhat parallel-ing the road to the right. In about 100 yards, follow the trail as it turns away from the road at a creek running through an oak-speckled hillside. Even after rain, your crossing of this creek, coming up in a few minutes, will be easy. Your trail will soon veer slightly to the right as Cache Creek Ridge Trail heads left.

In this wet area, wildflowers jump out at you: larkspurs, lupines, Chinese houses, wally baskets, clover, and irises adorn the trailside and streamside banks. The next mile will boost your elevation from about 1,700 to about 2,200 feet— heading up the side of a slope to meet the ridgeline. After that, the trail will head largely downhill to the creek. Blue-oak limbs adorned with moss add a brilliant yet diffuse glow around the trees as you make the pleasant walk uphill.

In 0.5 mile, the entire slope takes on a parklike appearance, covered with a stand of blue oak. This well-crafted trail meanders through it, taking your mind off the fact that it's momentarily uphill. You will emerge from the cool shade just shy of the ridge after exactly 1 mile. The exposure remains southerly and sunny for the rest of the hike, with periodic respite found among stands of blue oak. The primary veg-etation along the trail is chaparral—mostly yerba santa, chamise, and manzanita.

As you look southwest, your trail appears as a distinct tan line through the green chaparral. Other trails are visible, but yours takes a definite tack southwest. The next trail junction, a jeep road, enters from the right. Join it for the next 0.3 mile by continuing left, slightly downhill, past the burned gateposts and their downed gate, to the last signed junction on this trail.

Curiously, the signpost, 1.5 miles from the trailhead, indicates that Cache Creek Ridge Trail leads left. Almost as an afterthought, a handwritten sign—now lying sideways in the greasewood on the right—indicates that the Judge Davis Trail, marked with an arrow, leads to the right. Neat or not, southwest is the way to go.

No trails intersect the Judge Davis Trail other than Cache Creek Ridge Trail, which you just passed, so you won't have to make any navigational decisions. Despite the very invasive Asian star thistle, this wide trail has been well main-tained and, in several places, has been redesigned to make it more manageable and less prone to erosion. Keep a watchful eye for downed wood, which has been placed across the closed trail to block it off. Over the next 2 miles, there will be six of these trail reroutes.

Chaparral, the dominant biozone along your trail, consists of many species of shrubs: manzanita, rabbitbrush, buckbrush, sagebrush, ceanothus, tobacco brush, Scotch broom, chamise (often known as greasewood), and at least a dozen others that fall into this broad category. The dominant chaparral shrub along your trail is greasewood, which comprises pure stands in some areas, denying access to other plants and large mammals. These areas support large numbers of smaller mammals and reptiles. Don't be surprised by a fat lizard drowsing beside the trail or the occasional garter snake lounging in the middle of these dense shrubs.

You can depend on a few well-placed stands of blue oak for shade when you traverse the north side of the ridge. One such stand occurs just before the 4-mile point. From there you have a clear vista encompassing the Wilson Valley. Continue on, being alert for the reroutes. About 0.25 mile after the final workaround, with only 0.5 mile to go to the creek, a tempting side trail heads downhill to the left (southeast), just like a reroute. Your trail, however, will continue southwest over the ridge until it makes a definite turn west and enters the area above Wilson Valley.

When you are 0.25 mile above the creek, vistas of Wilson Valley below will start to open up. Just before the trail makes its final descent to the creek, you will reach a fairly flat, open space in the trees. This 100-foot area has a perch overlooking the creek, the meadow, and a bald-eagle nest straight ahead. If you arrive at dawn or dusk with binoculars and you have an hour to sit, your chance of observing wildlife will be greatly enhanced. If you don't have the patience or time, take a photo or two before descending to the creek on a winding singletrack.

At creek level, you will emerge right next to a tall foothill pine, which has a distinctive huge branch that curves in the opposite direction to the rest. Use this as your marker of the correct trail location for your return.

The trail ends at a broad, flat area next to the creek. Other hikers have camped beside the creek here, as evidenced by the rock-enclosed fire ring and paths leading to the creek. Although it looks possible to cross Cache Creek near this spot, you'll have to do so during low water flow.

When you're well rested and ready to face the uphill return, remember to thank the trail crews for their work in "moderating" the trail along the way. After taking farewell photos of Wilson Valley, you'll look forward to entering the shade of oaks, about 1 mile from the trailhead.

12 REDBUD TRAIL

KEY AT-A-GLANCE INFORMATION

LENGTH: 15.5 miles

CONFIGURATION: Out-and-back

DIFFICULTY: Hard

WATER REQUIRED: 4–5 liters

SCENERY: In spring, the wildflowers are magnificent. Broad, open meadows are ringed by oak and pine.

EXPOSURE: More exposed than shaded. Wear a floppy hat.

TRAIL TRAFFIC: Light

TRAIL SURFACE: Dirt, duff, rock

HIKING TIME: 8.5 hours

SEASON: Year-round, but access is restricted during periods of high water flow.

ACCESS: No fees. Downstream irrigation requirements tend to increase through the summer, limiting foot travel across Cache Creek. Hikers must check water-flow rates at ycfcwcd.org/waterinfo.html for access across the creek.

MAPS: USGS Lower Lake, Wilson Valley

WHEELCHAIR ACCESS: None

FACILITIES: Pit toilet, trash receptacle, and picnic table at trailhead

DRIVING DISTANCE: 84 miles

SPECIAL COMMENTS: The extraordinary wildlife-viewing opportunities demand binoculars and a camera.

GPS TRAILHEAD COORDINATES

Latitude   N38° 59.221´

Longitude   W122° 32.376´

IN BRIEF

Redbud Trail offers a strenuous hiking experience, an opportunity to observe wildlife, and seclusion along a trail surrounded by wildflowers. So head out on an early-spring morning, generally southeast, across Cache Creek and two of its drier tributaries, over two ridges and a few smaller bumps, ending in a picturesque 1-mile-long valley meadow. You will almost assuredly encounter most of the flora and fauna briefly mentioned. You deserve a reward on this trek, with its 4,500-plus feet of elevation gain and loss. If quiet is your companion, have your camera at hand—it'll get plenty of use.

DESCRIPTION

Redbud Trail takes advantage of both State of California and federal Bureau of Land Management lands, providing easy entry for wildlife-viewers and wilderness hikers into a primitive area where the habitat is managed for wildlife and plants. In the northwest corner of the 70,000-acre Cache Creek Natural Area, the Redbud Trail gives hikers access an area that supports two extraordinary species: tule elk and bald eagles.

Your trail, almost 8 miles long if you walk to the end of Wilson Valley, winds along the North Fork of Cache Creek through a riparian

Directions

From Sacramento near Arco Arena, take I-5 North 55 miles to Williams and take Exit 577/ CA 20 West. Take CA 20 West 31 miles to the crossing of the North Fork of Cache Creek. About 0.2 mile after the bridge, turn left at the BLM sign and drive 0.1 mile to the signed trailhead.

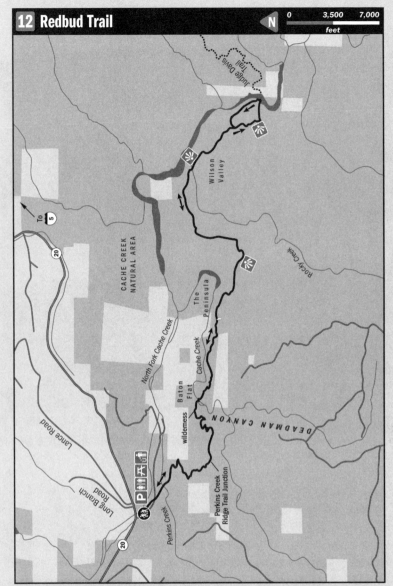

12 Redbud Trail

N

0   3,500   7,000
feet

To 5

20

CACHE CREEK
NATURAL AREA

Judge Davis Trail

Wilson Valley

Rocky Creek

The Peninsula

North Fork Cache Creek

Cache Creek

Baton Flat

wilderness

DEADMAN CANYON

Lance Road

Long Branch Road

Perkins Creek

Perkins Creek
Ridge Trail Junction

20

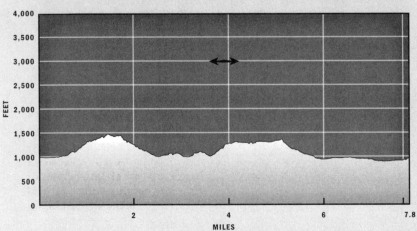

FEET

4,000
3,500
3,000
2,500
2,000
1,500
1,000
500
0

2   4   6   7.8

MILES

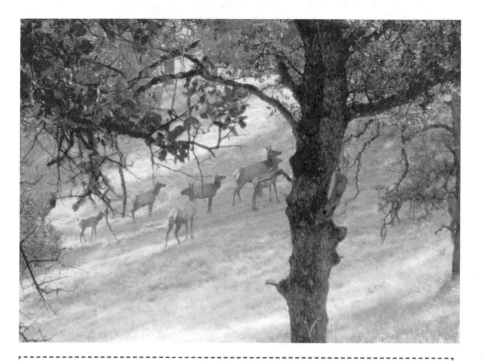

Females and young elk precede the male who observed them from a distance. A stable population of Tule elk roams the Cache Creek Natural Area in three or four separate herds.

zone—live oak, alder, cottonwood, grass, and sedge—that supports an abundant community of wildlife. Wild turkey, black-tailed deer, black bear, and three or four of the few free-roaming herds of tule elk make this area home and share it with migrating waterfowl, upland birds, and the magnificent bald eagle, which winters here. The Cache Creek Natural Area also exhibits a display of wildflower color and scent that makes a visit here an experience to anticipate.

Your trailhead starts at the parking lot just to the left of the pit toilets. The sign will direct you left, away from the gravel road, to a trail that passes the information kiosk and picnic table, crosses the creek, and heads southeast across the meadow.

Follow the trail sign as you begin an uphill trek to Perkins Creek Ridge. First, cross oft-dry Perkins Creek, which can be up to 50 feet wide during the rainy season. As you walk through live oak, manzanita, foothill pine, buckbrush, and alder, you'll be escorted by a squadron of tiger swallowtails moving from one nectar feast to another.

The smaller flora and fauna are—counterintuitively—far easier to see. The butterflies and moths flutter all around you; the alligator lizards, tree frogs, and common king snakes scurry under your feet; and the blue wally baskets, yellow pretty face, white globe tulips, and purple irises just sit there looking good. The larger flora—spreading blue oak, smooth-barked manzanita, and fragrant buckbrush—provide shade for hikers and other mammals.

Observing the larger fauna, such as elk, deer, and turkey, is a bit trickier, despite their size. On this hike, carrying a pair of compact binoculars will help. You will greatly increase your chances of sighting wildlife if you hike at dawn or at dusk. Otherwise, just find a spot that looks across a meadow or down on the creek, and wait patiently. The meadows are full of tracks, laydowns, and other signs of large mammals.

Water or a treatment/filtering method is a must on this hike, especially in the summer. Don't forgo sunscreen, and be aware that this hike is rife with poison oak.

After walking through a spacious, very mature manzanita grove, you'll have a nice vista of Al Slides and the Peninsula. Your trail climbs some easy switchbacks through manzanita and oak groves. At about 1.5 miles, you'll emerge into a pleasant grove of blue oak atop a knoll. Look directly in front of you here: a trail sign indicates that Perkins Creek Ridge Trail heads right and your trail heads left (east).

Look down to the slow pools of Cache Creek on your right just before they enter the rapids and Deadman Canyon some 300 feet below. Use-trails off to the right reveal the paths leading down to the pools. Just about the time you're seriously considering a swim down there, your trail begins a gentle downhill to Baton Flat. As you wind down past blue oak and foothill pine, the trail's smooth surface is interrupted only by the foothill pine's cones. Heft a fresh one and compare it with the core left by squirrels, and you'll see why these squirrels are sometimes mistaken for elk.

Shortly after passing a sign indicating entry into designated wilderness, your trail crosses the algae-laden rocks in Cache Creek. Frogs, lizards, and snakes are all common in this creekside area. Look carefully before you step, because some spend their downtime in the middle of the trail. On the other side, your trail is a distinct doubletrack in a parklike area.

At the next fork, a trail sign will direct you uphill, to the right. On a path winding in and out of lupines, irises, and yellow-star tulips, you ascend to cross one creek, drop down to Cache Creek again, and ascend again to oak-covered hillsides. Roughly paralleling the creek below, your trail through the trees will be interrupted by large meadows extending uphill from the margin of the creek. These spots afford excellent wildlife-viewing opportunities.

Trail markers guide your way across a small stream with milky-looking water—or clear water in a milky-looking streambed. Then the trail turns really scuddy and becomes an uphill slog next to a rutted-out four-wheel-drive road. Blue wally baskets are the only joy that this short stretch brings.

Notice the amount of rock debris strewn in this area. Large outcrops of rock are scattered, with one monolith appearing completely out of place on the left side. A blizzard of yellow poppies engulfs the trail as you top out in a moist, grassy spot that sports a couple of seasonal runoffs protected by culverts. Look for Chinese houses adorning the trailside here.

Head toward a huge blue oak on a four-wheel-drive road around 4.4 miles into the hike, and prepare for another viewing opportunity before you emerge from the forest cover. The oak up in the middle of the meadow is a common laydown for black-tailed deer and tule elk. Turkey hens move through the grass, heads high and scanning the terrain, with their broods stumbling along behind. Blue-eyed grass and paper onions are everywhere among the grasses. Indeed, the foxtail varieties will remind you of the gaiters that protect your socks and boots from collecting seeds and pebbles along the trail. That thought is interrupted by a California quail within feet of you that starts up at 90 miles an hour.

At the end of this open area, around 4.5 miles, your rock-and-dirt trail widens, thanks to excellent treatment by trail crews. The walk through this chaparral, free of poison oak, reveals an abundance of other mammal "signs," so watch where you step. As this section of the trail heads uphill, it becomes somewhat indistinct and appears to end. Keep walking straight, then left. You can see a copse of oak in the middle distance. It looks like a nice place for a shady respite, but before you know it, the trail has bypassed it.

Your downhill trail, with its rocky slope to the right, flanks a hilltop of dense chaparral. Descending a grassy slope sprinkled with dark-purple larkspur, the distinct trail heads directly toward two tall foothill pines, which mark the beginning of more doubletrack.

The map says "Rocky Creek." It's hard to imagine that it could be named anything else. Short, tumultuous, and untamed Rocky Creek empties its liquid load into Cache Creek just below your crossing. As you cross this wide stream, the dry gravels along its margins will reveal clusters of white whorl lupine.

Turn southeast as you enter Wilson Valley; the trail climbs slightly. When you arrive at the next stream crossing, your choice will depend on the time of year. A jumble of trails or shortcuts confuses the situation somewhat, but you can take one of them southeast to the creek and walk along the lower side of the meadow. In wetter months, you can head about 150 feet southwest and cross a small stream, allowing you to skirt the upper edge of the meadow and enjoy a view down to the creek.

In late April, a late-staying pair of bald eagles was nesting in the foothill pine at the far south end of Wilson Valley. Lingering to take advantage of the solitude and plentiful food in Cache Creek, this pair would soon be ready to continue its northward migration. Take care not to harass the birds—especially when they're nesting. Approaching no closer than 500 feet to their nesting spot is a responsible approach. Your telephoto lens or binoculars will give you an excellent view without stressing the raptors.

If your destination is Cache Creek, you have arrived. If you continue across the creek, you can join the Judge Davis Trail (see previous profile). Follow your tracks and take your memories back to the trailhead.

PERKINS CREEK RIDGE TRAIL 13

IN BRIEF

Hiking this trail in the winter, spring, or fall is highly recommended because this is a hot, exposed route that can be blistering during the late summer. The wildflowers and green grasses are so spectacular in the spring that they eclipse the beauty of the woodland and chaparral. However, in the summer, the blue oaks and foothill pines contrast with the sun-browned stems and seeds to yield a unique beauty best enjoyed early in the day. This route follows the Redbud Trail to its junction with the Perkins Creek Ridge Trail, about 1.5 miles from the trailhead, where it turns southwest and begins ascending and descending along the ridge to a final vista of Clear Lake.

DESCRIPTION

The initial 1.5 miles of this hike follow the Redbud Trail (see previous profile) from its trailhead up to the point of the junction with the Perkins Creek Ridge Trail.

Head southeast across the large meadow, which is filled with pretty face, wally baskets, and poppies in the spring; then cross the normally dry, 50-foot-wide Perkins Creek before you enter a woodland of blue oak, manzanita, foothill pine, and toyon. Switchback to the southwest through a stand of mature white-leaf manzanita bushes, then head southeast as

---

i KEY AT-A-GLANCE INFORMATION

LENGTH: 12.4 miles

CONFIGURATION: Out-and-back

DIFFICULTY: Hard

WATER REQUIRED: 4–5 liters

SCENERY: Foothill woodland and chaparral with ridgetop views

EXPOSURE: Barely a mile of trail is shaded; wear a hat and sunscreen.

TRAIL TRAFFIC: Light

TRAIL SURFACE: Dirt and rock

HIKING TIME: 6–8 hours

SEASON: Year-round

ACCESS: No fees or permits

MAPS: USGS Lower Lake

WHEELCHAIR ACCESS: None

FACILITIES: Pit toilets, interpretive kiosk, trash receptacles, and picnic table at trailhead parking lot

DRIVING DISTANCE: 84 miles

SPECIAL COMMENTS: Great views are the rewards for those hikers who ascend and descend this chaparral-covered ridge. There is no drinking water at the trailhead. Binoculars and a camera are almost essential on this trek.

Directions ⟶

From Sacramento near Arco Arena, take I-5 North 55 miles to Williams and take Exit 577/CA 20 West. Take CA 20 West 31 miles to the crossing of the North Fork of Cache Creek. About 0.2 mile after the bridge, turn left at the BLM sign and drive 0.1 mile to the signed trailhead.

GPS TRAILHEAD COORDINATES

Latitude   N38° 58.486´

Longitude   W122° 31.778´

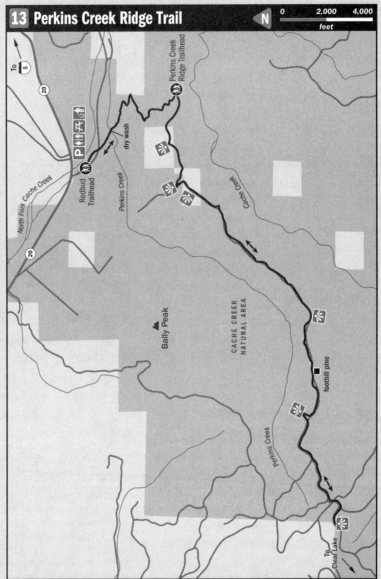

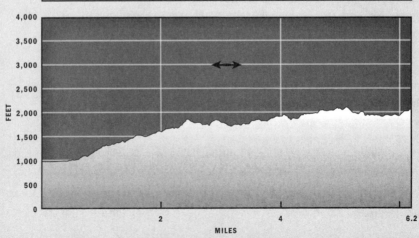

blue oaks become the dominant flora, with foothill pines adding colorful accents above the oaks' dark leaves. The berries of the manzanita, which is the Spanish word for "little apple," become ripe and red in late summer, adding more color.

After gaining almost 500 feet, you reach the signed junction at the top of an oak-laden hill. Notice the sign facing backward at your left shoulder as you near the top; it directs your return to the trailhead. This is a pleasant point at which to catch your breath and take pictures of Deadman Canyon and Baton Flat below. The scattered blue oaks make this shaded and breezy spot a welcome respite after your first 45 minutes of hiking.

After resting and checking maps, turn right (southwest) and head up a short, steep hill through the thickening chamise bushes. Often called greasewood, chamise is the dominant shrub in these chaparral-covered hills. After another short, steep hill, you will reach a very steep hill. You could hustle up the steep pitch and take some pictures from this excellent vantage point. A more amenable idea: circumnavigate this hill by taking the trail to the left, at the exact base of the hill. There is another misleading trail to the left 75 yards before this hill, so be patient.

At this point you're about 150 feet above the junction, and you will ascend some 600 more feet over the next few miles. However, you will also descend frequently. At many of the high points on the ridge, you'll notice a trail leading off to the side, at the base of the slope. These wonderfully energy-saving trails generally contour around the hill. The junctions are all fairly evident. There are about ten of these walk-arounds that lead to the right and about three that lead around to the left.

As you walk along, you will surely notice, and perhaps try to avoid, the signs of a few of the more territorial animals in Cache Creek. Footprints of turkeys and quail are clustered randomly in the dust, where it looks as if a happy hour was held. Raccoon, coyote, and even mountain-lion signs are evident. With the forage diminishing in the late summer, eating requires animals to do a bit more traveling, and so game trails intersect your route constantly.

In the next mile of this dirt-covered trail, you will notice—perhaps when you slip on their small acorns—that the blue oaks have become the dominant species of flora. By late summer, the blue oak has reached its full complement of foliage, so it presents a nicely rounded blue-green profile against the golden dried grasses. In contrast, the gray-green of the foothill pine dazzles in the bright sun in the canyon below and on the ridge above the trail. For the next 40 minutes or so, you can see down to Cache Creek on the left. Bally Peak is about a mile north. Chamise still crowds the trail, which continues southwest, following the ridge up and down.

You can just begin to see Clear Lake in the distance by the time you have reached a vista point at the 5-mile mark. Trails are clearly visible against the chaparral, which also includes bush monkeyflower and buckbrush. From a knoll with a solitary foothill pine, you can see trails in all directions. Some of these—OHV trails used by the Bureau of Land Management and the California Department of Fish and Game—head northwest. Continue along the ridge another 1.2 miles to the southwest.

If you get buzzed by vultures every now and then, it's because they're sizing you up for later. Take heart just about when the chamise is joined by the tiny-leaved scrub oak. An OHV road makes a U-turn at a flat spot about 10 minutes before you reach your destination, barely a mile from Clear Lake's border and a scant 3 miles from its shore. Although it's up a hill, you'll find it easily, because X literally marks the spot. To the northwest sits the flattened knob of Quackenbush Mountain. Clear Lake is about 600 feet below to your west, glinting in the sun, and the head of Perkins Creek sits idly dry about 250 feet below you.

From this serene viewpoint, game trails and laydowns are visible on the slopes below you. Apparently, deer and tule elk seek solitude in the same areas that hikers do. The breeze is refreshing and the view is excellent, but there is a distinct lack of shade at this spot, which encourages you to hasten into the shade of the oaks back down the trail. Retrace your steps to the trailhead.

NEARBY ACTIVITIES

Cache Creek is popular among kayakers and rafters of all skill levels. All-inclusive package trips are available from a number of travel companies in the area. White-water Adventures in Sacramento can be contacted at 800-977-4837 or **gotwhite water.com**; contact Cache Creek Whitewater River Trips of Rumsey at 530-796-3091 or **cachecanyon.com**.

JOHNSON RIDGE–
GUNSIGHT ROCK TRAIL 14

IN BRIEF

No other vista overlooking the Sonoma Valley is as broad as the one that you have from atop Gunsight Rock. Hikers can reach this lookout on an easier trail; in fact, this route is used by those training to climb Mount Shasta. Wildlife, wildflowers, and wild views en route to the summit make this one wild hike.

DESCRIPTION

Drop $6 into the self-register pay station, check out the maps and natural-history information on the kiosks, pick up an area trail map from the dispenser, and stretch a bit; then take off along the pole-fence next to the road. Fifty feet up, under a live oak, is the trailhead. Here a sign indicates distances to various destinations and lists some safety rules.

The Hood Mountain Regional Park and Open Space Preserve stretches from the Santa Rosa Creek to the summit of Hood Mountain,

----

Directions

From the junction of the Capital City Freeway and I-5 South, which soon merges with I-80 West, continue on I-80 West toward San Francisco. Drive 45.5 miles to Exit 39B/CA 12 West toward Napa/Sonoma, then head 6.2 miles west on Jameson Canyon Road. Turn right on CA 12/29 West, driving 1.4 miles, then keep left on CA 12 West for 2.6 miles. Turn left at the traffic light onto CA 12/121 and drive west 12 miles, up Broadway, to West Napa Street. Turn left and drive 0.9 mile to CA 12, where you turn right. Drive 12 miles on the Sonoma Highway to Pythian Road, which is on the right, next to the St. Francis Winery. Drive 0.2 mile to where Rancho Los Guilicos Road bears left and Pythian Road bears right. A marker at the junction informs you that the park and trailhead are 1 mile ahead.

KEY AT-A-GLANCE INFORMATION

LENGTH: 9.2 miles

CONFIGURATION: Out-and-back

DIFFICULTY: Challenging

WATER REQUIRED: 3 liters

SCENERY: Foothill woodland, wildflowers, broad vistas

EXPOSURE: Mostly shaded, with some southern exposure

TRAIL TRAFFIC: Light

TRAIL SURFACE: Dirt and duff, dirt and rock

HIKING TIME: 3–4 hours

SEASON: Year-round, 8 a.m.–sunset

ACCESS: $6 fee

MAPS: USGS Kenwood; park trail map at trailhead

WHEELCHAIR ACCESS: None

FACILITIES: Parking area has water, toilet, maps, pay station, information kiosks, benches, and a creekside picnic table.

DRIVING DISTANCE: 82 miles

SPECIAL COMMENTS: Awesome view of Sonoma Valley from the aptly named Gunsight Rock. There's water at the trailhead, so stay hydrated and safe.

GPS TRAILHEAD COORDINATES

Latitude   N38° 27.135´
Longitude   W122° 34.455´

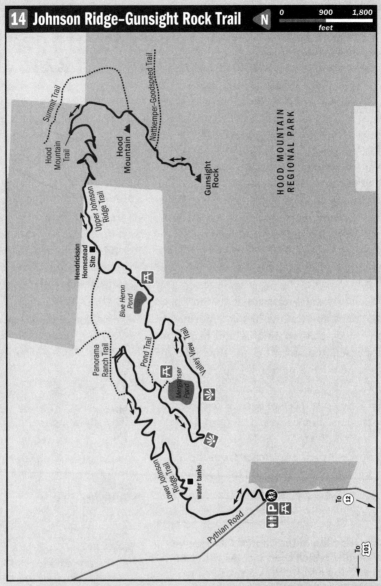

14 Johnson Ridge–Gunsight Rock Trail

N

0   900   1,800
feet

HOOD MOUNTAIN REGIONAL PARK

Summit Trail

Hood Mountain Trail

Nattkemper-Goodspeed Trail

Hood Mountain ▲

Gunsight Rock ▼

Upper Johnson Ridge Trail

Hendrickson Homestead Site ■

Blue Heron Pond

Pond Trail

Valley View Trail

Panorama Ranch Trail

Merganser Pond

Lower Johnson Ridge Trail

water tanks ■

Pythian Road

To 12

To 101

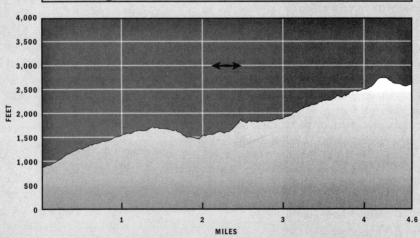

at the crest of the Mayacamas Mountains. It connects with Sugarloaf State Park on the east and has a 1,200-acre addition to the north. Your 4.5-mile trail gains 1,750 feet from the trailhead to a spot on Hood Mountain.

This route combines six excellent trails to create a trek that mirrors the Bay Area Ridge Trail on the park map. You'll start on the Lower Johnson Ridge Trail and then join the Pond and Valley View trails and finally the Upper Johnson Ridge Trail to reach the Hood Mountain Trail and the Gunsight Rock Trail.

Walk along, with the board fence to your right, and cross the open space on a gravel path. Throughout the park, look for 6 by 6–inch wooden posts bearing trail names and directional arrows. You are currently on the Lower Johnson Ridge Trail, which passes the second house and climbs to meet the road, where the park boundary lies.

Tighten your bootlaces. As the PLEASE DISMOUNT sign suggests, the next 0.3 mile of paved road is seriously steep. Shaded by madrone, live oak, sycamore, and Douglas fir, the path—and your uphill grind—end when you reach the gated residence on the right. Your trail is 100 feet on the left, beyond the gate. Under the shade of bay-laurel trees, hike the switchbacks past boulders and then snake past three wooden water tanks. The pipes leading from the spring to the tanks border your trail to the right. Walk along the left side of the road, then cross to the right along a path next to a park-boundary fence. Walk up the road, with boulders to your left, and turn right at the next trail marker. The posts can sometimes blend with their surroundings, but all the trail junctions are marked on this route. Live oak and madrone have shaded this rock-and-dirt trail from the trailhead on, and occasional manzanita crowds the junctions. A few switchbacks lead to the next junction.

This junction calls for you to turn right and head toward Merganser Pond. A turn to the left would lead you away, on Panorama Ranch Trail. So take a right on Johnson Ridge Trail as it climbs a bit from the 1.3-mile mark. Cross a culvert over a small runoff, then continue uphill on the right-hand trail as it turns to a gravel causeway that crosses a hillside meadow thick with Santa Barbara sedge, accented by blue-and-yellow, purple-and-white, and green-and-silver flowers mobbed by bees and butterflies.

As you step across the rock culverts of two more drainages on the way to Hood Creek, you'll see a jumble of downed trees that speaks of the torrents and winds that can rip through this canyon. Cross the bridge over Hood Creek, then head up to the right toward Pond Trail. The sound of the cascades to your right fades as you move away from the creek and start descending on a singletrack.

Avoid the old trail to the left; your trail winds along in total shade. Head around a knob from the north side to the south on this rocky section, with the creek to your right. At a junction, the Pond Trail heads both left and right. Heading left takes you about 1,500 feet over, to the Blue Heron Pond. But this shortcut misses the Valley View Trail.

So take the right-hand fork downhill toward the Valley View Trail, then continue downhill, where you will see a NO sign off to your left just as you reach

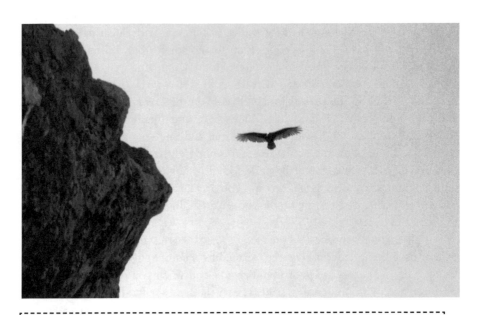

Social and quite aerobatic, turkey vultures boast wingspans of 5–6 feet. The distinct black T of the bird's feather pattern is visible as this one eyes me at Gunsight Rock.

Merganser Pond. If you want to picnic, you can walk up the road about 500 feet past the NO sign, where there is a table at the pond's edge. Your route keeps on going along the Valley View Trail, past the fenced culvert to your right. Another Valley View Trail sign is up ahead; here you will turn left and walk past the pond, with a view of Merganser Island on your left.

A huge outcrop of rock imposes itself on the opposite side of the pond as you walk through the grass on the doubletrack. At the end of the pond, walk to the right, down the trail and past a rock outcrop. You're now on the Valley View Trail as it descends under Douglas firs and bay laurels. Start skirting the hill and then turn southeast up a 150-foot road to a wonderful vista point overlooking the valley at about the 2-mile point. Wind uphill again to a shady spot, where you'll have another nice vista if you climb to the trail's right a bit.

Descend to another broad vista point, descend some more, and then climb on a broad doubletrack with a steep slope to your left. After 2.5 miles, the trail flattens a bit at the junction where you head right on Pond Trail on the way to Upper Johnson Ridge Trail. On your left, beyond the California nutmegs, is small Blue Heron Pond; a picnic area sits just past the pond's northern end. The road remains flat as you pass over another culvert with water cascading across it.

The next junction sees Orchard Meadow Trail going left; you'll head to the right on the Upper Johnson Ridge Trail. A scant 200 feet ahead on the left is the fenced-off Hendrickson homestead site, for which the county is conducting a historical survey in order to best preserve and present the site.

A 0.25-mile uphill stretch of doubletrack leads you to a junction with the Knight's Retreat Trail, which heads to the right in front of you. The Upper

Johnson Ridge Trail turns left under the shade of live oak, sycamore, and bay laurel. Foothill pine and manzanita crowd the trail as you use six switchbacks to ease your trail up some 300 feet to the junction with the Hood Mountain Trail. As you near the junction, you'll discover a small, isolated stand of cypress trees.

Now, well exposed to the sun, you reach the Hood Mountain Trail, which leads 0.3 mile up to the summit of Hood Mountain. This ranch road leads southward to a broad, flat area at the summit. It can be combined with the Panorama Ranch Trail for a loop route, or it can be hiked all the way here from the Los Alamos Road trailhead.

This section is steep, so it may seem like an unpaved version of the 0.3 mile you climbed at the outset. The leaves, duff, and pebbles on this section make this steep trail slippery. Watch your footing on both the uphill and the return (no sudden stops going downhill).

After you catch your breath at the summit, look around as you enter this broad clearing. To your left is a trail sign for the Summit Trail. This trail does *not* lead to the summit; rather, it descends to Azalea Creek alongside the Hood Mountain Trail. Look across the clearing and you'll see a trail marker for the Gunsight Rock Trail and Sugarloaf Ridge State Park. The summit is beyond the break in the manzanita, to the left of the trail sign. A large marker here provides some local historical background. A summit register is usually hidden in a coffee can among the rocks.

After marking your summit, descend on the rocky Gunsight Rock Trail and squeeze through the volcanic-rock outcropping before coming to the junction with the Nattkemper–Goodspeed Trail, which leads to Sugarloaf State Park. Gunsight Rock Trail turns right here; walk the final 0.1 mile to the overlook.

It's not too hard to understand how the trail got its name. Climb the left- or right-hand boulders by easing around to the front of the rock. The vultures take off from their perches below you and soar up and around your lofty seat while you look out over the Sonoma Valley landscape. Orchards, hills, vineyards, and fields spread out below and before you. Your vista includes three state parks, famous wineries, and the valleys and towns in which they lie, from Napa to Santa Rosa.

After the picture-snapping is finished, turn back and retrace your steps 4.6 miles to the trailhead. You can opt to return to the trailhead via the Orchard Meadow and Panorama Ranch trails or the Pond Trail. Both of these well-signed routes will offer you new vistas and a slightly shorter return route.

NEARBY ACTIVITIES

The towns of Kenwood, Agua Caliente, Glen Ellen, and Oakmont have excellent wineries and tasting rooms.

Jack London State Historic Park, Annadel State Park, and Sugarloaf Mountain State Park have additional hiking trails to explore. All are within 10 miles to the east, south, and west of the St. Francis Winery.

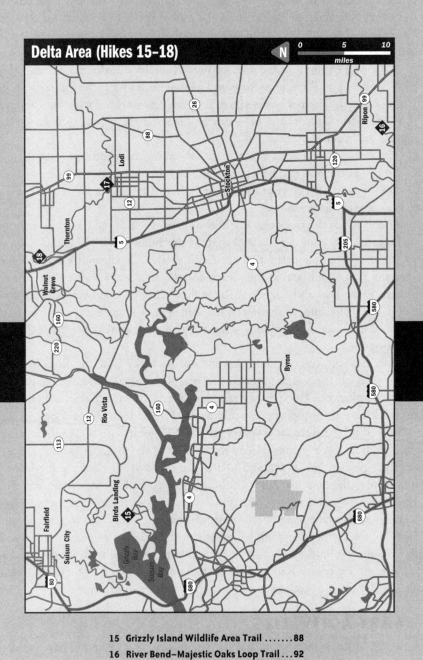

Delta Area (Hikes 15–18)

0   5   10
miles

N

Ripon · 99 · 16

26

88

Lodi

99

17

Thornton

12

Stockton

120

5

5

18

Walnut Grove

205

160

220

580

Byron

580

Rio Vista

12

160

4

4

113

Birds Landing

Fairfield

Suisun City

4

680

Grizzly Bay

15

Suisun Bay

680

680

DELTA AREA

15 GRIZZLY ISLAND WILDLIFE AREA TRAIL

KEY AT-A-GLANCE INFORMATION

LENGTH: 4.5 miles

CONFIGURATION: Balloon

DIFFICULTY: Easy

WATER REQUIRED: 1 liter

SCENERY: Delta marshland

EXPOSURE: Fully exposed to sun and wind. Ear protection, hat, windbreaker, and gloves may be needed any time of year. The temperature here will be several degrees lower than in the valley.

TRAIL TRAFFIC: Minimal

TRAIL SURFACE: Dirt and grass

HIKING TIME: 2 hours

SEASON: Feb.–July, sunrise–sunset

ACCESS: $4 day-use fee; free with an annual DFG Lands Pass (see dfg.ca.gov/licensing/landpass for details). Open for hunting; call ahead (707-425-3828) for hiking dates and closures.

MAPS: USGS Honker Bay; area map in office or at dfg.ca.gov/lands/wa/region3/grizzlyisland/index.html

WHEELCHAIR ACCESS: None

FACILITIES: Pit toilet at trailhead

DRIVING DISTANCE: 57 miles

SPECIAL COMMENTS: This is an unsigned route on levee roads, which may lead to dead ends or small adventures. Do not leave the levee roads, even for short distances.

GPS TRAILHEAD COORDINATES

Latitude   N38° 06.679´

Longitude   W121° 56.297´

IN BRIEF

Carved out of the Suisun Marsh, the largest contiguous saltwater marsh on the West Coast, the Grizzly Island Wildlife Area offers an abundance of wildlife and botanical diversity. This short hike lets hikers walk slowly enough to quietly observe amphibians, reptiles, and fish; waterfowl, songbirds, and raptors; and burrowing mammals, grazing mammals, and predatory mammals. At any given moment along this trail, the alert hiker will be able to spot easily identified specimens, whether turtles, frogs, otters, or skunks. Your challenge is to not miss the next three while identifying the first—there are that many species to see.

Directions ⟶

From the junction of the Capital City Freeway and I-80 West, drive 42 miles on I-80 West to Exit 44A/Suisun Parkway in Suisun City. Take Suisun Parkway to CA 12/Rio Vista Road, follow Rio Vista Road 3.8 miles to Grizzly Island Road, and turn south. This turn is directly across from the shopping center at Sunset Avenue. As you drive south around the Potrero Hills, you may notice an immediate change of scenery from valley to delta. About 5.5 miles from your turn south onto Grizzly Island Road, you will turn right, across the bridge and boat-launch ramps at Montezuma Slough; the transition is unmistakable.

   Another 3.5 miles and you will be greeted by signs requesting that you register at the DFG office. After registering and looking at the displays inside, continue 5.6 miles straight ahead on the gravel-and-dirt road (bear left whenever you get a choice) until you see the towering eucalyptus tree at the signed Parking Lot 3. There is plenty of parking here and a portable toilet, but no water.

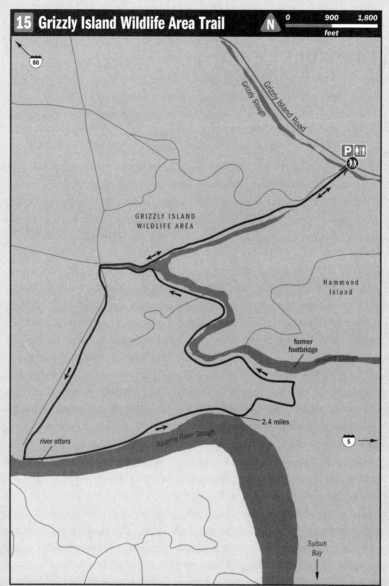

15 Grizzly Island Wildlife Area Trail

N

0   900   1,800
feet

80

Grizzly Slough

Grizzly Island Road

P

GRIZZLY ISLAND
WILDLIFE AREA

Hammond
Island

former
footbridge

Howard Slough

2.4 miles

5

river otters

Roaring River Slough

Suisun
Bay

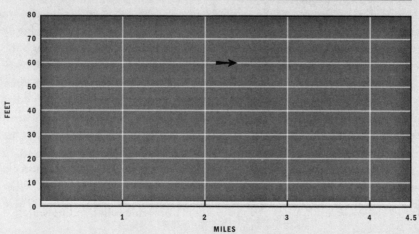

80

70

60

50

40

FEET

30

20

10

0

1   2   3   4   4.5

MILES

DESCRIPTION

The informative kiosks at the DFG Field Office provide a good overview of the area. Inside the office are more displays that hint at the diversity of wildlife here. The Suisun Marsh Natural History Association website, **suisunwildlife.org,** includes lists of species found on Grizzly Island, making it easy to recall all you have viewed.

Binoculars will help the patient hiker spot a surprising number of species. Mornings and late afternoons are best, because most animals tend not to move during the heat of the day. Hikers will need a hat with a brim, sunglasses, sunscreen, and a wind jacket or soft-shell top. Light gloves also help, even when the valley is quite warm. Insects abound, and the trail is uneven thanks to burrowing mammals.

Starting at the large eucalyptus tree at the parking lot, cross the gravel road to the wooden footbridge. Stop along the bridge and take a moment to look around. You may have spotted several raptors while driving to the trailhead. You will see harriers swooping from field to field, kites hovering just above their prey, and hawks soaring even higher. For no apparent reason, an entire flock of mallards, egrets, or any of a dozen other waterfowl may churn the water and air to get somewhere else fast.

Walk across the bridge, heading toward Mount Diablo, about 15 miles due south from the trailhead eucalyptus. Legend holds that Grizzly Island was so named because bears from Mount Diablo used to make an annual trek to feast on the island's blackberries.

At the end of the bridge, zig to the right and then zag to the left on the obvious levee road, heading southwest toward Roaring River Slough. At 0.6 mile, a levee road will enter from the left. (You can take an alternate route from this point. Turn left and follow this road, taking two left turns to get back to the trailhead.) This hike continues 0.2 mile farther down the trail to another junction. Your choices are to cross the canal and turn left, make a U-turn to the left, or turn left over the culvert pipe and continue on the dirt tracks.

The hike described here turns left over the pipe and heads slightly southwest on the dirt tracks. Mount Diablo, to the southeast, can act as your guide. More directly east are the large wind turbines that harness the constant gusts to busily churn out electricity. Tule elk are commonly spotted in the highlands around the island. They were successfully reintroduced to the marshes in the late 1970s.

Along this short stretch of dirt trail, travel may be difficult in wet weather. Take the next left 0.7 mile, noticing the steep edges of the slough. In midday, none were active, but the signs of river otter and their slides were everywhere. Tracks and signs of other mammals were also frozen in the muddy margins of the sloughs and shallow ditches.

Sometimes our own senses provide us all the clues we need to identify a mammal. Very close encounters with very active skunks are a real possibility. Let your nose be your guide in turning away whenever the odor intensifies. These trails are choked with tall grasses and weeds or have grass-constricted margins that can conceal any manner of creatures. Keep a sharp lookout for a T-intersection just before you walk into the slough.

Another left turn and another 0.7 mile—to the east this time. Your left-turn marker is the point at which you are directly south of the trailhead eucalyptus. So far you've traveled 2.4 miles. It is just a short walk north to another T-intersection; take a right there. When a pheasant cock takes flight along here, try to stay on the trail and in your boots—this bird goes from 0 to 60 right underfoot.

Navigation is easy, and you can see your trailhead, so spend some time crawling along the margins of the slough, where the amphibians and reptiles spend their days. Western pond turtles enjoy warming in the sun along a log or on a muddy bank. The two-tone green Pacific tree frog may surprise you with its voice, but if you're sharp enough to spot one, you'll see that its call far outweighs its body.

Turn left at the next intersection, then make another left before you run into the water at the dilapidated footbridge. You will now be heading generally northwest. Your winding trail parallels the trail along the opposite shore of Hammond Island. (That is the alternate trail mentioned previously.)

Your next intersection is a repeat of your confusing first turn. Cross the culvert and turn right, toward your trailhead tree. If you prefer a longer hike from this point, in just 0.2 mile you can turn right to follow the margins of Hammond Island, circumnavigating it back to the trailhead parking lot. Just turn left twice and you'll be back at the trailhead with more stories.

The great thing about Grizzly Island is its concentration of wildlife and its network of levee roads, all of which are open to hikers. And remember, dead ends are just a reason to enjoy your trail twice.

NEARBY ACTIVITIES

Nearby Rush Ranch is a 2,070-acre open space that protects important brackish tidal marshes. For details on its many offerings, including hiking, see **rushranch.org**.

The Delta region has several preserves and parks with interpretive nature trails. The Cosumnes River Preserve (Hike 18, page 101) and Caswell Memorial State Park (see next profile) both have excellent interpretive trails.

16 RIVER BEND-MAJESTIC OAKS LOOP TRAIL

KEY AT-A-GLANCE INFORMATION

LENGTH: 3 miles

CONFIGURATION: Loop

DIFFICULTY: Easy

WATER REQUIRED: 1 liter

SCENERY: Riparian forest

EXPOSURE: Shaded trail

TRAIL TRAFFIC: Light

TRAIL SURFACE: Duff and dirt

HIKING TIME: 1.5 hours

SEASON: Year-round, 8 a.m.–sunset

ACCESS: $8 day-use fee

MAPS: USGS Ripon; local map at entry kiosk

WHEELCHAIR ACCESS: Access on Gray Fox Trail and part of River Bend Trail

FACILITIES: Trailhead toilets and water; picnic tables; camping

DRIVING DISTANCE: 63.5 miles

SPECIAL COMMENTS: This is a great trail for children on a hot day. It's wide, shaded, and surrounded by wonderful plants and animals.

GPS TRAILHEAD COORDINATES

Latitude   N37° 41.624´

Longitude   W121° 11.035´

IN BRIEF

These easy trails loop through the magnificent valley oaks and towering cottonwoods of this rare riparian forest. A hike through this forest, draped with wild grapevines and filled with the song of various birds, will be remembered even by children for a long time. Excellent interpretive signage also makes this an educational trip for hikers of all ages.

DESCRIPTION

Only about 5 percent of California's original Central Valley riparian forest remains. On the Stanislaus River, Caswell Memorial State Park (MSP) has preserved an impressive expanse of woodland: 258 acres of this rare California ecosystem, which once stretched for miles toward the mountains.

If you begin at the restrooms, your trailhead is at the end of the walkway leading west past the picnic tables and the seating area. An information kiosk at the trailhead displays a general map of the park, along with descriptions of the flora and fauna one might encounter here.

Directions ⟶

From the intersection of CA 99 and the Capital City Freeway, drive 58 miles on CA 99 South toward Stockton. Just past CA 120, exit at Austin Road, turn left, and drive less than 100 yards to make a right turn to cross the railroad tracks. Then drive south 5.1 miles on Austin Road, cruising through orchards to reach the Caswell Memorial State Park entrance. The entry kiosk is 100 feet ahead. After paying your entry fee and picking up a map, drive 0.4 mile to the end of the shaded road. Turn left into the parking lot. Restrooms are at the east end of the lot, and the trailhead is toward the west end, near the information kiosk.

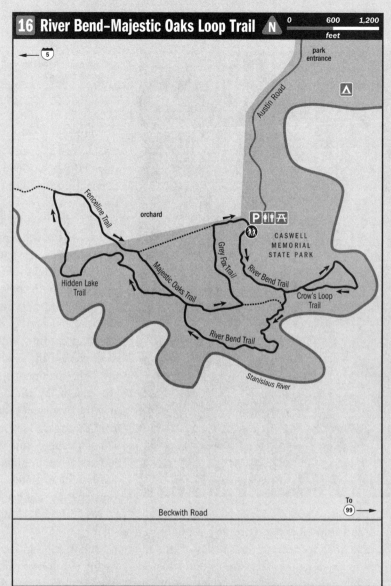

N

0   600   1,200
feet

← 5

park entrance

Austin Road

orchard

Fenceline Trail

P

CASWELL
MEMORIAL
STATE PARK

Hidden Lake
Trail

Majestic Oaks Trail

Grey Fox Trail

River Bend Trail

Crow's Loop
Trail

River Bend Trail

Stanislaus River

Beckwith Road

To
99 →

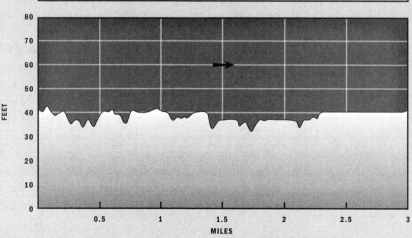

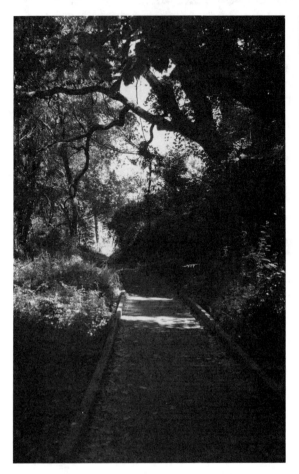

Black oaks shade this well-placed causeway.

Hikers in wheelchairs can access the first 0.25 mile of the River Bend Trail. Connect to the Gray Fox Trail for a 0.7-mile loop. These trails are unpaved—made of smooth, packed dirt—so those in wheelchairs may need some assistance along both trails.

Past the signs for the trailhead, towering valley oaks and cottonwoods cast shade across the trail, and any light that might sneak in is caught by the curtain of wild grapevines draped from the trees. The sounds of owls calling and woodpeckers hammering are muffled immediately. Your footsteps are almost silent as you proceed along this dirt-and-duff trail on the way to the next interpretive sign.

Rather than just listing the species of this riparian habitat, the signs in Caswell MSP relate a natural scenario in terms that are easy for everyone to remember. You will pass an area close to the river, where a sign cautions hikers to stay back from the eroding bank. After that, the trail is wide and there is not too much poison oak.

Get on the Crow's Loop Trail by taking the next two left turns. Blackberries and sedges both thrive in this floodplain, growing amid the poison oak. There are some nice vistas of the river here as long as you stay on the trail. Although it's not as manicured as the interpretive section, this 0.4-mile loop gives one some insight into the variety of this ecosystem's wildlife. Raccoons, foxes, skunks, weasels, and squirrels have all left evidence of their presence. Most of the smaller mammals, such as the riparian brush rabbit and the riparian wood rat, take up residence in the thick understory and rarely venture farther than 50 feet from their burrow or nest. And for good reason: sitting at the bottom of the food chain, they are meals for raptors such as great horned owls, osprey, and Swainson's hawks; they're also on the menu for all the mammals listed above. They're even taken by snakes. No wonder they live in seclusion.

When you're halfway around this loop, valley oaks fill the sky above your trail and block the horizon. Pass through a grove of young sycamores to finish the loop. Take the same two left forks you passed previously to return to the River Bend Trail. Every intersection in this thickly forested park is marked with a brown wooden post signed with trail names and directional arrows, so you should have no worries about becoming disoriented.

In about 100 feet, you will stay on River Bend Trail by turning left at the intersection with the Gray Fox Trail. Follow the River Bend Trail with the river on your left as you head south. As you walk in and out of the shade, your path is interrupted by a horizontal oak that offers no options other than scrambling through its broken limbs and over its trunk, as the blackberries on the other side beckon and the wild rose perfumes the air. The poison oak reminds you to watch what you grab.

There are plenty of side trails over to the edge of the Stanislaus River. Here you can watch for the occasional turtle as it suns itself on a stick poking out of the mud bank. The trail remains a wide doubletrack despite the overgrowth of sedges. More frequently now, cottonwoods tower 75 feet over your track. You are totally shaded for the next 5–10 minutes on even the sunniest day. Look down for a bit to spot the next two turns. Take a left at the intersection that puts you on Majestic Oaks Trail. (Straight ahead would take you to the parking lot.) Walk just 100 feet and take another left back onto River Bend Trail.

Geese can be heard arguing over on the river as you walk through the wild grapevines, but you'll be unable to see past the greenery to the water. Continue to the junction with Hidden Lake Trail. Make a left on this trail, heading southwest. (From this point, you can reach the Fenceline Trail by walking 50 feet ahead.) As you walk along Hidden Lake Trail (it could have been called "Active Raccoon Trail" for the plentiful markings of these nocturnal mammals), you will encounter another fallen oak where a trail enters from the right. Signed as the Mosquito Trail, it does not appear on the park map. Our route goes forward in search of Hidden Lake.

Perhaps there is a lake hidden in the thick forest that this trail skirts, but light does not penetrate far enough to reveal any sort of secret fishing spot here. Regardless, the trail is soft, the shade is cool, and the wild rose is relaxing. Notice that some small areas of the forest have been thinned by burning; the Yokut people did the same thing when they lived in this area under the leadership of Chief Estanislao. Look for green or brown narrow fiber tubes standing in these thinned areas: they protect valley oak seedlings as they gain a foothold in the forest. Hike onward to a right turn at Fenceline Trail, where Rabbit's Run Trail leads left, then hike along Fenceline Trail about 0.25 mile. The duff-covered road is bordered by the orchard to your left and valley oaks to your right. You can see many more of the seedling tubes here as you approach a junction with River Bend Trail. Continue on to your left and pass a wood-chipping area. In a moment, you will take a right

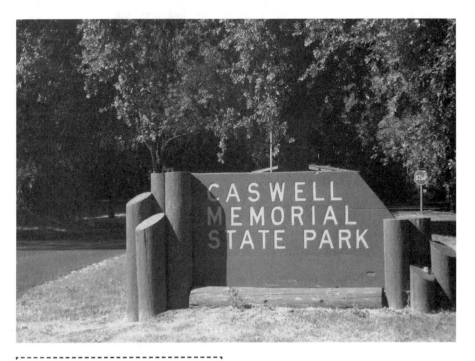

A hidden gem at the end of an orchard road

onto Majestic Oaks Trail. Aside from the huge valley oaks with their spreading canopies, there are numerous seedlings planted and protected here for future generations to enjoy.

Pass the next two intersections; they are both part of the River Bend Trail. Your task is to take in the vast numbers of valley oaks that grow here. They are magnificent and will be here for a while, thanks to the care of this park and the Caswell family.

Turn north on Gray Fox Trail, where the interpretive signage continues. Blackberries and roses on one side and grapes overhead bound your trail an hour into the hike. When you reach the fence line, turn right toward the parking lot. The corner of the orchard is to your left, and the trail enters the parking lot at the northwest corner.

LODI LAKE NATURE TRAIL

IN BRIEF

The nature trail joins the exercise trail to form a pleasant loop that lets hikers experience the wonderful sights, sounds, and scents of the Mokelumne River riparian area.

DESCRIPTION

Rarely does a small town take such care to preserve an important ecological site as the city of Lodi has done with this 58-acre nature area. You know this place is special as soon as you see the murals at the trailhead. Walk straight ahead on the asphalt-paved pathway to the Nature Trail, which will take you generally northeast 0.5 mile. You could actually turn around at this point, satisfied that you've seen most of what the park has to offer, but the hike continues on the exercise trail to make a loop around the park and along the former river channel.

Walk past an outdoor theater set amid a grove of majestic coast redwoods. They may be the most obvious of the trees that are not native to the Central Valley, but they are not the only nonnative species. The Himalayan blackberry

- -

Directions ⟶

From the junction of CA 99 South and the Capital City Freeway, drive 32 miles on CA 99 South to Lodi and take Exit 267A/West Turner Road. Turn left on West Turner and drive 1.7 miles to the park entrance on the right, just past Laurel Avenue and directly opposite Superburger Drive-In. Enter the park and turn right to drive through the parking lot. When the lane narrows, drive slowly past the large oaks in the road and turn at the next right, at the large sycamore. Park inside the fenced area. Your trailhead is in the northeast corner of the small lot.

KEY AT-A-GLANCE INFORMATION

LENGTH: 2.5 miles

CONFIGURATION: Loops

DIFFICULTY: Cakewalk

WATER REQUIRED: 0.5 liters

SCENERY: Riparian area with nice views of the Mokelumne River

EXPOSURE: Shaded trail; little exposure

TRAIL TRAFFIC: Light on weekday afternoons

TRAIL SURFACE: Asphalt and packed dirt

HIKING TIME: 1.5 hours

SEASON: Year-round, sunrise–sunset

ACCESS: $5 fee

MAPS: USGS Lodi North

WHEELCHAIR ACCESS: Yes, on the paved nature trail

FACILITIES: Restrooms near swimming area

DRIVING DISTANCE: 34 miles

SPECIAL COMMENTS: Docent-guided tours can be arranged by contacting Lodi Lake Park, 1101 W. Turner Road, Lodi, CA 95242; 209-333-6742. Bicycles are prohibited on the trails, and dogs must be leashed. Your canine hiking partner may appreciate a run at the dog fields over near the swimming area.

GPS TRAILHEAD COORDINATES

Latitude   N38° 08.911´

Longitude   W121° 17.517´

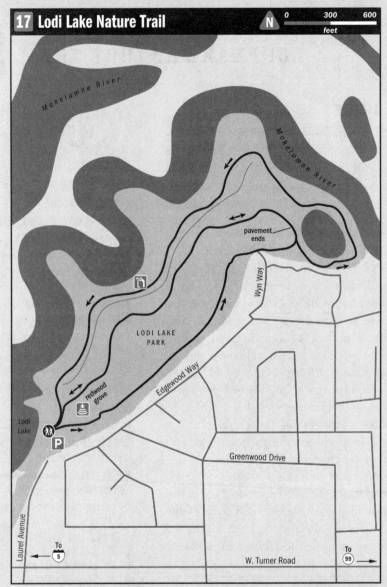

N

| 0 | 300 | 600 |

feet

Mokelumne River

Mokelumne River

pavement
ends

Wyn Way

LODI LAKE
PARK

redwood
grove

Edgewood Way

Lodi
Lake

P

Greenwood Drive

Laurel Avenue

To
5

W. Turner Road

To
99

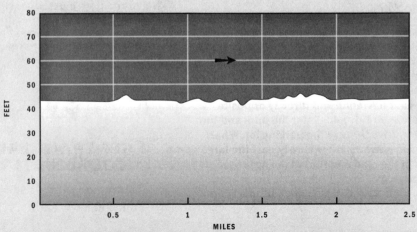

| | 0.5 | 1 | 1.5 | 2 | 2.5 |

FEET

80
70
60
50
40
30
20
10
0

MILES

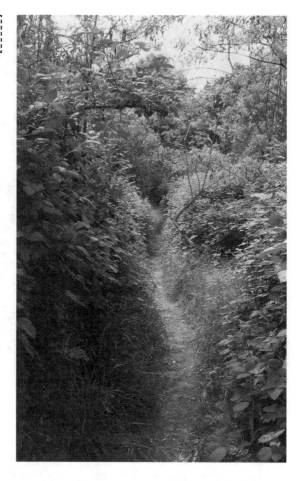

Blackberries abound on the
Lodi Lake Nature Trail.

(not a foreign handheld device) and black locust (not an insect) are two other introduced species that have adapted well to the sandy loam of the valley's riparian environment.

The grasslands that you soon pass display both native and nonnative species. There are informational placards in the ground that have suffered some flood damage, but they are generally well placed. Markers attached to the trees seem to last longer.

Valley oaks stand like huge, ponderous ancestors of the area, but even they look up to the noisy foliage of the cottonwoods. When the explorer John C. Fremont came through here in 1844, he made special comment about the musical rustlings of the leaves of the cottonwoods and oaks. Just about the time you're thinking about relaxing while listening to the trees yourself, nice benches will start appearing like poppies.

Casual trails lead to the water's edge or across the area between trails, but the Nature Trail continues on the pavement until a substantial yellow metal post. Continue past the post, and your dirt-and-duff trail will lead left around a small pond, which is excellent for spotting frogs, turtles, mallards, and wood ducks amid the dozen birds hiding in the understory and sprinting along the pond's edge. As you exit the pond area, you'll walk past a tree dedicated to the anonymous "E"—perhaps indicating an invitation to eat the mountain of blackberries along here.

The cattails and their resident frogs line the trail as it traces a small creek formed by river water that has soaked the ground. Hummingbirds and a variety of understory-dwelling songbirds and dozens of little brown birds join the frogs just after you pass the viewing platform.

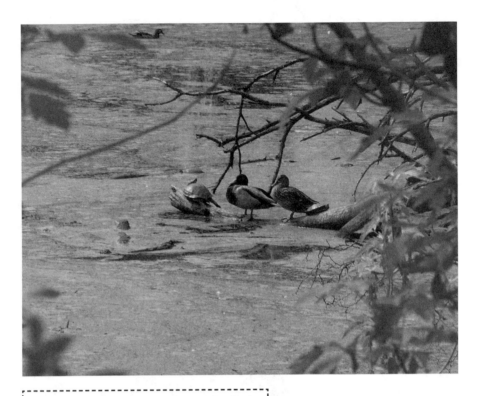

A pond turtle shares its perch with a pair of mallards.

Back at the trailhead, this half of the trail and loop has covered about 1.5 miles. If you want, continue around to the other half of the exercise trail and walk with the outdoor theater and redwood grove on your left. There is some exposure along here, where your trail runs close to the neighborhood. The unexpected feature of this hike is not that it's so quiet along the trail, but that it's so noisy—but just noisy with the sounds of trees, wind, and animals.

At 1.9 miles, you will plunge back into the woods once again just before the path joins the nature trail at the yellow post. Turn left here and follow the nature trail back to the trailhead and the parking lot.

NEARBY ACTIVITIES

The Lodi Lake Discovery Center natural-history museum has excellent displays. Near the dog fields and picnic area at the far end of the parking lot, it's open Saturdays between Memorial Day and Labor Day, and admission is free. (See Special Comments for contact info.)

COSUMNES RIVER PRESERVE TRAILS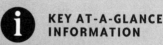

IN BRIEF

The River and Wetlands walks at the Cosumnes River Preserve showcase the plant and wildlife communities of the largest free-flowing river entering the Great Central Valley. Close to town and accessible to all, these trails offer tranquility, beauty, and a sense of what the area once looked like to settlers.

DESCRIPTION

The trails at the preserve guide hikers through two of the Central Valley's diminishing plant communities. Here, hikers can stroll through a riparian forest, past a freshwater marsh and vernal pools, and along annual grasslands at a leisurely pace. The preserve is subject to—and celebrates—the natural changes that occur seasonally in this fragile ecosystem. From time to time, whether it's beavers or spring snowmelt that overwhelms the culverts and floods the trails, nature has its own methods of causing temporary trail closures. Hopefully, these will offer opportunities to view the area from a new perspective.

The Cosumnes River Preserve is managed by The Nature Conservancy, the U.S. Bureau of Land Management, Ducks Unlimited, the California Department of Fish and Game, the

KEY AT-A-GLANCE INFORMATION

LENGTH: 1–4.1 miles

CONFIGURATION: Connected loops

DIFFICULTY: Easy

WATER REQUIRED: 1 liter

SCENERY: Open savanna and riparian woodland

EXPOSURE: Bright in the meadows

TRAIL TRAFFIC: Light

TRAIL SURFACE: Grass or dirt trail; concrete sidewalk

HIKING TIME: 2 hours

SEASON: Year-round, sunrise–sunset. Visitor center hours vary; call ahead (916-684-2816) for information.

ACCESS: No fees or permits

MAPS: USGS Bruceville

WHEELCHAIR ACCESS: Yes; the Wetlands Trail is a level sidewalk with observation platforms. Check out the waterfowl from the wetland-observation decks on the west side of Franklin Boulevard from the Boardwalk.

FACILITIES: Pit toilets in the parking lots on both sides of Franklin Road

DRIVING DISTANCE: 22 miles

SPECIAL COMMENTS: Excellent hands-on displays are included in the visitor center exhibits. Pets are prohibited in the preserve.

Directions ⟶

From Sacramento, take I-5 South 20 miles to Exit 498/Twin Cities Road. Turn east, driving 1 mile to make a right onto Franklin Boulevard south. In 0.4 mile, you will see the Cosumnes River Preserve sign on the right. The visitor center is on the left, another 1.2 miles down Franklin Boulevard. The trailheads are next to the visitor center, on the left.

GPS TRAILHEAD COORDINATES

Latitude   N38° 15.959´

Longitude   W121° 26.373´

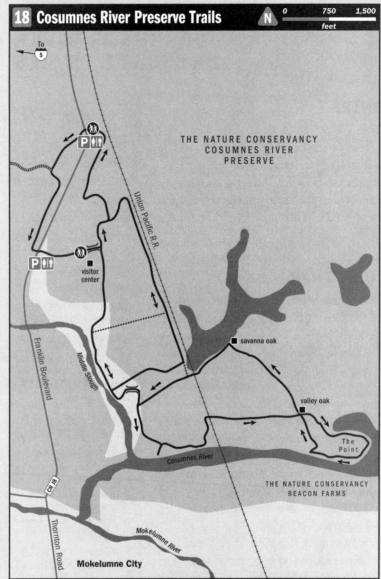

18 Cosumnes River Preserve Trails

N   0   750   1,500
feet

To
5

THE NATURE CONSERVANCY
COSUMNES RIVER
PRESERVE

Union Pacific R.R.

P

visitor
center

savanna oak

valley oak

The
Point

Franklin Boulevard

Middle Slough

CR 18

Cosumnes River

THE NATURE CONSERVANCY
BEACON FARMS

Thornton Road

Mokelumne River

Mokelumne City

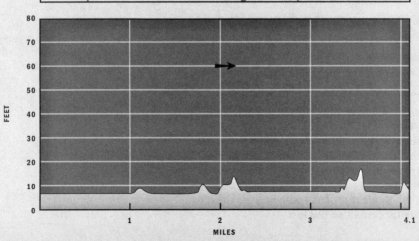

FEET
80
70
60
50
40
30
20
10
0
     1   2   3   4.1
              MILES

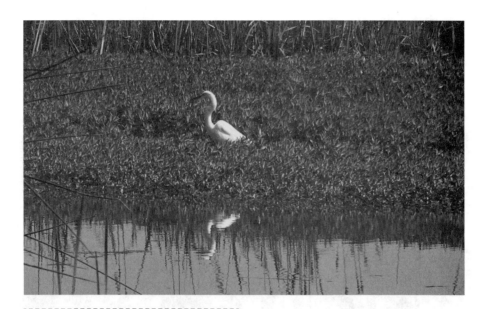

The great egret patiently hunts frogs and fish.

State Lands Commission, the California Department of Water Resources, Sacramento County, and private landowners.

If your party includes children, the visitor center should be your first stop: let them acquaint themselves with the plants and wildlife they're about to see. Hands-on displays encourage everybody to touch, feel, and learn about the elements of this unique and diminishing environment. Pick up trail maps and interpretive information for the area.

The annual grasses and flowers surrounding the visitor center hint at the flora along the trails. Trailheads for both trails are to the left of the visitor center, at the top of a wooden ramp that descends to Willow Slough. The benches and observation points at each end of the bridge are nice spots for reflecting on the posted interpretive material and touch signs.

When you cross the bridge, you have two choices. One is to turn left onto the concrete sidewalk of the Lost Slough Wetlands Walk. One mile long, Wetlands Walk shares the trailhead with the Cosumnes River Walk. Wetlands Walk can be also started at the parking lot across Franklin Boulevard.

The trail described here turns right onto the Cosumnes River Walk, following its dirt path south along Middle Slough. A warning sign at the trail's start relates the danger that mountain lions pose to humans. For more information on this very serious animal hazard, see page 11.

This dirt trail can be flooded at times, but when dry it is smooth, soft, wide, and shaded. Himalayan blackberries line the path on the left, and songbirds exercise both lungs and wings. Flashes of color and whistles follow you along as you pass each of the interpretive-sign markers.

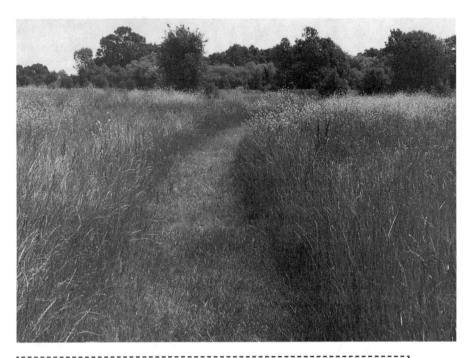

Broad savannas dotted with valley oaks are an important habitat for birds of prey such as hawks, falcons, kites, and owls.

The trail has been planned so that hikers are treated to a bit of everything the preserve has to offer. Well marked at every turn, the path even allows for whimsical side trips or loops to let you see all its features.

The marshland to the east of the trail was restored through the efforts of Ducks Unlimited. Mallard ducks and egrets, red-wing blackbirds, and even slow pond turtles move among the tall grasses and reeds. Turn left and head to the footbridge on the marsh's south side. Another 200 feet along, head up the wooden step to your right.

A boulevard of majestic valley oaks shades your way as you walk toward the river to the south, then head east along it, listening to acorn woodpeckers. These beautiful trees shaded the Miwok people, who used Santa Barbara sedges to create the intricate baskets they cooked the abundant acorns in.

The scent of the wild California rose becomes stronger as you approach the Cosumnes River 0.5 mile above its mouth at the Mokelumne River. The Cosumnes flows about 80 miles from its source high in the El Dorado National Forest to join the Sacramento–San Joaquin Delta. The river and sloughs here are subject to the same tidal forces as those in the San Francisco Bay. The Cosumnes is the spawning grounds of Chinook salmon and is home to muskrat, beaver, mink, and river otter.

Now it's time to turn north before passing under the railroad trestle. A pair of interpretive signs tells of the work involved in identifying and managing nonnative species. Your grassy trail is exposed as you parallel the Union Pacific tracks. As soon as you turn under the tracks, you'll see that the extra sun is worth it.

Immense valley oaks are the highlight of this grassland savanna. The color surrounding you depends on the season, but the lush grasses, wildflowers, and oaks are a backdrop for wonderful memories.

Continue walking east across this vast meadow. At the next trail crossing, turn right or go straight, as this route describes. The nesting boxes in the trees are for wood ducks. Kites soaring and spotted towhees scrambling underfoot are hints of the 200 identified species of birds that visit or live here. House finches and sandhill cranes, swans, ducks, geese, and coots flock to this wetland annually.

Complete this mini-loop by walking south and west past The Point, where you may enjoy a rest on the benches placed here as part of a Boy Scout project. Then it's on to a lonesome live oak, where you'll turn left and head northwest to the oak-marked junction you passed earlier.

Continue northwest across the meadow toward a grand savanna oak at the edge of a tule marsh. Linger in the shade here and take a moment to use your binoculars while under cover. You won't have to wait long to observe several species from this cool spot.

Now head southwest to follow the trail signs under the tracks and across an old doubletrack; then make a right at the wooden stairs that you ascended previously. Cross the bridge, turn left, and follow the path back to the visitor center.

When you reach the concrete sidewalk, you'll have traveled 3.1 miles. The Lost Slough Wetlands Walk is 1 mile long. Within 200 feet, an observation point and benches entice you to rest. The trail continues to the right, past the native ryegrasses.

After crossing the bridge, you'll see the uniform growth of the grove of valley oaks planted as acorns in 1988. Brush your hand lightly across the fennel to release more of its fragrant scent as you pass. Butterflies are all over this and other blossoms along the path.

An observation point is conveniently located along the slough, just before the trail crosses the road. The Boardwalk extends from the parking lot into the wetland on the west side of Franklin Boulevard. There are interpretive signs in the parking lot. The ponds to your right are wet year-round, although they grow and shrink. Another observation deck awaits at the southernmost end of this section of the walk. Cross Franklin Boulevard to return to the visitor center.

NEARBY ACTIVITIES

Excellent home-style meals are prepared at Giusti's, near the Walnut Grove Marina (14743 Walnut Grove–Thornton Road; 916-776-1808; **giustis.com**). Drive 2 miles south on I-5 to Walnut Grove–Thornton Road. Drive west to the second bridge and turn right for good food and good company.

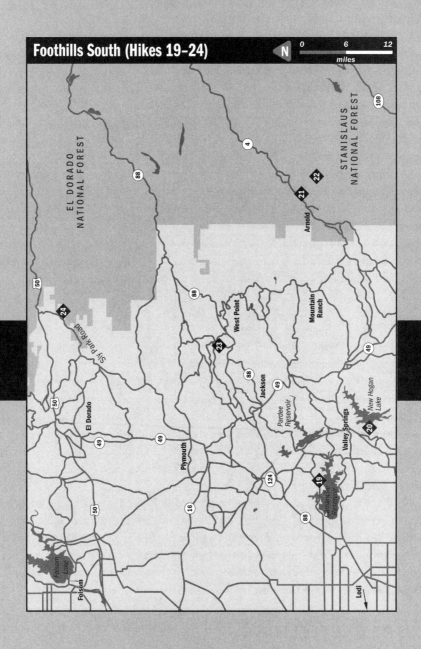

Foothills South (Hikes 19–24)

N

0   6   12
miles

EL DORADO
NATIONAL FOREST

STANISLAUS
NATIONAL FOREST

108

4

88

22
21

Arnold

50

24

Sly Park Road

88

West Point

Mountain
Ranch

23

49

88

Jackson

49

El Dorado

Pardee
Reservoir

New Hogan
Lake

50

49

49

20

Valley Springs

Plymouth

124

19

Camanche
Reservoir

50

16

88

Folsom
Lake

Lodi

Folsom

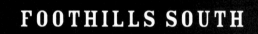

FOOTHILLS SOUTH

19 CHINA GULCH TRAIL

KEY AT-A-GLANCE INFORMATION

LENGTH: 11 miles

CONFIGURATION: Out-and-back

DIFFICULTY: Challenging

WATER REQUIRED: 3–4 liters

SCENERY: Blue oak and open grassland meadows overlooking lake

EXPOSURE: Exposed to the sun for most of the route

TRAIL TRAFFIC: Light

TRAIL SURFACE: Dirt and gravel

HIKING TIME: 4 hours

SEASON: Year-round, sunrise–sunset

ACCESS: $2.50 day-use fee for parking at trailhead only

MAPS: USGS Wallace; EBMUD trail map at entry kiosk

WHEELCHAIR ACCESS: None

FACILITIES: Parking lot with two pit toilets and trash receptacles; water at trailhead

DRIVING DISTANCE: 46 miles

SPECIAL COMMENTS: The blue-oak-studded meadows are overflowing with wildflowers in spring. No dogs permitted. Unless you are hiking in the spring or early summer, water is unavailable on this trail after the trailhead.

GPS TRAILHEAD COORDINATES

Latitude   N38° 14.287´

Longitude   W120° 56.492´

IN BRIEF

This hike takes wildflower lovers through vast meadows of colorful blossoms every spring. The rolling hills are sprinkled with handsome blue oaks that contrast with the light-blue sky. This equestrian and hiking trail is easy to follow, but it is exposed to the sun all day. A hat is a must.

DESCRIPTION

The China Gulch Trail is an equestrian path that traces the north lakeshore past China Gulch to the area of Lancha Plana, then returns to the equestrian-assembly area. Your track takes advantage of the wide horse route as it meanders around, over, and down small hills and knobs, all decorated with uniformly spaced blue oaks and alive with colorful wildflowers in spring.

Once you've parked, find the trail, which begins at the north end of the staging area, and start walking north on the gravel road next to the board fence. When you round the first curve, a sign-in kiosk, which is the official

Directions

From the junction of CA 99 South and US 50, drive 25 miles on CA 99 South, past Galt, to the Liberty Road exit. Drive 12.5 miles east on Liberty Road to the junction with CA 88. Continue straight across on Liberty, which will become North Camanche Parkway, driving another 7.5 miles. After the village of Camanche, turn right onto Camanche Road; the entry kiosk is about 1 mile on. To reach the trailhead, follow the road to the left after the kiosk, and the sign will point to the trail, which is about 0.2 mile ahead, to the left of the mobile-home park. The trailhead is reached from the north end of the equestrian staging area.

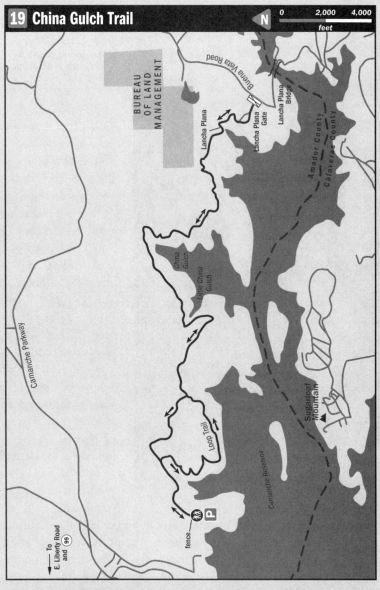

0   2,000   4,000

N

feet

BUREAU
OF LAND
MANAGEMENT

Buena Vista Road

Lancha Plana

Lancha Plana Gate

Lancha Plana Bridge

Amador County
Calaveras County

China Gulch

Little China Gulch

Camanche Parkway

Loop Trail

Sugarloaf Mountain

Camanche Reservoir

P

fence

To
E. Liberty Road
and 99

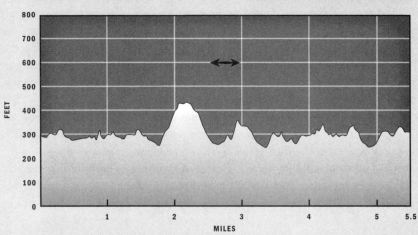

800
700
600
500
400
300
200
100
0

FEET

1   2   3   4   5   5.5

MILES

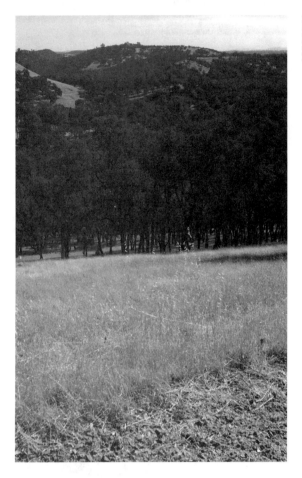

The rolling, forested grassland is typical of the southernmost Foothills.

trailhead for the China Gulch Trail, comes into view on the other side of a gated fence. Make sure to close the gate across the trail after you pass through.

If you picked up a trail map at the entry kiosk, you'll see a narrow-gauge trail leading to the south and then looping back to join the main trail. Your route follows this extra loop. If, however, you feel like taking only a short trail, you can return to the trailhead after rejoining the main trail, and your trek will have covered just 3 miles. The described hike goes outbound via the loop trail and returns by way of the main road, making an 11-mile round-trip.

Your first scenic vista pops into view within 0.25 mile of the trailhead. When you finish taking pictures here, you may notice one of the first few watering stations for horses over on the right. Descending this larkspur- and buttercup-lined road northeast, you might stop, turn around, and take in the broad blue-oak meadow on both sides of the upcoming drainage.

A trail sign on the right indicates the loop trail—"narrow gauge" on the map—which approaches the lake for a 1.5-mile diversion before rejoining the main trail. Your route turns southeast at this point and crosses a seasonal drainage. Then it takes another 90-degree right turn as you parallel the trail you descended, now visible across the meadow.

The path is covered by horses' hoofprints, which have erased the previous night's wildlife tracks. So if you're on this trail early in the day, pay close attention to the animal tracks in the dust. They were all made overnight. These prints tell little stories about the wildlife here: A cluster of quail prints midtrail that lead off at an angle into the grass might be an interrupted meeting. Raccoon prints that change from a walk to a run, crossing the many large tracks of a trailside turkey convention, followed by a small pillow of down in the grass, bring to mind a frantic but brief chase. A careful coyote's prints at the margin of the trail tell of a search for other nocturnal travelers.

Blue oak is certainly the dominant tree species of this open chaparral. No other tree is visible here as you overlook the small bay to your west. This trail will generally skirt the knoll, which crests about 100 feet above the trail. Reverse direction again and travel east, with the lakeshore on your right. The broad hillside to your left is topped by distinctive blue oaks and is filled with butterflies and bees, mauling every one of the thousands of flowers like ants at a picnic.

As the ridge dwindles out on the east end, cross a seasonal drainage and then angle right, across the wash, where you can see the junction with your original trail. If you're returning to the trailhead, keep left on the wide trail to rejoin your track. Otherwise, keep right, across the meadow. If you embarked on this trail without a hat, this is about the point at which you'll start to think about fashioning a *chapeau* from just about anything: kerchief, T-shirt, sandals, maybe a snack wrapper. It's hot and exposed along the entire route.

Camanche Reservoir, which straddles the San Joaquin, Amador, and Calaveras county lines, fills the lower valleys along the path of the Mokelumne River. While the land in the vicinity of the Mokelumne was being settled during the Gold Rush years of 1849 and 1850, Campo Seco and Mokelumne Hill were thriving towns, and even Camanche had a population of up to 1,500 people who hailed from all over the world. Hydraulic mining moved the course of the river, dried it completely at times, altered its looks, polluted it, and returned enormous monetary profits, until flood control, irrigation, and electricity production became more profitable and important than gold. Developed and operated by the East Bay Metropolitan Utility District (EBMUD), Camanche Reservoir is the largest in its system of lakes in the southern Foothills.

There are differing accounts regarding the naming of Camanche. The one thing all agree upon is that its original name was Limerick and that it was subsequently changed to the current misspelled version, either deliberately, in memory of a town in Iowa, or inadvertently, after a frustrated postmaster proposed two other names that were rejected. Either way, the town now lies silently beneath the lake's waters.

Turn right and head uphill, where you have a nice vista to the south and east. Another watering trough sits amid the blue oaks and small displays of irises and lilies. Spend the next 5 minutes walking along the ridgeline toward the southeast. Enter the shade of another blue-oak grove, and the trail heads down.

Enter this next ravine—Little China Gulch on the maps—and then exit it while climbing northeast, with trees to your right, where your trail becomes gravel-covered after it crosses the small drainage. Continue uphill, probably following turkey tracks, and it changes to dirt again. For the first time on this route, a few foothill pines appear on the knoll ahead that separates Little China Gulch from China Gulch.

When you gain about 50 feet, the trail will contour across the face of this hill and then descend again into China Gulch. Just as you begin heading downhill, you'll see the crowns of about a half-dozen gray pines sticking out above the blue oak on the hill to your right. A close look reveals another few dozen spread out across the hill.

Cross the rock culvert at China Gulch, where a ranch house looks down on your trail. In wet years, the lake sneaks up to this crossing. When it's dry, you can track raccoons as they travel along this dirt trail. Leave China Gulch behind as you ascend the hill and cross another small drainage. In a short distance, live oaks briefly provide shade as you climb up and over another low ridge to Lancha Plana.

A parklike setting awaits you as you enter the signed Lancha Plana. The low-canopied trees grow close enough together to block the sun and keep the grasses from scorching. This is a great spot for a relaxing break. Lancha Plana, meaning "flat boat" in Spanish, was the name of the ford in the Mokelumne River where a ferry operated in 1850, reportedly at the site of the Lancha Plana Bridge on Buena Vista Road.

Head uphill and cross another small culvert, also signed Lancha Plana, on your way to the trail's end about 0.5 mile away. A small pond sits atop the next hill. Your trail skirts it to the right, then drops downhill to the right. You'll see an irrigation ditch from the trail. This may be part of the old Poverty Bar Ditch, which the lakes and reservoirs later replaced. You can trace portions of this, or some other irrigation ditch, at various points along your route.

The trail winds around until it comes within sight of Buena Vista Road. The end of this hike is along the road at a gate marked LANCHA PLANA GATE—AC 49. You can walk past this gate down to the trees alongside the lake, then return via your previous route. When you reach the LOOP TRAIL sign on your return, you can retrace your steps exactly onto the 1.5-mile loop, or you can continue straight for 0.8 mile to the staging-area parking lot.

NEARBY ACTIVITIES

The Mokelumne Watershed and Recreation Division maintains 21 miles of hiking, equestrian, and jogging trails. Call 209-772-8204 for permit information.

RIVER OF SKULLS TRAIL 20

IN BRIEF

In about an hour, you can walk through two of the valley's important ecosystems—foothill woodland and increasingly vanishing riparian forest. The entire family can learn about the major flora while cruising along this mile-long rock-lined path.

DESCRIPTION

Nature trails are wonderful vehicles for learning about natural history and are fun places to hike. River of Skulls Trail is an important part of the riparian-conservation effort. (Less than 5 percent of the original riparian area in the Sacramento Valley and Foothills remains today.) This trail is fun and informative for hikers of all ages.

Although the name of the trail is a bit macabre—*calaveras* is the Spanish word for "skulls"—children seem naturally drawn to it for just that reason. Apparently, the large number of human skulls found along the lower reaches of the river was the inspiration for the river's name. Regardless of the name, this trail has been expertly laid out to make the most of the small area's diverse flora.

Directions ———————————⟶

From the junction of US 50 East and CA 99 South, drive 31 miles on CA 99 South to the CA 12/East Victor Road exit in Lodi. Then drive 5 miles east on CA 12, where it will join CA 88 for 7 miles. Continue 15 more miles east on CA 12 to the town of Valley Springs. Turn right onto CA 26, drive 3 miles south to Silver Rapids Road, and turn left. In 1.5 miles, turn right onto Hogan Dam Road. Cross the bridge over the Calaveras River, and immediately turn left into the equestrian parking lot at the Monte Vista Day Use Area. The trailhead is on the left, at the far end of the parking area.

KEY AT-A-GLANCE INFORMATION

LENGTH: 1 mile

CONFIGURATION: Loop

DIFFICULTY: Cakewalk

WATER REQUIRED: 1 liter

SCENERY: Riparian and foothill woodland

EXPOSURE: Mostly shaded trail

TRAIL TRAFFIC: Light

TRAIL SURFACE: Dirt and duff

HIKING TIME: 1 hour

SEASON: Year-round, sunrise–sunset

ACCESS: No fees or permits

MAPS: USGS Valley Springs; New Hogan Lake Trail map

WHEELCHAIR ACCESS: None

FACILITIES: Pit toilet, parking area

DRIVING DISTANCE: 62 miles

SPECIAL COMMENTS: Pick up a trail map and interpretive trail booklet at the headquarters building before you drive to the trailhead. Turn left at the sign 0.4 mile south of Valley Springs, and follow the signs to the headquarters. You can reach the trailhead from here by turning left at the end of the parking lot onto Hogan Dam Road, then following this road to the left after 1.2 miles.

GPS TRAILHEAD COORDINATES

Latitude   N38° 08.917´

Longitude   W120° 49.410´

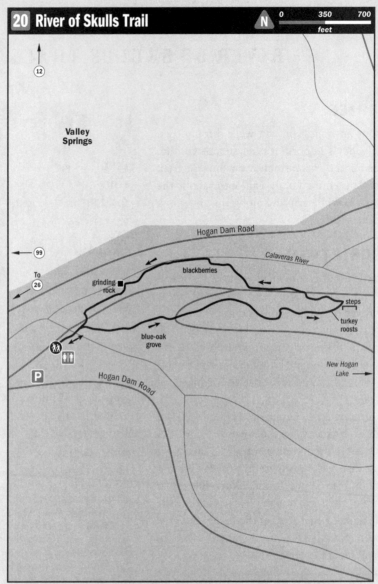

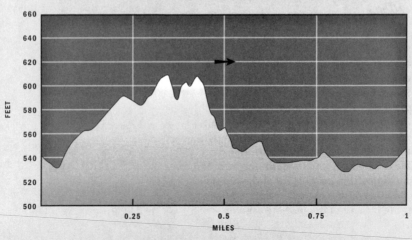

The trail covers two ecosystems. The first half of the path encompasses the upland area, which highlights the foothill-woodland flora. Then the trail descends to the river, where riparian flora flourish. That the two are so close is not uncommon in Central California.

With your interpretive trail booklet in hand, walk over to the northeast corner of the parking lot, where posts mark the trailhead. Follow the wide gravel path over the bridge, then bear right as the next trail sign indicates. Bear right again, then follow the rock-bordered trail to the left, up to a group of benches at the beginning of a blue-oak grove.

The dominant hardwood of the upland area is blue oak. Its small acorns were gathered by the Miwok, the Native Americans who occupied this area for thousands of years before settlers arrived en masse during the Gold Rush era. You will see a variety of oaks on this trail. Besides the blue oak, there are also valley, black, and live. All supplied large quantities of acorns, which were an important staple to the Miwok. As you identify each of these trees, notice the size differences among their acorns and leaves.

The upland area is also noted for its chaparral, which consists, in this area, of chamise and buckbrush. These offered the Miwok a good area in which to hunt for deer and rabbit. Walk beneath the dying foothill pine's one massive limb, which reaches out and down to the ground. Colorful in any season, poison oak is plentiful here—enough to keep you on the trail as you continue along under foothill pine and live oak.

The trail emerges onto a wildflower-encrusted hillside after you pass the knoll above you to the right. Reenter the shade of pine, toyon, and manzanita as the trail continues eastward. Manzanita, whose name is the Spanish word for "little apple," was another food source of the Miwok, who used the red berries for tea and stored the dried berries for winter.

There are several turkey roosts among the black oak and its large pointy-lobed leaves. As you walk toward a set of steep steps, look trailside for feathers. Carefully avoid the poison oak as you examine the different types of feathers discarded here by preening turkeys.

From the bench at the stairs, you can hear the rushing of the water as it exits the dam about 1,000 unseen feet from your position. Continue down the steps, where you will see black oak, elderberry, toyon, coffeeberry, and valley oak. Another nice grouping of benches offers a great place to sit in the shade and read about what you've seen so far. Head west on the trail and skirt the base of the short slope that you traversed moments earlier.

The trail crosses a dirt-and-gravel road on its way to the river. There is never any doubt about which way to travel on this well-marked route. The trail does become rockier as you near the river, which grows louder despite the thick trees lining its banks.

Riparian trees and bushes close in tightly on the trail, which often looks like nothing more than a break in the vegetation. Blackberries grow in profusion here,

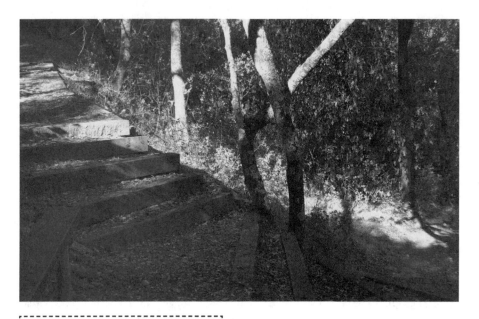

A perfect spot for an impromptu classroom

and there are signs that other berry lovers, including birds, skunks, and raccoons, have stopped by for a snack. A large buckeye on the opposite shore leans out over the river and nearly touches the trail as you walk by. Another huge buckeye actually has half its large trunk in the water and half on the shore. Several small clearings allow access to the swiftly flowing river to the west. Fremont cottonwood trees, an important part of the riparian zone, can grow to heights of 100 feet.

As the trail moves away from the river, it passes over ancient sedimentary rock, formerly ocean floor, which has been upended and now forms much of the exposed bedrock in this complex geological area. As you near the trail's end, notice a small rock outcrop, nearly covered by brush, which has a few Miwok grinding holes in it. These mortar cups were used to pound the acorns that were so highly prized. Even in ancient times, food processing was done on-site, just as it is today.

In another minute, you'll arrive back at the bridge leading to the trailhead.

NEARBY ACTIVITIES

If you want a bonus trail, follow the 8-mile Equestrian Trail. It's sunny, with only a little shade, but it is an interesting hike, with huge wildflower displays and plenty of fishing opportunities. The trailhead is across the parking lot next to the toilet.

Several excellent hike-and-bike trails begin near the headquarters parking lot but can also be accessed from many of the campgrounds along the way. The bike trail has sections rated for all skill levels from easy to difficult.

BIG TREES NORTH GROVE TRAILS 21

IN BRIEF

The interpretive trail through the North Grove of giant sequoia trees offers hikers of all ages and abilities a detailed, up-close, and inside view of these impressive giants. Clearly signed and well designed, the trail through these spectacular trees is a pleasure to hike in almost every month.

DESCRIPTION

Discovered in 1852, these trees have, incredibly, avoided the fate of other groves throughout the state, many of which were destroyed by logging. Your trailhead through these centuries-old trees is signed NORTH GROVE TRAIL, RIVER TRAIL, THREE SENSES TRAIL, GROVE OVERLOOK TRAIL. If you didn't pick

- -

Directions ⸺⸺⸺⸺⸺⸺⸺⸺⸺⸺→

From the junction of US 50 East and the Capital City Freeway, drive 3 miles on US 50 East and take Exit 19/Howe Avenue toward Power Inn Road. Turn at the first left onto Folsom Boulevard. In 0.5 mile, bear right onto CA 16 East/Jackson Road; after 30.5 miles, turn right at the junction with CA 49 South, then drive 7.8 miles through Drytown toward Jackson. Turn left onto CA 49 South/CA 88 East, and continue on CA 49 through Jackson 16.3 miles to San Andreas. Follow CA 49 South 11.8 miles to Angels Camp and turn left onto the CA 4 East bypass. Drive 21 miles to Arnold and look for Calaveras Big Trees State Park on the right, 3 miles east of town. Stop at the entry kiosk to pay your daily fees and pick up a map. Bear right and then turn left into the main parking lot. The trailhead is currently at the far end, past the restrooms and next to the Warming Hut. You can start your hike right away or use the path to head a few hundred feet southwest to the visitor center.

KEY AT-A-GLANCE INFORMATION

LENGTH: 3 miles

CONFIGURATION: Loops

DIFFICULTY: Cakewalk

WATER REQUIRED: 1 liter

SCENERY: Old-growth forest

EXPOSURE: Totally shaded trail

TRAIL TRAFFIC: Moderate

TRAIL SURFACE: Duff and dirt, boardwalk

HIKING TIME: 1.5–2 hours

SEASON: Year-round, sunrise–sunset

ACCESS: $8 day-use fee

MAPS: USGS Dorrington

WHEELCHAIR ACCESS: The Three Senses Trail

FACILITIES: Visitor center, picnic tables, restrooms, telephone, campgrounds

DRIVING DISTANCE: 95 miles

SPECIAL COMMENTS: This is an excellent interpretive trail among gigantic old-growth trees. Guided hikes are conducted every Saturday. Snowshoe hikes are conducted in winter. Dogs are prohibited on California State Park trails.

GPS TRAILHEAD COORDINATES

Latitude   N38° 16.743´
Longitude   W120° 18.433´

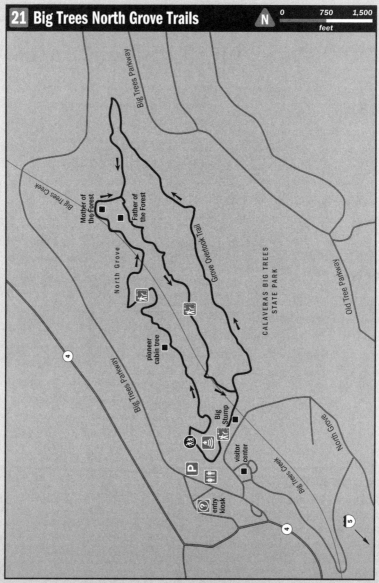

N

0   750   1,500
feet

Big Trees Parkway

Big Trees Creek

North Grove

Mother of
the Forest

Father of
the Forest

Grove Overlook Trail

pioneer
cabin tree

CALAVERAS BIG TREES
STATE PARK

Old Tree Parkway

Big Stump

Big Trees Parkway

visitor
center

Big Trees Creek

North Grove

entry
kiosk

P

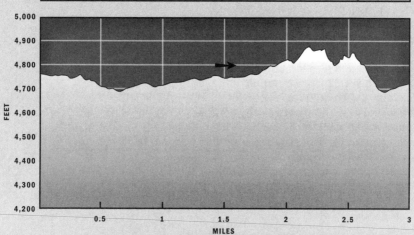

one up at the visitor center, purchase a guide to the Calaveras North Grove Trail at the trailhead for 50 cents. It contains an excellent map and helpful, informative notes about the area's natural history.

"Wow!" and "That's huge!" are the most common words heard on these trails. And how could it be otherwise? These trees *are* huge. The loop trails wind around the giant sequoias and other old-growth trees, such as ponderosa pine, white fir, sugar pine, and incense cedar. We are familiar with these trees, but they certainly are an order of magnitude larger due to their having been protected from logging.

This hike takes in two of the trails in the North Grove: the North Grove Big Trees Trail, which is the interpretive loop, and the Grove Overlook Trail. This does require repeating a short segment of the trail—but that is no drawback, considering the awesome scenery. The interpretive loop is highly recommended if you prefer a shorter hike. The Grove Overlook Trail is unsigned and a bit less tame than the loop.

From the trailhead, you will follow a path that, like the entire trail, is bordered and signed the whole way. Pass the campfire center, with its outdoor theater, on your way to the Big Stump. The Discovery Tree had stood for more than a millennium when this 300-foot Sierra redwood (giant sequoia) was discovered in 1852. One year later, it had been stripped of its bark and toppled, and its stump had been turned into a dance floor and later a saloon. Interpretive signs and descriptive kiosks ring the Big Stump, where docents or rangers are on hand to answer questions. You can walk up on the stump and get a view of the area, too.

Look for the trail sign just past the downed log of the Discovery Tree; it points you toward the Grove Overlook Trail. Take the right-hand path and ascend slightly. Then turn left and continue an easy yet steady slant up the hillside. Douglas squirrels may flash by you along here as they retreat from the activity along the main trail. These squirrels are undoubtedly well fed, judging by the massive amounts of nuts and seeds evident in this old-growth forest.

The trail is made of the softest duff, part of a deep layer of organic material in which the redwoods spread their roots, keeping them from toppling onto random hikers. The path traverses the hillside through stands of incense cedar, which also has a soft, reddish bark. But even as the view through the trees changes along this trail, the unmistakable red of the giant sequoia glows in the sunlight from the grove. When you look toward the grove from this elevation, you're looking at the midsection of the sequoias.

Although the trail along here is fairly clear, watch out for the cones of the many old-growth sugar pines in this forest. For the most part, there are very few exposed rocks along the trail. Thick duff of tree bark, cones, and needles overlays almost every mineral outcropping. Some of the young giant sequoias along here play host to woodpeckers, which seem to work their way down in search of their next snack. On this quiet, lightly traveled trail, the woodpecker's rapid hammering is muted and muffled by the redwood's soft, fibrous bark.

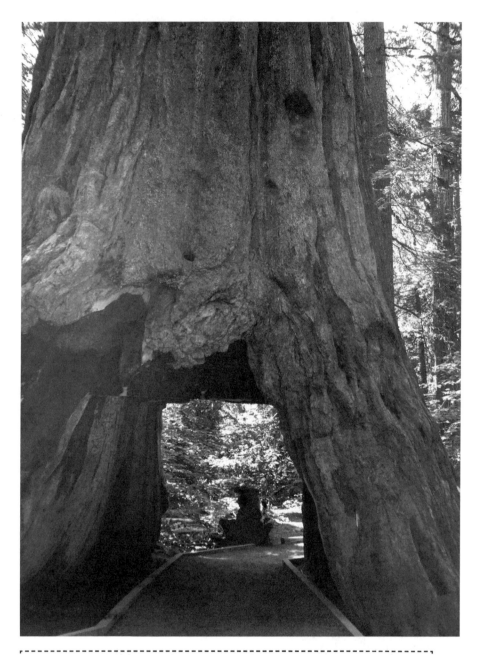

The tunnel through the Pioneer Cabin Tree was carved in the 1880s to create a tourist attraction to compete with a similar one—the Wawona Tree, in Yosemite's Mariposa Grove.

You will spend so much time looking up that you may miss some of the groundcover, especially the lupine. But you needn't worry about missing a junction or trail directions: they're posted at every point where you might wonder which way to go. In fact, the location of the trails was reworked during the summer of 2007, although it appears that the general layout will remain as is, with minor modifications from time to time.

At the end of the overlook trail, turn left (west) and descend somewhat to the main loop trail. When you rejoin the loop trail, turn left and proceed clockwise along the loop, or head straight to go counterclockwise along the second half of the loop before walking the first half. Either way, you can repeat any of the three legs to return to the trailhead.

Benches are liberally scattered around the grove, not only for resting but also for lining up that difficult photo. Wherever the understory is thick or the terrain uneven, either a wood-lined pathway or a boardwalk will assist you.

This trail has an even more magical appearance in winter, when the crowns of the trees are topped with snow. The trail is passable on foot except after a heavy snowfall, when it is open to cross-country ski travel.

NEARBY ACTIVITIES

If you have time, the South Grove Trail (see next profile) is another wonderful stroll, with fewer hikers sharing the trail.

Want to get off your feet? Take a break at the Oak Leaf Spring Picnic Area or the River Picnic Area, on the Parkway about 6 miles from the North Grove. Want to get back on your feet? Hike the Arnold Rim Trail for 10.5 view-laden miles. Visit **arnoldrimtrail.org** for more information.

22 BIG TREES SOUTH GROVE TRAIL

KEY AT-A-GLANCE INFORMATION

LENGTH: 5.4 miles

CONFIGURATION: Out-and-back

DIFFICULTY: Moderate

WATER REQUIRED: 2 liters

SCENERY: Awesome old-growth forest

EXPOSURE: Nothing but shade

TRAIL TRAFFIC: Light

TRAIL SURFACE: Duff and dirt

HIKING TIME: 3 hours

SEASON: May–October, weather permitting

ACCESS: $6 entry fee

MAPS: USGS Stanislaus, Crandall Peak

WHEELCHAIR ACCESS: None

FACILITIES: Pit toilet and benches in parking area

DRIVING DISTANCE: 91 miles

SPECIAL COMMENTS: Bring a wide-angle lens and a sit pad to kneel on to frame these spectacular giant trees. Dogs are prohibited on the trails.

GPS TRAILHEAD COORDINATES

Latitude   N38° 14.804´

Longitude W120° 16.078´

IN BRIEF

More than 1,000 giant sequoias tower over you and everything else in this natural preserve. The trail leads you through and around more than 100 individual giant sequoias, including one of the largest trees on Earth.

DESCRIPTION

The South Grove Trail leads hikers through a mixed-conifer forest, dominated by towering old-growth sugar and ponderosa pines, to the grove of giant sequoias that straddle Big Trees Creek. The South Grove is within the Calaveras South Grove Natural Preserve, which contains more than 1,000 of these giant trees. Known commonly as the giant sequoia, the Sierra redwood is a species distinct from the coast redwood. Discovered by settlers in the 1850s, the trees in this grove have been protected since 1954 from being disturbed by extractive industries.

Directions ⟶

From the junction of US 50 East and the Capital City Freeway, drive 3 miles on US 50 East and take Exit 19/Howe Avenue toward Power Inn Road. Turn at the first left onto Folsom Boulevard. In 0.5 mile, bear right onto CA 16 East/Jackson Road; after 30.5 miles, turn right at the junction with CA 49 South, then drive 7.8 miles through Drytown toward Jackson. Turn left onto CA 49 South/CA 88 East, and continue on CA 49 through Jackson 16.3 miles to San Andreas. Follow CA 49 South 11.8 miles to Angels Camp and turn left onto the CA 4 East bypass. Drive 21 miles to Arnold and look for the Calaveras Big Trees State Park on the right, 3 miles east of town. Stop at the entry kiosk to pay your daily fees and pick up a map. Signs ahead of you will direct you to the South Grove.

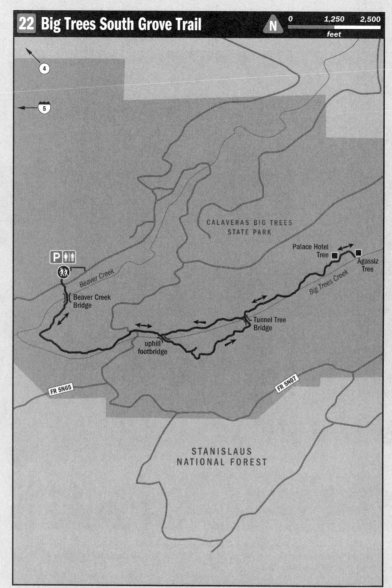

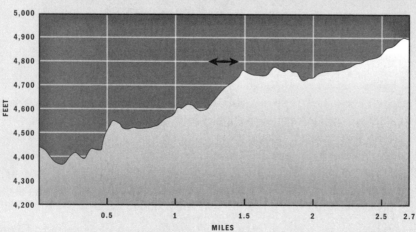

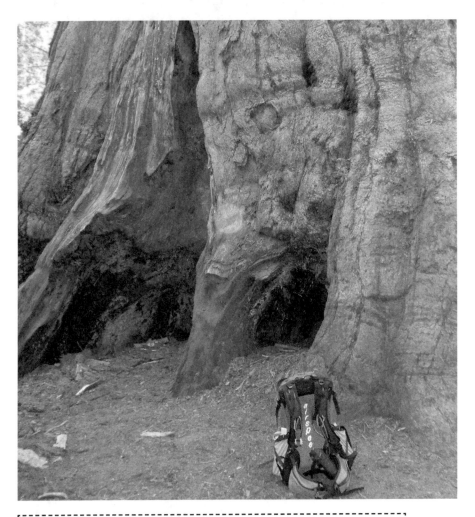

The Agassiz Tree—about 25 feet in diameter and 250 feet tall—was named in honor of the renowned American naturalist.

The trail here is, in a word, sweet. Duff and dirt are so thick in this preserve that rocks, boulders, and outcrops are rarely seen. This is good for hikers who spend considerable time looking up at the treetops and do not enjoy tripping over rocks. Highly visible and distinct in all parts of the preserve, the trail winds around noteworthy trees. Although an excited populace felt compelled to name the trees, very few have the kitschy-sounding names that are popular in many caverns. Pick up an information pamphlet and trail map at the visitor center. Complete with tree names, the pamphlet is an informative guide that will add to your understanding of the special forest you're visiting.

Start on the south side of the parking area, opposite the toilets, near the trash receptacles. A clearly signed trailhead marks the start of your trek. An information kiosk about 300 feet down the winding trail tells hikers a bit about the memorial groves that are eternal thank-you notes to the benefactors of this site. Continue around a small meadow of bunchgrasses and descend to the Beaver Creek Bridge. The trail eases off to one o'clock at the end of the bridge and begins gently gaining elevation. In a matter of moments, you'll pass the trailhead for the Bradley Grove Trail, which takes interested hikers to a grove of Sierra redwoods that were planted in the 1950s by the preserve's caretaker. You may already be dizzy from looking at these huge trees surrounding the trail. And not one of them is a giant sequoia.

This entire preserve is full of old-growth trees, all of them familiar—sugar and ponderosa pine, incense cedar, and white fir. The difference in these trees is that most of them are a few hundred years old. Their size reveals it: these trees are huge. Seeing a ponderosa pine with a trunk more than 3 feet wide or a sugar pine with one more than 5 feet wide is not uncommon along this trail. The firs and cedars are similar in size and proportion.

Continue slowly gaining elevation for about a mile. When you leave the Beaver Creek drainage, your direction will change from generally southwest to somewhat southeast, now trekking along Big Trees Creek, which empties into Beaver Creek after its approximately 3-mile course. At a junction with a dirt road, cross and bear slightly left on the obvious trail, past a blackened stump and a burned-out standing snag. The trail is now sloped at a somewhat gentler angle.

Keep on the lookout for the point at which the trail splits. The sign is difficult to see, but the split is marked by an unusual-looking white-fir stump next to its healthy-looking twin. Keep right at this split, but first turn and look back into the forest. You may have missed a tree or two, but a glance will reveal the overlooked, distinctive, red-barked goliaths. There will be so many more in the next mile. Even the standing snags, bereft of their bark, are majestic-looking.

Big Trees Creek can be heard on your right as you head upstream. In a short while, you'll cross a footbridge that slants uphill. Take a left at the end of the bridge and allow yourself a moment to look around. You'll likely comment out loud when the giant sequoias come into view. Look all around. Take a few steps. Stop. Look around again. More trees are visible every time your aspect changes, and it changes with every step. Walking gradually uphill to the southeast, you are surrounded by more than 30 of these massive trees.

The trail is flawless soft duff, but the egg-shaped giant-sequoia cones often collect themselves into a cone-puddle, which when stepped on has a ball-bearing effect on unwary hikers. The trail is incredibly distinct throughout the preserve. As you walk northeast, you are somewhat crowded by bush chinquapin and Pacific dogwood. This is the only thing close to a hindrance on this stretch. It would be hard to complain about it for long, though: look around at these trees. Whether they're standing or fallen, dead or alive, with bark or without, they are impressive. When you see a tree down on the ground, look more closely. It might be just a limb from the sequoia 30 feet from you.

Even in death, these trees are spectacular. Fallen trees are neatly cut through to ease your travel along the trail. That's true for the smaller trees like the fir; the downed sequoia, however, is not so accommodating. When your trail reaches a giant sequoia on its side, broken and hollowed out, you will recross Big Trees Creek on a footbridge. Walk around, through, and past this tree. Its immense root system is above ground now. As it decays, it has become home to a variety of plant and animal life—including a giant sequoia growing from the top.

Turn left after the tree and walk about 50 feet to another well-signed junction. Turning left at this point will lead you back to the parking lot. A right turn will take you about 0.5 mile uphill to the end of the trail, where you'll find the famed Agassiz Tree. Trees that you pause and inspect, perhaps even photograph and discuss, will have a distinctly different appearance on your return trip. One of these trees is about 0.1 mile along on the right. You will certainly notice that it has an uncommonly large amount of burn damage. Indeed, its trunk has burned through completely. Incredibly, this tree has also burned through its top—that is, the place where its top used to be—revealing sky where the crown once was. How the crown came off is unknown. Strong winds are probably responsible. However these calamities occurred, the tree remains alive. On your return, you'll think you had never seen this tree. From the opposite direction, the crown's disappearance is obvious. But in place of the tree's original *chapeau* are two limbs the size of normally large trees, growing straight up.

Sequoiadendron giganteum has a few unique survival techniques. One is the ability, as you can tell from the charred scars on most Sierra redwoods, to resist fire, its thick, fibrous bark acting as a barrier. "Self-healing" is another tactic that can be observed on one of the upcoming twin trees. As the trail leads around the tree, notice how the bark has grown over the deep fire scar to repair itself. Another survival strategy: its cones open and its seeds are released following hot, debris-clearing fires.

The trail leads gradually uphill to a broad, flat area with a stand of young firs and giant sequoias. Listen as the Douglas squirrels (chickarees) jabber at you, then try to figure out what might prompt their verbal tirades. A fir, fallen across the trail, has become a racetrack for gray squirrels that appear far too well fed. Walking through the cut in the downed fir reveals a nearly perfectly circular hole to a depth of 3 feet in place of the tree's heartwood.

Continue a short way to the signed Palace Hotel Tree. Its trunk has been burned out so evenly that it makes a nice room; early visitors to the grove were reminded of the San Francisco hotel that is the tree's namesake. A few hundred feet away is the famed Agassiz Tree. Named after renowned zoologist and naturalist Louis Agassiz, it may be one of the ten largest trees in the world. Many of the trees in this grove have been here for as long as 2,000 years.

In the 1940s, the grove was purchased by a logging company and slated to be harvested, starting with its sugar pine. Like many other groves left to extractive industries, this one came close to ruin. Through the heroic efforts of the Save the

Redwoods League, California State Parks, and individuals such as Frederick Law Olmsted and John D. Rockefeller, the grove was purchased for posterity in 1954 and became part of Calaveras Big Trees State Park.

The preserve continues another 2 miles to the northeast. Hikers with good navigational skills are welcome to explore further. The unmaintained use-trail leads past the sign at the Agassiz Tree. I have not hiked this path, and so I have not described it here. But if you do decide to explore it, budget plenty of time, bearing in mind that maintained trails are easier to travel and therefore take less time for equivalent distances.

If you're returning after visiting the Agassiz Tree, retrace your steps to the junction near the tunnel tree, but this time follow the sign toward the parking area. Lustrous copper butterflies dance along the trail's edges as you walk downhill past the Kansas group of trees. Woodpeckers, pounding their beaks at jackhammer speed, make a muffled noise as they look for insects in the soft, fibrous bark. Rejoin the main trail at the junction with the odd stump. The balance of your trail heads largely downhill until the Beaver Creek crossing.

NEARBY ACTIVITIES

The Beaver Creek Picnic Area, just past the South Grove trailhead, offers great swimming holes in which to cool off.

There are a number of interesting spots to visit in nearby Murphys and Arnold. Stop in at the Snowshoe Brewing Company (209-795-2272; **snowshoe brewing.com**), on CA 4 in Arnold, for several varieties of excellent beers. While in Murphys, check out Ironstone Vineyards and all the other great wineries in the area at **calaveraswines.org**.

23 INDIAN GRINDING ROCK LOOP TRAILS

KEY AT-A-GLANCE INFORMATION

LENGTH: 1.8 miles

CONFIGURATION: Connected loops

DIFFICULTY: Cakewalk

WATER REQUIRED: 1 liter

SCENERY: Foothill woodland and grassland

EXPOSURE: Shady, except at midday

TRAIL TRAFFIC: Moderate

TRAIL SURFACE: Dirt and duff, asphalt

HIKING TIME: 1 hour

SEASON: Year-round, sunrise–sunset

ACCESS: $8 day-use fee

MAPS: USGS Pine Grove; local map in park brochure

WHEELCHAIR ACCESS: Some, near grinding rocks and other exhibits

FACILITIES: Restrooms, water, camping

DRIVING DISTANCE: 55 miles

SPECIAL COMMENTS: The Indian Grinding Rock has the most mortar holes of any grinding rock in North America.

GPS TRAILHEAD COORDINATES

Latitude   N38° 25.499´

Longitude   W120° 38.464´

IN BRIEF

The trails around the 135-acre Indian Grinding Rock State Historic Park pass exhibits, plants, reconstructions (including a Miwok village and a ceremonial round house), and the famous Indian Grinding Rock, Chaw'se. Having nearly 1,200 mortar cups on its bedrock limestone, it encompasses the largest number of bedrock mortars anywhere in North America. Still visible next to some of the mortars are 2,000-to-3,000-year-old petroglyphs.

DESCRIPTION

The two trails—the North Trail and the South Nature Trail—can be joined conveniently to create a loop that takes in all the park's sights. No route-finding is necessary, because all the trails are well marked and easily identified. This loop starts at the trailhead in front of the museum.

Head up the stone steps and walk along the trail as it trends northeast above the

----

Directions ⎯⎯⎯⎯⎯⎯⎯⎯⎯⟶

From the junction of US 50 East and the Capital City Freeway, drive 3 miles on US 50 East and take Exit 19/Howe Avenue toward Rancho Murieta. Drive southeast 18 miles on Jackson Road to Rancho Murieta, then about 13.5 miles to the CA 49 junction (the second right turn); drive 7 miles south to Sutter Creek and another 4 miles to Jackson. Turn left on CA 88 and drive 8 miles to Pine Grove. Turn left onto Pine Grove–Volcano Road toward Volcano. In about 1 mile, a sign on the left indicates the campground. The park entrance is 0.25 mile past this on the left. The trailhead, marked by a directional arrow, is at the end of the sidewalk that leads into the museum.

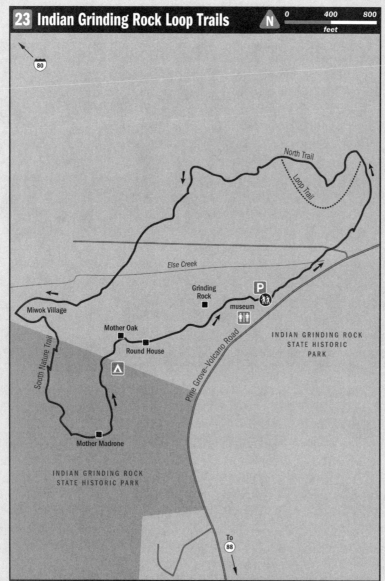

N

0   400   800
feet

80

North Trail

Loop Trail

Else Creek

Grinding
Rock

Miwok Village

museum

P

Mother Oak

Round House

INDIAN GRINDING ROCK
STATE HISTORIC
PARK

Mother Madrone

INDIAN GRINDING ROCK
STATE HISTORIC PARK

South Nature Trail

Pine Grove-Volcano Road

To
88

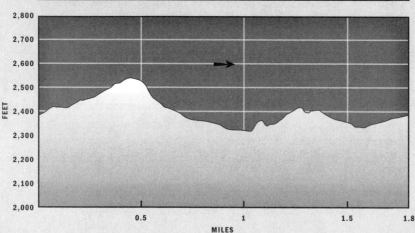

2,800
2,700
2,600
2,500
2,400
2,300
2,200
2,100
2,000

FEET

0.5   1   1.5   1.8

MILES

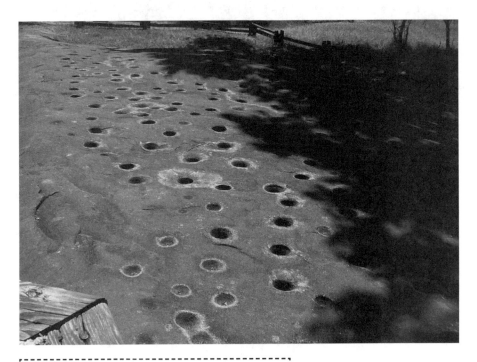

The Chaw'se (Grinding Rock) was used for three millennia.

parking area. Walking between the road and the entrance drive, you will pass under incense cedars, foothill pines, and live oaks. Some faint-purple brodiaeas add color to the trailside. A footbridge keeps your feet dry as you cross the head of Else Creek, named for one of the original farming families. Look ahead for the hole in the wooden fence, where you'll cross the road.

The farmhouse to your right was an original pioneer homestead. In the late 1880s, the land here was sold to Serafino Scapuccino, who protected the grinding-rock area and whose family sold the farm to the state in 1958 to be used as a park. The orchards here provided fruit for miners in Volcano and elsewhere. Continue your northward walk under some huge madrone and whiteleaf manzanita.

A junction offers hikers a choice between the lower Loop Trail or the upper North Trail. Both trails feature foothill-woodland and grassland ecosystems. Small clearings between manzanita display colorful irises and lupines; buttercups, monkeyflower, and brodiaea border the trail. Towering overhead are Douglas fir, ponderosa pine, incense cedar, and foothill pine, interspersed with live oak and black oak. But none of these specimens shines like the majestic valley oak—of which there are huge examples here.

Head slightly uphill on the North Trail, a packed-dirt path that winds in and out of the madrone and pine. The scent of needles baking in the sun fills the air. A grove of live oak provides some cool shade at midday, when the sun breaks through onto the trail just before the Loop Trail rejoins the North Trail.

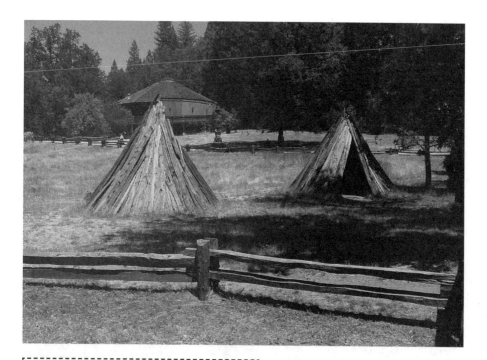

Miwok bark dwellings in front of Chaw'se Museum

Meander down some easy switchbacks through the manzanita on this rock-lined section of the trail. Fence lizards are the only critters scurrying about in the heat of the day, and they reveal their every step in the dry duff littering the forest floor. Cross a small runoff stream and head down some improvised steps.

Your trail takes a distinct left turn downhill toward the first valley oaks to come into view. Cross the gravel road, making a slight jog to your right, and continue walking, now through the tall grass bordering a much narrower trail. A sign displays the distance to junctions and park features.

Ahead of you on the right is a grove of valley oaks in which all of the trees are more than 300 years old. With the support of their enormous trunks, they spread majestically across the meadow, creating a shaded, parklike setting. A small footbridge helps hikers across Else Creek at the end of the meadow. Incense cedars and native grasses lead hikers up to the Miwok village reconstruction, at the junction with the South Nature Trail.

The Miwok settled a broad area between the Cosumnes River to the north and the Calaveras River to the south. Because acorns were a staple food crop, the Miwok were attracted to this area, which has groves of valley oaks and a broad, flat rock on which to grind the nuts into flour. One wonders if the trees were here before the rock was discovered, or if their proliferation was a result of the grinding rock's use.

After inspecting the round cedar-bark dwellings in the village, turn right onto the South Nature Trail and start looking for interpretive-marker posts—about 3 feet tall, brown, numbered, and hard to spot. The interpretive guide for sale in the museum will guide you along.

Towering incense cedar, Douglas fir, ponderosa pine, sugar pine, and valley oak shade your downhill trail as you cross a creek and enter a rather open area right up against fenced-in private property. Blackberry, iris, and columbine grow in this moist, cool area, along with ferns and kit-kit-dizze, which crowd the trailside. Iris and lupine surround a formerly majestic madrone as it begins another phase of its life cycle. Continue winding through the trees, soon passing a trailside bench on your way north.

The trail borders the campgrounds to their left and passes a grand incense cedar whose imposing split trunk reaches 8 feet in diameter. Trail markers will keep you on track when you're about to walk into the picnic tables. Jog slightly left and stay close to the fence around the campsites. Watch for signs directing hikers to the park's features. The grandest living feature of the park is the Mother Oak—a 600-year-old valley oak that spreads across the meadow. It is an awesome natural wonder and an imposing presence not found in most parks.

Valley oak also shades the entrance to the ceremonial Round House, which is one of the largest in California. Continue along the walk to the grinding rock itself. A bedrock formation of marbleized limestone with 1,185 individual grinding holes, the grinding rock is the largest such collection of mortars in North America. The rock's use has been dated to 2,000–3,000 years ago. Beside some of the mortars are petroglyphs—pictorial representations carved in the stone—which show everyday important objects such as nets, the sun, and man himself. A viewing platform allows for up-close views of the entire rock.

Return to the museum trailhead by walking past the bark houses and the metal sculpture of a Miwok Indian dancer.

NEARBY ACTIVITIES

Next to the trailhead, the Chaw'se Regional Indian Museum has excellent Miwok and natural-history exhibits and is especially oriented to children, with many hands-on displays. The Black Chasm Cavern, in the town of Volcano, is listed as a National Natural Landmark.

JENKINSON LAKE TRAIL 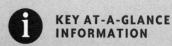 24

IN BRIEF

This easy loop is enjoyable any time of year. You hike through Douglas-fir and incense-cedar forest, where you can seek solitude and visit crystal-clear pools. Continuing along the north shore and past the campgrounds requires a determination to exercise and see new flora.

DESCRIPTION

Jenkinson Lake—formerly Hazel Canyon—was formed by damming the outlet of Hazel Creek and bringing water through a tunnel from a drainage to the south. A popular destination for picnics and family camping, the lake has campsites and picnic tables on its north side.

Your trail begins at the second dam, on the south side of the lake. Park in the wide dirt patch on the right. The official "tale of the tape": 8 miles around the lake, 3 miles to Park Creek, and 4 miles to Hazel Creek. Your mileage may vary. Mine did.

Southshore Trail is a multipurpose trail serving hikers, horse riders, and bike riders. With few exceptions, the horse trail is separate

- -

Directions ⟶

From Sacramento, take US 50 East 47.5 miles to Sly Park Road in Pollock Pines. Drive 4.5 miles south on Sly Park Road, passing the entrance to Sly Park Recreation Area, and turn left on Mormon Emigrant Trail, just 0.5 mile past the entrance station. Your trailhead is 1 mile from this turn. Cross Dam 1 and continue to the south end of Dam 2, where you can park on the right side, directly across from the trailhead. More parking is available at the north end of the dam; you can also park for a $5 fee at the Bumpy Meadows Trailhead. That parking area, with pit toilets, is 100 yards beyond your trailhead on the left.

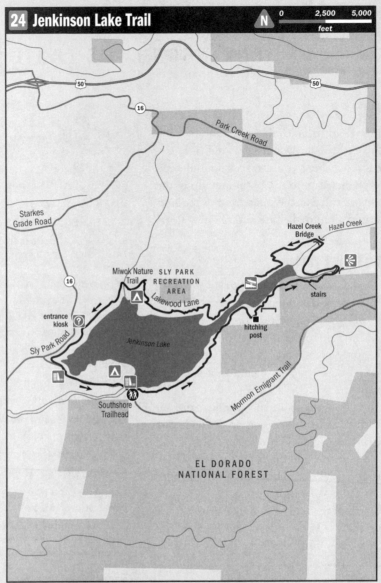

N

| 0 | 2,500 | 5,000 |

feet

50

16

Park Creek Road

Starkes
Grade Road

16

Hazel Creek
Bridge

Hazel Creek

Miwok Nature
Trail

SLY PARK
RECREATION
AREA

Lakewood Lane

stairs

entrance
kiosk

Sly Park Road

Jenkinson Lake

hitching
post

Southshore
Trailhead

Mormon Emigrant Trail

EL DORADO
NATIONAL FOREST

50

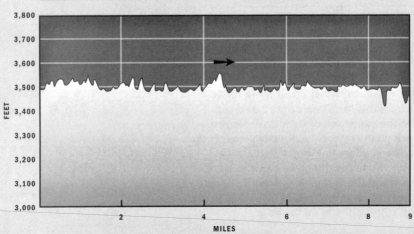

3,800								
3,700								
3,600								
3,500								
3,400								
3,300								
3,200								
3,100								
3,000								

FEET

2   4   6   8   9

MILES

from and above the hike-and-bike trail. A number of trails lead to reach favorite fishing spots at the lake's edge. These trails are usually easily distinguished from the hiking trail proper.

After passing a black 500-foot-long security fence and a lakeside bench or two, your trail heads somewhat downhill and turns left at the large incense cedar, where the horse trail heads uphill to the right.

The terrain on your right rises steeply, lifting the Douglas fir, ponderosa pine, and white fir—giants on level ground—even higher. Black oaks are randomly distributed, but more grow toward the lake, surrounded by buttercups.

Shortly after the lake narrows, you will encounter a split: take either track. Turning generally southeast into a secluded cove with a convenient bench, you can sit for a moment to contemplate. You may have company because this bench is the intersection of the horse trail, the hiking trail, and a biking trail. Notice the hitching post and the bike bridge over the puddle. Another nice bench, among trees marked with interpretive signs, overlooks the cove.

The generally flat terrain is interrupted by a brief uphill beneath towering firs. As you approach and then parallel the inlet creek, bikers get a sweet ride down an easy ramp, while hikers descend left down wet stairs. Back down to a broad, flat area, a jumble of driftwood floats against the willow-choked lakeshore. The trail widens here, where the hiker and equestrian trails diverge. A bridge appears just as you bear left toward the creek.

The Park Creek Bridge across Sly Park Creek marks the end of your third mile. Before crossing the bridge, you can explore ahead on the trail leading uphill to the outlet of the Bureau of Reclamation tunnel, which diverts water to the lake. Across the bridge and to the right is a path that leads upstream about 100 feet to a rocky bench on the creek, where a waterfall comes directly at you.

After taking a rest or a snack or just a moment to cool your heels in the creek's pool, walk past the kiosk, heading west to circumnavigate the peninsula formed by the ridge dividing the two creeks. It is about 0.75 mile to the next drainage, Hazel Creek. The dirt-and-pine-needle trail meanders along the shore under a changing canopy. The firs have diminished, and manzanita flourishes waterside along the open ground. Hikers bear left where horses are directed right.

Cross the road coming in from the right, and continue on the upper side of the road through a ponderosa-pine grove. This is a comfortable trail with nothing to break your stride—unless you enjoy kicking pinecones. Stay on the main trail, ignoring trails heading down the bank. Continue straight on the wide four-wheel-drive road as the horse trail joins from the right. At 4 miles, you'll cross the bridge over Hazel Creek leading to the group camping area and bear left, following the trail signs southwest past the pit toilets and observation point.

You are at the halfway point. If you don't mind the sudden increase in trail users, continue as described. The hiker is presented with a different aspect of the lake's ecosystem here. Also, the trail is much more urbanized from this point. Whether you head forward or back, it's the same distance. You choose.

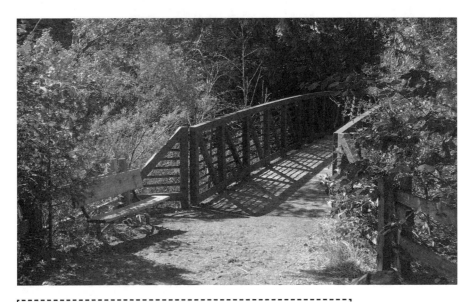

> The Park Creek Bridge has interesting features to visit upstream at both ends:
> a waterfall, a water tunnel, and a mellow pond.

The trail skirts the shore, along the picnic area, then continues on or near the road as it heads west 0.4 mile toward the Chimneys Campground. At Campsite 132, you will pick up the Sierra–Chimney Trail and follow it on dirt for a mile to the next small campground. Looking back from your lakeside trail, you can see the chimney ruins.

When you reach the boat ramp with boat rental, parking lot, and pit toilets, you'll have hit the 5-mile mark. When you next approach the shore, turn around to take in the vista to the east. In a brief 0.5 mile, you'll reach the other end of the Sierra–Chimney Trail. This trail continues through the campground and exits at Site 66 for another 0.25 mile of dirt track.

You again join the road as you reach the 6-mile mark, moseying along it for just 0.4 mile. As before, watch for trail signs on or alongside the road. Among the picnic areas, you'll see a sign indicating that the Miwok Nature Center is a scant 0.2 mile ahead. Once again on dirt, as you near the nature center you will encounter four picnic tables among the tall Douglas firs. Hidden from one another, these secluded tables are the best four seats in the house. Your vista takes in the marina and the dams as well as the hills and canyon beyond. Enjoy your solitude in this cool shade.

The Miwok Nature Center is near Pinecone Campground. A kiosk on the road displays information on the self-guided figure-eight trail. The nature trail has a tread of thick forest duff—spongy in places—in a surprisingly dense section of forest. A mellow creek makes for a contemplative moment among the tall trees. Thoughtfully, the interpretive signage is thorough and plentiful. Check out the Eagle Scout project at the entrance.

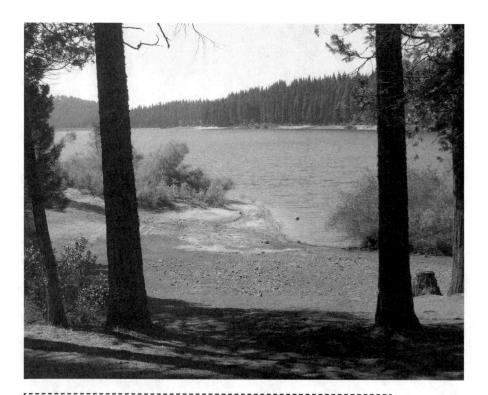

From pine-shaded picnic tables, hikers can enjoy a beautiful view and seclusion too.

After that pleasant diversion, follow your trail 0.3 mile to a signed junction with the Acorn Trail. You will remain on this trail through the upcoming picnic areas, so watch for its nutty logo. Follow the trail through the picnic grounds and down to the main marina and launch site.

Once you reach the boat launch, walk to the far-right corner of the parking lot and resume the trail just after the wheelchair-accessible picnic tables. Before reaching Dam 1, ascend the steps at the Walter Jenkinson Monument and continue on the road across the dam. Your trail is still on the lakeside, just after the chain-link fence. Step up off the road and turn right at the boulder in the trail. Now walk parallel to the road, crossing a driveway that leads to a group campground. At the next campground road, turn left and go 50 paces, then turn right to resume your trail through the woods.

Emerge from the woods at the north end of Dam 2. You should be able to see your car at the trailhead parking area.

NEARBY ACTIVITIES

You can hike the trails of Fleming Meadow, which lies on the downstream side of the dam. A map is available online at **tinyurl.com/fleming.pdf**.

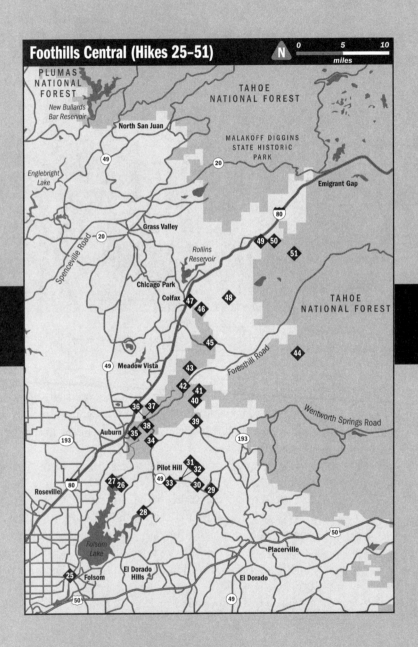

Foothills Central (Hikes 25–51)

N   0   5   10
miles

PLUMAS NATIONAL FOREST

New Bullards Bar Reservoir

North San Juan

TAHOE NATIONAL FOREST

MALAKOFF DIGGINS STATE HISTORIC PARK

49

20

Emigrant Gap

Englebright Lake

80

Grass Valley

49   50

Spenceville Road

20

Rollins Reservoir

51

Chicago Park

Colfax

48

TAHOE NATIONAL FOREST

47   46

45

44

Foresthill Road

49   Meadow Vista

43

42

41

40

Wentworth Springs Road

36   37

39

38

Auburn

35

193

34

193

Pilot Hill   31   32

49   33   30   29

27   26

Roseville

80

28

50

Folsom Lake

Placerville

25   Folsom

El Dorado Hills

El Dorado

50

49

FOOTHILLS CENTRAL

25 PIONEER EXPRESS TRAIL

KEY AT-A-GLANCE INFORMATION

LENGTH: 9.5 miles

CONFIGURATION: Out-and-back

DIFFICULTY: Moderate

WATER REQUIRED: 3 liters

SCENERY: Excellent views of Lake Natoma and Folsom bridges and Nimbus Dam; revegetated mining site

EXPOSURE: Some shade, some sun; sunscreen advisable

TRAIL TRAFFIC: Light on described route, active on the bike path

TRAIL SURFACE: Duff and dirt, rock and gravel

HIKING TIME: 3.5 hours

SEASON: Year-round, sunrise–sunset

ACCESS: $10 day-use fee; self-register with cash, credit, or debit card

MAPS: USGS Folsom

WHEELCHAIR ACCESS: Yes. This route roughly parallels an excellent 2-lane bike path that wheelchair users can avail themselves of.

FACILITIES: Toilets at the parking area, water at the trailhead kiosk, picnic tables near the beach

DRIVING DISTANCE: 21 miles

SPECIAL COMMENTS: This hike can be altered easily by hiking the bike trail rather than the Pioneer Express Trail. The bike path is far more exposed to the sun, however.

GPS TRAILHEAD COORDINATES

Latitude   N38° 40.737´

Longitude   W121° 11.416´

IN BRIEF

Once the site of intense gold mining and dredging, this former riparian area has been revegetated by the Teichert Corporation in cooperation with California State Parks, allowing native plants to be reestablished and creating an ideal environment for creatures from butterflies to egrets and mud turtles to deer. Your trail wanders across terrain that affords an up-close view of the geology—the ancient river gravels and sands—that beckoned miners of different eras, and ends with a bird's-eye view of Nimbus Dam.

DESCRIPTION

Pioneer Express Trail, which is part of the coast-to-coast American Discovery Trail, runs from Auburn to Sacramento and generally

----

Directions

From the junction of US 50 East and the Capital City Freeway, take US 50 East for 16 miles to the Hazel Avenue exit, then drive north on Hazel Avenue to Madison Avenue. Turn right and drive 3 miles on Madison, which will join with and become Greenback Lane just before the Negro Bar Recreation Area. Turn right at the sign and drive to the entry kiosk, where you may self-register before entering. Turn right a few hundred feet past the kiosk and take another right immediately to turn into the boat-launch parking lot; head toward the southwest corner of the parking lot. Drive on and pass the horse-assembly area on the right and continue on to a space in the beach parking lot. Look for an information kiosk at the top of the open field, which is usually occupied by Canada geese, and directly on the bike path. Standing with your back to the restroom doors, you can see the kiosk across the field. An overview map and water are available at the kiosk.

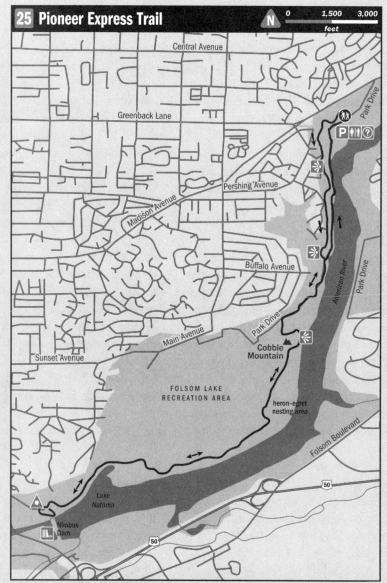

0   1,500   3,000
feet

Central Avenue

Greenback Lane

Pershing Avenue

Madison Avenue

Buffalo Avenue

Park Drive

Park Drive

Park Drive

American River

Main Avenue

Cobble
Mountain

Sunset Avenue

FOLSOM LAKE
RECREATION AREA

heron–egret
nesting area

Folsom Boulevard

50

Lake
Natoma

Nimbus
Dam

50

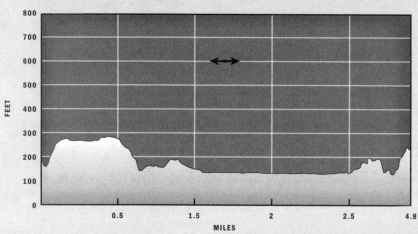

800

700

600

500

400

300

200

100

0

FEET

0.5   1.5   2   2.5   4.8

MILES

follows the American River. Twenty-one miles of this trail wind through Folsom Lake State Recreation Area (FLSRA). Your trail stretches from the horse-assembly area at the historic Negro Bar downstream to Nimbus Dam at Mississippi Bar.

When you finish reading the information on flora and fauna and fill your water bottles, turn around and look across the bike path for the sign pointing the way to Pioneer Express Trail. At the top of this brief trail stands the Pioneer Express Trail mileage sign. It is the 28.2-mile point, and your hike will take you 4.7 miles to the Nimbus Dam overlook.

If you'd like to take the cakewalk version of this hike, stay on the bike path all the way from the kiosk to the dam. Just as enjoyable a hike as the described route, it does have different vantage points but a bit less solitude and far less shade.

The Pioneer Express Trail heads southwest and almost immediately joins the bike path for 150 feet. This is a good spot to make your route decision. To avoid a passel of weeds, you could just turn left (southwest) at the trailhead kiosk and walk about 500 feet to this point along the bike path. Turn right uphill at the next opportunity to begin the climb to the cliff top—a bit more than a 100-foot ascent will gain you an excellent view of Lake Natoma. Look back over your shoulder to three of Folsom's bridges: Lake Natoma Bridge, Rainbow Bridge, and the historic truss bridge. And what a history the truss bridge has. Designed in 1893 for horse-and-wagon traffic, it was replaced by the Rainbow Bridge in 1917. In 1930 the truss bridge was bought and then sold by the State of California. This bridge gets around: it was moved to Siskiyou County, where it served as a Klamath River crossing until 1998. Then Folsom bought it, and the bridge was returned to the site of its original footings.

As you reach the 0.5-mile point, you should have excellent views of all three bridges. There is a protective chain-link fence on your left because the cliffs are sheer, but the views are impressive nonetheless. Walk along the fence line for another 0.5 mile and then begin to descend. There is an unobstructed viewpoint at the end of the fence. To reach it, stay on the higher trail rather than taking the gently descending trail, which curves around to the right. The two trails join at the base of the hill; on your way down, they will cross each other at a telephone pole. Continue straight ahead to a small pond, which is well worth a short pause to look for wildlife.

The pond sits at a junction of the trail to Snowberry Creek, where the Pioneer Express Trail crosses the bike path as you head toward the river. The trails in the FLSRA are well signed; that is, the signs are both accurate and frequent, so you shouldn't have any difficulty navigating this path. Depending on the time of year, you may have trouble staying on the path—you walk past some huge blackberries. Look for signs of raccoon, opossum, and skunk along here; they love these like some folks love a dessert bar.

Walk along to the left of the bike trail, which comes in and out of view for just about 0.5 mile. Your track continues southwest for 0.25 mile until it zigs right, then zags left, and so forth for another 0.25 mile. A slight course correction to the south, and a small pond on the left signals a sharp left turn coming up in about 500 feet as you cross a cobble pile. After that, you'll have another, much larger pond on the left as you walk in the shade of live oak and toyon. A large hill, composed entirely of river gravels, rises above you to the right. After you ascend this revegetated "hillside," turn to your right for a full view of Cobble Mountain (officially, The Volcano).

There is an excellent view of the lake from the prominent, bare area to the east. This spot marks the beginning of Mississippi Bar—an area of intense gold dredging until the late 1880s, and later the site of aggregate mining until the 1980s. Thanks to revegetation efforts, California poppy, larkspur, monkeyflower, and lupine are everywhere. Buckeye blossoms fill the air with their sweet scent all along the trail, and native trees like toyon, black oak, foothill pine, and valley oak dot the open areas and hillsides.

The bike path is again in sight as you parallel it briefly. Before you reach the path, turn directly left, away from it, 100 yards to the southeast. You will make a slight jog to the right again when you encounter the sign for the heron–egret nesting area. Continue generally southwest for almost 0.5 mile, at which point you'll cross the bike path, only to recross it 500 feet later. The trail will remain obvious, meandering through some ponds as it passes between a power-line pylon and an out-of-place palm tree.

Follow the trail as it crosses the bike path and stays on the north side of it. Pass the turnoff to Snowberry Creek. After just about 0.5 mile of flat walking to reach the dam, walk toward the apex of the curved asphalt, where you'll find the trail to the overlook. At the base of the overlook hill, you can see the ancient alluvial gravels and sandstones that signaled potential deposits of gold. The trail to the overlook is rocky, slick, and steep. It is also short. At the top of the trail, a walkway through the fence will give you access to the area overlooking the dam.

As an alternative, start your trip from this overlook trailhead and hike to Negro Bar. Or leave a car here and treat this as a one-way trip with a shuttle.

Retrace your route to the parking lot, but add an easy alternative. At the first pond on the route coming in, stay on the bike path rather than ascending. The exposed portions of the cliff face also illustrate the ancient river deposits and volcanic overlay.

NEARBY ACTIVITIES

The American River Bicycle Path lines both sides of Lake Natoma and will take you from Beal's Point to Sacramento. Complete with solar-powered call boxes, this is rated as one of the best bicycle paths in the country.

26 AVERY'S POND TRAIL

 KEY AT-A-GLANCE INFORMATION

LENGTH: 4.1 miles

CONFIGURATION: Out-and-back

DIFFICULTY: Easy

WATER REQUIRED: 2 liters

SCENERY: Foothill forest surrounding lake

EXPOSURE: Shaded, with patches of sun

TRAIL TRAFFIC: Moderate

TRAIL SURFACE: Dirt and duff

HIKING TIME: 2 hours

SEASON: Year-round, sunrise–sunset

ACCESS: $10 day-use fee

MAPS: USGS Pilot Hill

WHEELCHAIR ACCESS: None

FACILITIES: Gravel parking area; picnic tables and pit toilets at boat ramp

DRIVING DISTANCE: 21.3 miles

SPECIAL COMMENTS: The historic North Ditch parallels the trail. The Pioneer Express Trail crosses the main road and continues from Rattlesnake Bar to Horseshoe Bar, as described in Hike 25 (see previous profile). Bikes are not allowed on this trail.

GPS TRAILHEAD COORDINATES

Latitude   N38° 49.162´
Longitude   W121° 05.373´

IN BRIEF

The hike to Avery's Pond is a great adventure for children and parents who want a brief yet interesting hike. This route takes you past Avery's Pond and on past the Newcastle powerhouse at Mormon's Ravine. The trail guides hikers along remnants of the North Fork Ditch, which supplied water to mining camps and towns along the river.

DESCRIPTION

After gold was discovered in the South Fork of the American River in 1848, mining camps sprang up along both the South and North forks. The river was worked by men from every corner of the world: England, Scotland, Wales, New York, Virginia, Kentucky, New South Wales, Hawaii, and China. They stayed with their claims, camping right beside their river workplace. The camps turned to towns

----

Directions ⟶

From the intersection of I-80 and the Capital City Freeway, drive 15 miles on I-80 East to Loomis and take Exit 110/Horseshoe Bar Road. Turn left at the end of the ramp onto Horseshoe Bar Road; bear left and immediately take the next left turn to stay on Horseshoe Bar Road. Continue on Horseshoe Bar Road 3.4 miles to Auburn–Folsom Road. Turn left and drive 2.3 miles to Newcastle Road, where you'll turn right and go 1 mile to Rattlesnake Road. Turn right again and follow the road another mile until the pavement ends. Stop and self-register at the entry kiosk. Drive 0.2 mile to the sign for the horse-assembly area and boat launch. Turn left and drive 0.4 mile to the sign for the horse-assembly area, then turn left again, into the gravel parking lot. The signed trailhead is at the northeast end of the lot, beside two boulders.

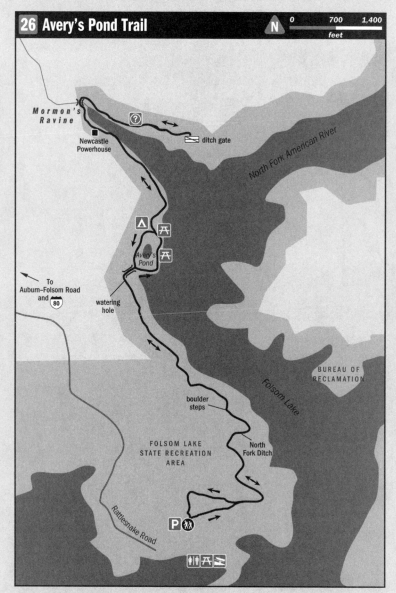

N

0   700   1,400
feet

Mormon's Ravine

?

◻ ditch gate

Newcastle Powerhouse

North Fork American River

⛺

⛏

⛏

Avery's Pond

To Auburn–Folsom Road and 80

watering hole

BUREAU OF RECLAMATION

Folsom Lake

boulder steps

North Fork Ditch

FOLSOM LAKE STATE RECREATION AREA

Rattlesnake Road

P 🚶

🚻 ⛏ 🛶

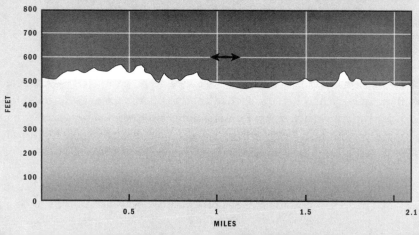

800
700
600
500
400
300
200
100
0

FEET

0.5   1   1.5   2.1

MILES

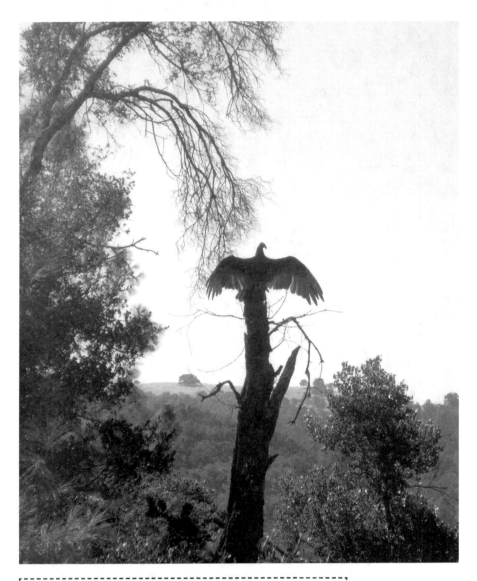

Turkey vultures begin their day with the sun, performing one long warm-up exercise before leaping into a warm-air current.

and, however small or large, these settlements were given names—colorful, descriptive names such as Rattlesnake Bar, Mormon Bar, Mormon's Ravine, Oregon Bar, and Manhattan Bar. Some establishments disappeared overnight, but others persisted. In 1865 Rattlesnake Bar was a town of more than 1,000 residents. Avery's Pond and some sights along the way are relics from the gold-mining days along the North Fork of the American River.

Leave the horse-assembly area at the signed trailhead at the northeast end of the parking lot. Your trail starts out as a dirt path that becomes a doubletrack in short order. When the wide track veers right, stay on the single path that leads left. The doubletrack will rejoin your path shortly. The meadow you are crossing is filled with wildflowers in the spring. A sign ahead proclaims that you are on the Pioneer Express Trail and indicates the distance to Avery's Pond and Auburn.

After you head generally east for about 10 minutes, the trail turns north to meander through live oak and toyon. Just as you near the 0.5-mile point, a sunny hillside offers a view of a nearly full Folsom Lake. Trees, with water climbing their trunks, were recently high and dry by several feet. This vista still shows some of the "bathtub rings" that will in future ages reveal the weather patterns that our area experiences. As you reach a sunny hillside, look to the opposite shore of the lake, where similar markings in the dirt bespeak the various lake levels over the years. With the lake in full view, you may be distracted by a turkey or two as they flash by, looking very intent on their way to somewhere. Above, foothill pines shade the trail while the manzanita blazes with bright-red berries, which are sticky—like its flowers—and are reported to be edible and sweet.

Walk along in the cool shade of black oak, live oak, and more manzanita until you come to an easy but steep downhill stretch. A large outcrop to your left leans out over the trail. Well protected by poison oak, these are not rocks that one would be enthusiastic about bouldering. The trail is crossed with smaller boulders that serve as stairs to help you clamber down the trail. Your path, now sand and pea gravel, contours along beside the lake about 50 feet above the shoreline. The trail runs right up next to a steep drop to the rocks below, just as you see the first signs of the North Fork Ditch. Along here you can see views of the lake as it disappears into the Foothills.

Cross a small drainage just before you come upon a large patch of blackberries at about the 1-mile point. The ditch is plainly visible for the next mile. Encrusted with blackberries, the ditch runs to your right. Below you is another section of the concrete wall that composed part of the ditch. Moisture-loving blackberries are the main ditch plant here, offering themselves to hikers at many points along the trail.

Under a nice cover of shade is a horse-watering trough fed by the spring just on the other side of the bridge at the pond. The wooden bridge crossing the aqueduct was restored in 1994 in an Eagle Scout project. Walk another 175 feet to cross another bridge, which signals your arrival at the pond. Turn right and head toward the lake. Look to the right of the trail and you will see Sierra iris growing among the live oak.

You will find a picnic table about halfway around the pond, next to a lonely live-oak tree surrounded by scant vegetation. This spot is totally exposed and might not be the best for a picnic, but the trails that lead to both the lake and the pond indicate that this might be a good fishing spot. Be careful: the bank surrounding the pond is steep, and the pond is unsuitable for swimming or wading.

For excellent shade while you picnic, there are tables farther along the pond trail just before the next junction on the left, and also just after it on the right. If you want to circumnavigate the pond, continue left at the next junction and make your way along the north shore of the pond. There is a bit more to see in the vicinity.

About 0.5 mile ahead is a small hydroelectric plant operated by PG&E. To get there, take the right-hand trail at the junction and you will walk roughly parallel to the road you see above you to the left. You will reach the road in a matter of seconds. Take notice of the mountain-lion warning posted on the tree. Follow the road down as it turns to gravel, and then follow it around the bend; you will see the small hydroelectric facility—the Newcastle power plant—ahead. Built in 1986, it produces electricity for up to 12,000 homes.

As you walk toward the power plant, you can see the point at which the North Fork enters the lake. The powerful stream creates a wide ravine here, dropping a jumble of rocks and debris in its wake. Look closely and you'll probably see deer feeding amid the willows and sedges growing in this tributary. The South Fork's entrance to the lake, near Salmon Falls, is 5.5 miles southeast of your current position; you can imagine the commerce that occurred between miners on both rivers. According to historical accounts, a bridge was built in 1862 at Rattlesnake Bar that served for almost 100 years, until a truck full of "fertilizer" sparked the bridge's collapse in 1954.

Pass the modern plant now and follow the trail across another bridge at Mormon's Ravine, just past the power plant. Turn right and continue through the wooded area above the river. Look below you on the right, and you can plainly see sections of the water ditch. Follow along the trail until, at the 2-mile point, you come to an information kiosk that highlights the hydro facility and provides some brief history regarding your trail.

The large, open field above you to the left fills with wildflowers each spring. Wally baskets, brodiaea, buttercups, and blue dicks sprinkle the hillside with color. Startle a deer from its afternoon slumber here and see who jumps higher. (Answer: the deer. Repeatedly.) This trail continues to Auburn, where it begins above the site of the proposed Auburn Dam. As you look right to the live oak about 10 feet off the trail, you may notice a concrete structure. A little investigation uncovers what appears to be a ditch gate, long since disused.

This is a convenient place to turn around. You've hiked 2 miles, and your small hiking companions are surely ready for refreshments back at the trailhead. Retrace your steps until you come to the pond, then take the right-hand fork at the junction. Walk through an environmental campsite with a few picnic tables. Just before you cross the bridge at the west end of the pond, look right to see more of the concrete sections of the ditch.

When you near the trailhead, you have a choice. Either retrace your steps exactly from the junction of the singletrack and the doubletrack, or take the fork to the right, startle some more turkeys in the woods, and then emerge at the kiosk adjacent to the trailhead.

RATTLESNAKE BAR—HORSESHOE BAR TRAIL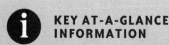

IN BRIEF

This trail leads hikers up, down, around, and through foothill woodlands nestled against a slim riparian zone along the fringe of Folsom Lake. The well-maintained trail lets walkers of all ages forget about the route and watch the flowers, birds, and butterflies. You can easily walk out to the lakeshore at two broad, unshaded bars.

DESCRIPTION

Hiking the Pioneer Express Trail affords you choices from among a number of embarkation points along the trail. This hike starts at Rattlesnake Bar, where Folsom Lake nears its upstream boundary and you can select your preferred endpoint: the near side or far side of Horseshoe Bar Road on the other side of this U-shaped route.

Directions ———————————————→

From the junction of I-80 East and the Capital City Freeway, drive 15 miles on I-80 East to Loomis and take Exit 110/Horseshoe Bar Road. Turn left at the end of the ramp onto Horseshoe Bar Road; bear left and immediately take the next left turn onto Horseshoe Bar Road. Continue on Horseshoe Bar Road 3.4 miles to Auburn—Folsom Road. Turn left and drive 2.3 miles to Newcastle Road, where you'll turn right and go 1 mile to Rattlesnake Road. Turn right again and follow the road another mile until the pavement ends. To the left is the boat-launch area; the right fork leads to your trailhead. Drive slowly over the chuckholed road, and keep right about 1,000 feet to reach a large dirt parking lot conveniently located in front of the trailhead. The trailhead sits behind some boulders about 10 feet inside the trees opposite the lake. A large sign indicates the mileage and directions on the Pioneer Express Trail.

KEY AT-A-GLANCE INFORMATION

LENGTH: 4.7 miles

CONFIGURATION: Out-and-back

DIFFICULTY: Easy

WATER REQUIRED: 1–2 liters

SCENERY: Great views of Folsom Lake

EXPOSURE: In and out of shade

TRAIL TRAFFIC: Light

TRAIL SURFACE: Sand and dirt

HIKING TIME: 2 hours

SEASON: Year-round, sunrise–sunset

ACCESS: $10 day-use fee

MAPS: USGS Pilot Hill

WHEELCHAIR ACCESS: None

FACILITIES: None at trailhead; toilet at boat ramp

DRIVING DISTANCE: 25 miles

SPECIAL COMMENTS: No water at trailhead or on trail. Bring plenty of your own.

GPS TRAILHEAD COORDINATES

Latitude   N38° 49.337´

Longitude   W121° 05.893´

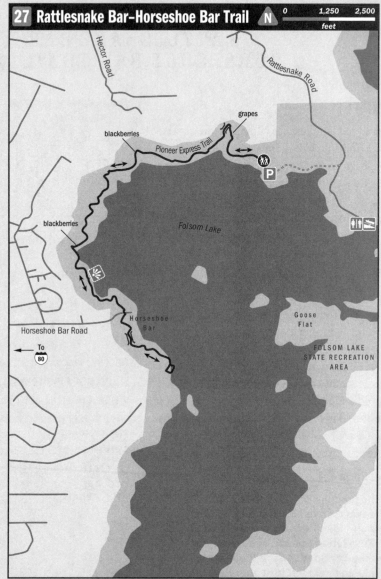

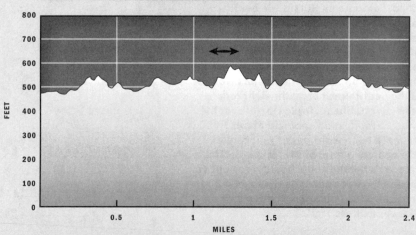

Rattlesnake Bar, covered with hundreds of houses, cabins, and tents in the 1850s, was one of several bars connected by trails from the river to the Auburn-to-Sacramento Road. Granite Bar, Whiskey Bar, Horseshoe Bar, and Rattlesnake Bar were all served by this supply route. One formerly successful miner of the Rattlesnake Bar area became infamous as "Rattlesnake Dick" after he robbed several stagecoaches along this pioneer road.

The trailhead is situated behind the boulders at the north end of the parking lot. Watch your step here: this trail is shared only with horseback riders. Start at the sign indicating your mile point on Pioneer Express Trail, heading west under towering foothill pines, which offer the most wicked hazard: they hurl 3-pound spiked, armor-plated cones from heights of 60 feet right onto the trail below. You may be saved by a well-placed manzanita, but keep your eyes open on windy days regardless.

The trail is well marked, as it is along its whole length, with signs at every junction, and it has been well maintained, mostly through consistent use. The trail has a comfortable surface of dirt and duff, which blend into sand or hard-packed dirt at times. An immediate opening to your left is a popular gathering ground for flocks of Canada geese.

Head north into and out of a ravine by crossing a footbridge, where live-oak boughs hang over a stream. When you begin to hear the stream on your left, you'll notice grapevines stretching along the trail and hanging from the live-oak and cottonwood trees. The grapes start to give way to blackberries around the bridge.

A grassy area below the trail comes into view as you encounter the 45-mile marker, where a trail from the right joins your route just as you descend a bit. A generous expanse of lake appears as you walk under the power line and enter a broad, sloping meadow.

Enter the woods again where bush monkeyflower grows beneath the foothill pines. A private-property fence borders the trail on the right for a short distance; several side trails head down to favorite fishing spots on the lake. A footbridge across a stream is a "blackberry magnet," and the next stream crossing is no exception. *Mmm-mmm-good.*

The trail is a bit ditchlike after the power tower, and then it turns to rock and dirt, making for unsteady footing. Another small stream awaits at the 44.5-mile marker. Just after this 1-mile point and a hill climb, you're rewarded with a nice vista. Toyon and oak still shade your trail. At the crux of the next ravine, your appetite for blackberries is sure to be sated by the fruit on these thick bushes, which are all within easy reach of the trail.

The trail moves closer to the lake, giving you another panoramic vista, with small islands in the view. Descend the short stretch of boulder-strewn path and head through a sandy S-curve before making a slightly longer ascent to the hilltop, where a trail joins yours from the right. Continue downhill and to the right, then uphill on a doubletrack section of rocky trail to reach a sign marking Horseshoe Bar. To your right are the boulders, blocking street access from the end of

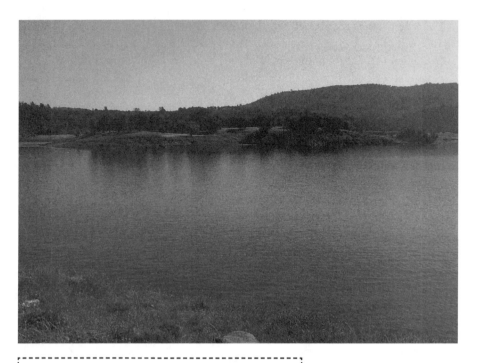

Folsom Lake below Rattlesnake Bar during a low-water period

Horseshoe Bar Road. To the left is a singletrack that loops nearer to the shore and then rejoins this main trail within minutes.

Continue to descend southeast and cross another footbridge near the wind-snapped ponderosa pine. Back on a singletrack for another 500 yards, you have a choice of side trails heading left to access the small beaches and expansive vistas.

Now that you've walked a pleasant 2-plus miles, you can linger at the water's edge or explore for more blackberries—jam on a stick—on the hillside above. The Pioneer Express Trail continues 6 more miles to Granite Bay, and beyond that it travels 37 miles to Discovery Park in Sacramento. Your route back retraces your path.

NEARBY ACTIVITIES

Avery's Pond Trail (see previous profile), in the horse-assembly area, leads to the north past the pond, all the way to Mormon's Ravine.

SWEETWATER TRAIL

IN BRIEF

This is a hike that you can cruise along on and get a good workout—never really climbing but always on an angle. Following the cool side of Folsom Lake's southern finger, the Sweetwater Trail begins just below the point where the South Fork of the American River meets the waters of the lake and curves around the low hills to the inlet of Sweetwater Creek (at Salmon Falls Road), slightly southwest of your trailhead. In 2007, the inlet filled by Sweetwater Creek was dry and rock-strewn. Now it's a pleasant haven for fish, frogs, and mosquitoes.

DESCRIPTION

Your hike starts out under the cover of shade on this multipurpose dirt trail. Little route-finding is necessary, since the south-trending trail is pretty distinct all the way to Sweetwater Creek. You will ascend and descend into and out of a few small ravines on the way south.

Foothill pine and live oak afford sparse cover. Stands of manzanita line the trail in places but barely cast any shadows. Before you cross the small runoff creek, stop to count the

KEY AT-A-GLANCE INFORMATION

LENGTH: 5.4 miles

CONFIGURATION: Out-and-back

DIFFICULTY: Moderate

WATER REQUIRED: 1–2 liters

SCENERY: Foothill woodland surrounding picturesque Folsom Lake

EXPOSURE: In and out of sun and shade

TRAIL TRAFFIC: Light

TRAIL SURFACE: Duff and dirt, gravel and sand

HIKING TIME: 3 hours

SEASON: Year-round, sunrise–sunset

ACCESS: $10 day-use fee

MAPS: USGS Pilot Hill

WHEELCHAIR ACCESS: None

FACILITIES: Pit toilet, trash, and pay phone in large parking area

DRIVING DISTANCE: 34 miles

SPECIAL COMMENTS: Early-morning hikes around the lake offer chances for bird- and wildlife-viewing.

Directions ⟶

From the junction of US 50 East and the Capital City Freeway, drive 24 miles on US 50 East to the El Dorado Hills Boulevard exit. Head north 4 miles, cross Green Valley Road, and then bear right onto Salmon Falls Road. Continue north 5.5 miles on Salmon Falls Road. Watch for the sign on the left, which reads SALMON FALLS–FOLSOM LAKE SRA, just before the Salmon Falls Bridge. Two parking areas for Skunk Hollow straddle the road just past the bridge. The signed trailhead for the Sweetwater Trail is at the south end of the Salmon Falls parking lot, next to the pit toilet.

GPS TRAILHEAD COORDINATES

Latitude   N38° 46.275´
Longitude W121° 02.593´

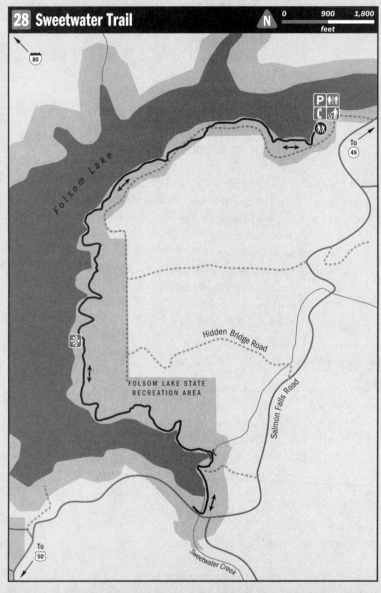

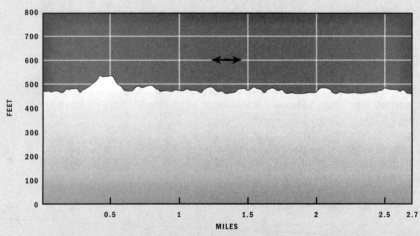

frogs pinging around the streamside. Blackberries are everywhere . . . except where there's poison oak. And that can be seen easily in the summer, because the poison oak is a beautiful red when everything else is still green or brown. Watch where you wander.

Within 0.25 mile you can turn for a look at the trailhead parking lot and view the secluded upper reaches of the lake. The trail becomes somewhat rocky but not too scuddy. Stone steps help you down the very distinct trail. You walk in shade for the next mile, as you slightly ascend one hillside, descend into a ravine, and then round another small ridge before heading straight south.

Depending on the temperature, you may feel fortunate to be on this side of the lake because the opposite shore appears to be continuously baking in the sun. Manzanita rises to the occasion, keeping you shaded when the trees thin out. The trail now feels more open and less rocky as you approach the 1-mile point.

After you've hiked for about an hour, you'll see more chaparral lining the trail. Step across a small stream onto a broad hillside dotted with widely spaced live oaks. Cross a grassy slope as soft breezes waft across the lake to cool you. A vista point lies just ahead as you reach 1.75 miles.

Your trail is now packed dirt. You will see a rocky jumble before a signed junction with a trail that enters from the left. Continue a bit to the right, across the rocky trail. You are following the shoreline, regardless of the water level. A blackberry magnet—any footbridge over a wet spot—is up ahead a bit.

Follow the tread into the trees as you generally trend in a southerly arc. Ignore the well-developed side trail coming in from Salmon Falls Road to the east. Another 100 paces will bring you to a three-way junction. The right fork will take you closer to the shore, and the left fork heads through the trees to the same destination: a faint trail to the right, just before you reach the gate at Salmon Falls Road.

Turn right on this overgrown track, immediately look to the left, and say, "Aww!" as you pass the grave of Cody, someone's family pet.

Ahead is a tangle of flowers, cobwebs, blackberries, and mosquitoes, which means you've arrived at Sweetwater Creek. Watch for fish in the shallows as the stream enters the lake. When you tire of swatting, it's time for a leisurely retreat to your car at Salmon Falls.

(Note: *In 2007, when I first hiked and described this trail, the lake level was distinctly lower than in 2011, when I hiked it for the second edition of this book. I've revised this pleasant track to be shorter by 0.7 mile. Assuming that the lake's level will again fall, exposing the inlet and the trail on the opposite shore, you can continue to follow these directions for a trek that's a bit longer. With water in the picture, however, these directions don't appear to make sense, so refer to the previous paragraph's last sentence for your trip's end.*)

Continue another 200 feet to a shady valley oak and a three-way junction, which on our hike was obstructed by a fallen foothill pine. Angle left and then look a bit right for another trail marker in the middle of the cobble mound. Head

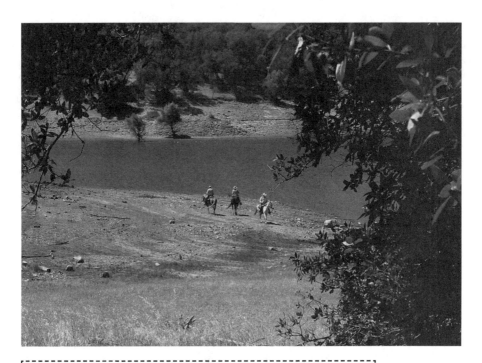

In very dry years, equestrians can take full advantage of the increased terrain and hikers can explore old trails.

toward it and stay on that line, heading west-southwest, as you cross the creek. If you bear just north of west, you may miss the trail.

The trail continues about 75 feet past the tree line. To get to it, look for a telephone pole up on Salmon Falls Road. Straight below that, at the tree line, is the trail opening, which is bordered by a foothill pine with two trunks—one skinny, one fat—on the left and a dead tree on the right. Follow this trail as it ascends toward the road. In about 100 feet, take a faint path that leads to the right through the chaparral.

Walk around the hill, briefly following a north-northwest track. Trails from the ranches above may join yours. Stay about the same distance above the lake as you work your way into and out of the next small ravine. The trail becomes less distinct, more like an informal use-trail, when it turns west to its terminus.

A parking lot with a pit toilet is a convenient turnaround point. The trail sign nestled among the valley oaks points out mileages for destinations to the west: Folsom Point, 15.5 miles; Folsom Dam, 17.5 miles; Brown's Ravine Trail, 17.5 miles. This is a great spot to take a splash before returning to the car at Salmon Falls.

NEARBY ACTIVITIES

The Darrington Bicycle Trail begins at the parking lot on the left as you cross the bridge at Skunk Hollow. Kayaks can be rented at the Skunk Hollow parking area.

MONROE RIDGE TRAIL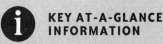

IN BRIEF

This pleasant, rolling trail gives hikers a beautiful overview of an area so important to the history of California. The cool, smooth, red skin and waxy leaves of the manzanita color your shaded path to the James Marshall Monument. On your return, you descend the Monument Trail back to the museum.

DESCRIPTION

Stepping onto a path that winds through forested hills, you also step back to the summer of 1847. Looking down from these formerly ponderosa-pine-covered hills, James W. Marshall surveyed the canyon below, gazing at a Miwok Indian encampment called *Culluma*, where he found the ideal location for a lumber mill.

By January 1848, having begun construction of a lumber mill the previous fall, James

----

Directions ⟶

From the junction of US 50 East and the Capital City Freeway, take US 50 East 41.2 miles to Placerville and turn left (north) onto Spring Street at the second traffic signal.

Follow Spring Street 0.1 mile and bear left (north) onto CA 49, Coloma Road. Enjoy this winding road for 7.7 miles to Coloma. Watch for fence posts topped with discarded boots and stray sneakers around 4.6 miles, and then for nectarine and pear orchards along the next mile.

You've reached Coloma when you turn right onto Main Street and take a gentle left curve at the old schoolhouse. Another 0.4 mile brings you to the park's visitor center and museum on the left (north), where you can park and/or pay the $5 fee. Trailhead parking is available another 0.4 mile along, on the south side of the highway. The trailhead is directly across the road from the parking lot.

KEY AT-A-GLANCE INFORMATION

LENGTH: 2.9 miles

CONFIGURATION: Loop

DIFFICULTY: Moderate

WATER REQUIRED: 1–2 liters

SCENERY: Foothill woodland with lush manzanita; panoramic view of historic gold-mining town

EXPOSURE: Wide trails with forest cover

TRAIL TRAFFIC: Light

TRAIL SURFACE: Forest duff; sandy in spots, mostly smooth and wide

HIKING TIME: 1.5–2 hours at a leisurely pace

SEASON: Year-round; hours vary, so check ahead (530-622-3470; parks .ca.gov/?page_id=484).

ACCESS: $8 parking fee

MAPS: USGS Coloma; Marshall Gold Discovery State Historic Park brochure and map available on-site

WHEELCHAIR ACCESS: None

FACILITIES: Generous parking, toilet, and picnic facilities throughout this small park

DRIVING DISTANCE: 49.5 miles

SPECIAL COMMENTS: Dogs are prohibited on California State Park trails.

GPS TRAILHEAD COORDINATES

Latitude   N38° 48.237´

Longitude   W120° 53.698´

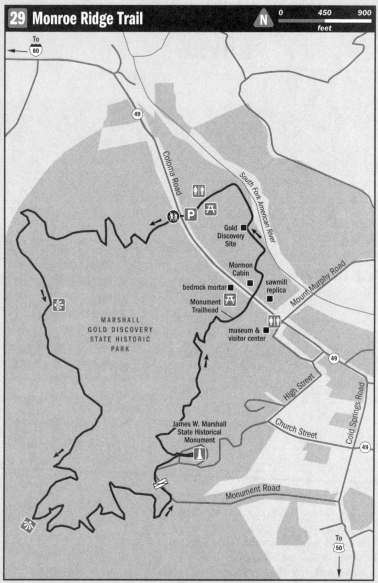

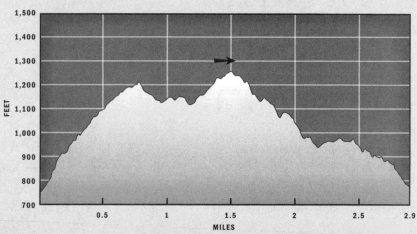

Marshall worked daily, troubleshooting the breaking-in of the mill. On the morning of the 24th, while inspecting a reworked tailrace, he spotted a few gold nuggets. He announced his find to his workers on-site and tucked the nuggets into the brim of his hat for the ride back to Sutter's Fort.

The trailhead for this historical hike is directly across from the southern end of the North Beach parking lot. A convenient break in the fence provides easy access from the parking area. Watch for traffic: it doesn't slow in this area.

Walk across the road to the sign marked MONROE RIDGE TRAIL; MARSHALL MONUMENT 2.3 MILES. The path passes through the original orchard site of the Gooch-Monroe family, freed slaves who settled here in 1849. You can learn more about this fascinating family in the museum.

At about the 150-foot point, a trail sign clearly directs you up to the right, leading you away from the doubletrack on the left. The hike's 600-foot elevation gain starts immediately, with a series of short switchbacks up a forested hillside. Well-placed stairs on this well-maintained trail facilitate your ascent. As you progress, the manzanita thickens all around you, but a brief view opens to give a peek to the north at Perry Mountain and Mount Murphy to the east above the American River.

About 0.75 mile from the trailhead, enter a cheerful clearing with a view overlooking the Coloma town site—from mill site to schoolhouse. This may be one of the views that James Marshall took in as he surveyed his mill site. His view may have been obscured, though, by towering ponderosa pines, which no longer grow here. Enjoy the view while you have a snack or lunch at the convenient picnic table.

Leaving the manzanita break, hike slightly downhill along the ridge while taking in the view. Dense jade-green manzanita and mixed-pine forest cover the rolling foothills to your south and west. This shady trail remains pleasant and cool throughout the afternoon. Within a few hundred feet, the fire road you encountered at the beginning of the hike again links up to the Monroe Ridge Trail, intersecting it from the left. Continue on your trail to the right, and you'll soon be rewarded with another excellent vantage point from which you can view the small town of Lotus. Again, a convenient picnic table offers a fine place to relax.

Continuing along the duff and dirt, within 200 feet or so there will be a trail marker with an arrow pointing toward your most significant waypoint: the Marshall Monument. At the 2-mile point, the trail takes a left at a long-abandoned and overgrown miner's cabin. Pass the gate at the end of the dirt trail, at the Monument Picnic Area parking lot. Continue across the parking lot and follow the signs on the paved path to the James Marshall Monument.

Now 2.3 miles into the hike, you arrive at the site where, in 1885, Andrew Monroe dug James Marshall's grave. Erected in 1890, this is California's first state historic monument. For a nice side trip, walk a few hundred feet farther up the paved path to the Marshall's Cabin Exhibit. Follow the signs there and back to the statue. Next, link up with Monument Trail to descend to the park's visitor center and museum.

While looking up at Marshall's face, turn right and, retracing your steps along the paved path, look for the arbor-covered drinking-water fountains near the park-employee residence. Just to your right, along the path, is the signed trailhead for the Monument Trail. This gentle leg ends in 0.6 mile, leaving you adjacent to the park's visitor center.

Watch for quail and deer in this area; both are plentiful. Signs will also warn hikers of rattlesnakes, poison oak, and mountain lions. The trails are plenty wide enough to accommodate walking side-by-side with young children.

A split-rail fence borders the entire trail down to the park's visitor center. Not only does it add charm but it probably provides some measure of safety for the many groups of schoolchildren who visit the park on weekdays. I was safely eyeballed by a six-point buck and two does as I walked past.

The trail crosses one of the many extant mining ditches along the way. Thousands of miles of ditches and flumes were dug to carry water to the placer-mining operations and were later used to irrigate orchards and farms. Entire companies were formed solely to dig such ditches—another way to extract gold from the miners. Essentially, more people became wealthy providing services to the miners than became wealthy from mining gold.

As you continue down the sandy, leaf-littered trail, the forest again yields to the town site and the trail ends, overlooking a picnic area where miners once camped. One hundred feet to the southeast is the park's visitor center.

To return to the North Beach parking lot near the Monroe Ridge trailhead, walk northwest along the Gold Discovery Loop Trail. Pass the bedrock mortar site and the Nisenan and Miwok dwelling displays, then continue 300 feet to cross the road. On your way to your car, you'll pass the Sutter Mill monument and the original mill site.

NEARBY ACTIVITIES

The park offers a short, somewhat accessible trail called the Gold Discovery Loop Trail, which you take to return to the trailhead. The sand-and-gravel path winds around several very interesting displays on the museum grounds, including an authentic miner's cabin and a Chinese store. California's first millionaire, Sam Brannan, owned a store less than 100 feet from here. Across the road and alongside the river is the most impressive display—a precise replica of Sutter's Sawmill. There are living-history interpretive displays throughout the town. If you're planning to stay awhile, the Coloma Resort offers a mile of riverfront camping and river activities.

DAVE MOORE NATURE AREA TRAIL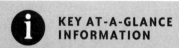

IN BRIEF

The loop trail at the Dave Moore Nature Area is a surprisingly all-inclusive treat. Historic mining remnants, riverside ecosystem and vistas, waterfowl and songbirds, foothill forest, displays of flowers in sun and shade—all are available to hikers of every age and ability, and all are packed into a 1-mile trail just off CA 49. The nature area was dedicated to David Moore, a former BLM conservation ranger, for his work on behalf of persons with disabilities (he was diagnosed with multiple sclerosis at age 35). Begin at either end of the parking lot, and enjoy this gentle trail to the river and back as it serpentines among the mining remains and stunning arbors. Picnic tables are well located for a quiet repast.

DESCRIPTION

When you have so much to see in such a small area, it's hard to know where to start. There are two possible trailheads; I took off on the one nearest the road at the east end of the lot.

Take your first step on this dirt track, and the pretty blue oaks immediately envelop you. Cross a footbridge within the first ten paces and pass a picnic table within the next ten, all

KEY AT-A-GLANCE INFORMATION

LENGTH: 1.1 miles

CONFIGURATION: Loop

DIFFICULTY: Cakewalk

WATER REQUIRED: 0.5 liter

SCENERY: Foothill-woodland and riparian zone along the South Fork of the American River. Evidence of old mining operations dots the area.

EXPOSURE: Shaded trail

TRAIL TRAFFIC: Light

TRAIL SURFACE: Dirt

HIKING TIME: 1 hour (including lingering)

SEASON: Year-round, 8 a.m.–sunset

ACCESS: No fees or permits; donations welcome

MAPS: USGS Coloma

WHEELCHAIR ACCESS: Yes

FACILITIES: Large dirt parking lot; pit toilet at west end of lot

DRIVING DISTANCE: 44 miles

SPECIAL COMMENTS: Watch for a hamburger-like boulder alongside the trail. Weak sandstone is sandwiched between harder rock in this boulder—likely a glacial erratic, possibly plucked from above the Yuba River and dropped in the American River drainage in relatively recent times.

Directions ⟶

From the junction of US 50 East and the Capital City Freeway, drive 31.1 miles on US 50 East and take Exit 37/Ponderosa Road. Then drive over the freeway bridge to the stop sign, turn right on North Shingle Road, and proceed 4 miles. Turn left at the Y onto Lotus Road and continue north 6.8 miles. Turn left at CA 49 and cross the bridge at the river. Continue about 1 mile along CA 49. The Dave Moore Nature Area entrance is on the left, at the cobblestone wall. The trailhead for this hike is at the east end of the parking lot.

GPS TRAILHEAD COORDINATES

Latitude   N38° 48.858´

Longitude   W120° 55.284´

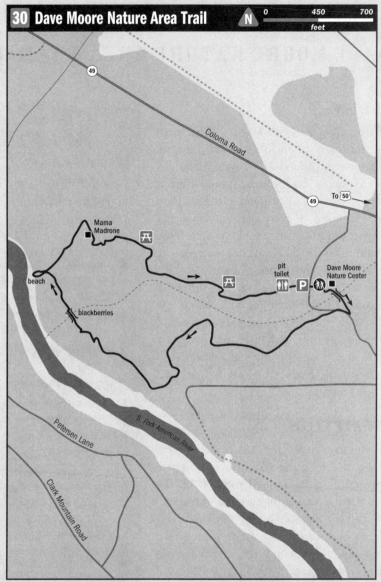

N

| 0 | 450 | 700 |

feet

Coloma Road

49

To 50

Mama Madrone

beach

blackberries

pit toilet

P

Dave Moore Nature Center

Petersen Lane

S. Fork American River

Clark Mountain Road

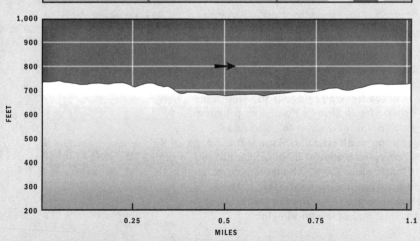

1,000		
900		
800		
700		
600		
FEET 500		
400		
300		
200		

| 0.25 | 0.5 | 0.75 | 1.1 |

MILES

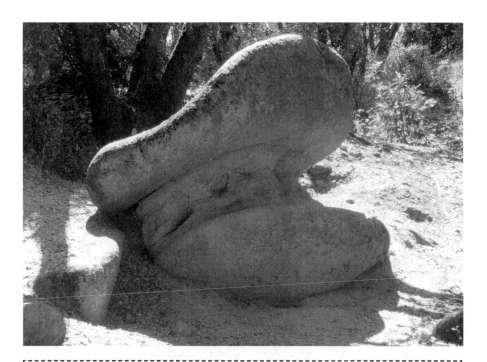

This boulder—weak sedimentary rock sandwiched between stronger igneous rock—was likely plucked from above Pyramid Creek in the Desolation Wilderness and deposited as an erratic during the last glaciation, and now temporarily rests as a big chunk of river gravel.

under cooling shade. The path turns sharply right just 75 yards ahead, whereupon you'll begin to see narrow game-trails zigzagging in and out of the manzanita. Birdsong emanates from the live oaks and foothill pines.

This pleasant track meanders past blue oak, crusted with oakmoss lichen and surrounded by patches of colorful poison oak (a reminder to stay on the trail). With no uphills, no navigating, no tricky junctions—just walking, looking, and listening—this trail becomes an almost instant pleasure. You may notice the distinctive line of a former water ditch just before you start seeing mounds and walls of river cobble.

Cross a creek and briefly navigate some of that cobble. The thick moss clinging to the stones on either side of the track looks to have been undisturbed for more than a century and a half. As the trail approaches the river, it winds through towering manzanita and 3-foot ponderosa pine, as well as toyon and incense cedar (the latter covered with twining brodiaea).

When the trail begins to parallel the river, it guides you through thick incense cedar as it heads northwest. After just a 0.5-mile walk, you'll come upon a footbridge crowded by streamside blackberries—all for hungry hikers. Yum! Eat up here or stop at the other blackberry magnet up ahead. The stream that feeds these berry bushes bisects the loop trail—entering where you crossed the first footbridge at the outset. You'll see this stream again after the next picnic table.

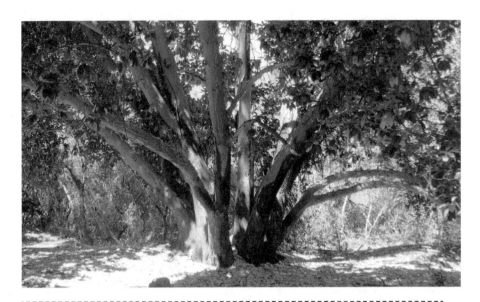

The Pacific madrone, also known as the refrigerator tree, spreads its cooling limbs across the trail.

At the next set of footbridges over a creek, head left to reach a placid beach on the river, or right if you want to continue walking. Left is a good choice: the beach here collects some driftwood, and you can safely sit as the water churns a hundred feet from you. The bedrock beyond it may hint at the cause for mineral hunting here a century and a half ago.

The rock-lined trail heads roughly northeast as it leaves the river, throwing in a zigzag to break up the easy hiking on this flat terrain, followed by a sharp right-hand turn. Cross another footbridge at a group of three ponderosa pines, and the path, bordered by rock walls, winds around to a magnificent tree—the "Mama Madrone"—whose branches span 75–100 feet across the forest.

Continue ambling eastward, passing a picnic table moments before you reach another blackberry magnet. Pretty yellow and scarlet madia dot the trailside as your route passes through some grasses, manzanita, and chamise. At the next footbridge, turn sharply to the right and pass a handicap-accessible picnic table as the rock-lined path persists.

Cross one last footbridge over the creek before reaching the end of the trail. The pit toilet to the right marks your return to the right spot.

NEARBY ACTIVITIES

Marshall Gold Discovery State Park is a mere 2 miles south on CA 49. There you can hike the Monroe Ridge Trail, Hike 29 (page 157). Or you can stick to the more historic parts of the park on the Gold Discovery Loop. Either way, this historic park should be seen and experienced.

SOUTH FORK AMERICAN RIVER– GERLE LOOP TRAIL

IN BRIEF

There is something magnificent about blue oaks standing on a hillside, glowing in the early-morning sun. Seeing the same sunlight glowing golden on a pristine river also offers some magic. Magnolia Ranch is one of those wonderful places where the trees, river, and hills also accompany some great hiking trails.

DESCRIPTION

The Magnolia Ranch trails are on land, like Cronan Ranch (Hike 33, page 174), that has been purchased by the American River Conservancy, the Bureau of Land Management, and other partners in order to preserve them for recreation and wildlife conservation.

This trail is so enjoyable that I had to do it twice, with a twist. I'll offer you both options here as well, although I'm pretty sure that most hikers would test both routes eventually on their own.

From the information kiosk, begin walking east at the base of this broad, squat mound to the south. You are heading directly toward the South Fork of the American River as it

KEY AT-A-GLANCE INFORMATION

LENGTH: 2.6 miles

CONFIGURATION: Loop

DIFFICULTY: Easy

WATER REQUIRED: 1–2 liters

SCENERY: Foothill woodland and riparian habitat with wildflowers on every hillside

EXPOSURE: Equally shaded and sunny

TRAIL TRAFFIC: Moderate; the trail is shared by runners, hikers, bikers, and equestrians.

TRAIL SURFACE: Dirt, duff, and river cobble

HIKING TIME: 1–2 hours

ACCESS: No fees or permits

SEASON: Year-round, sunrise–sunset

MAPS: USGS Coloma

WHEELCHAIR ACCESS: None

FACILITIES: Pit toilets in parking lot

DRIVING DISTANCE: 38 miles

SPECIAL COMMENTS: Ever hear the joke about the two-story outhouse?

Directions ⟶

From the junction of I-80 East and the Capital City Freeway, drive 25 miles on I-80 East toward Auburn and take Exit 119C/Elm Avenue. Turn left at the traffic light, onto Elm Avenue. At the bottom of the hill, turn left again, onto High Street. Drive under the railroad overpass before heading 2.3 miles downhill on CA 193 East/CA 49 South to the confluence and turning right. Follow CA 193 East/CA 49 South 10.7 miles through Cool and Pilot Hill to the Magnolia Ranch trailhead. Park on the west side of the lot. The trailhead is past the south end of the lot, at the information kiosk.

GPS TRAILHEAD COORDINATES

Latitude   N38° 49.539´

Longitude   W120° 57.321´

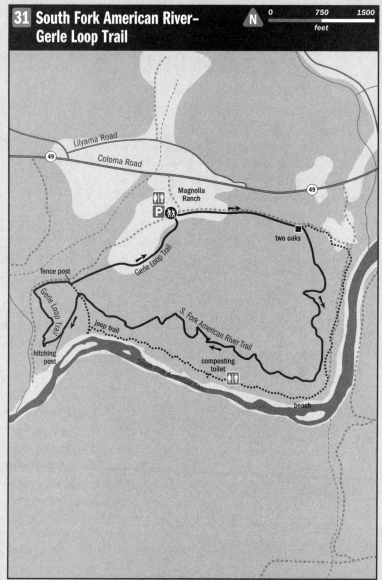

31 South Fork American River–
Gerle Loop Trail

N

0   750   1500
feet

Lilyama Road

49

Coloma Road

49

Magnolia
Ranch

P

two oaks

Gerle Loop Trail

fence post

Gerle Loop Trail

jeep trail

S. Fork American River Trail

hitching
post

South Fork American River

composting
toilet

beach

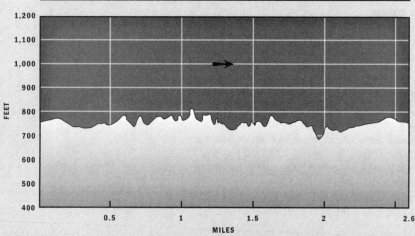

1,200

1,100

1,000

900

800

700

600

500

400

FEET

0.5   1   1.5   2   2.6

MILES

flows south. If you get here around sunrise, the eastward walk is quite warming. Your first junction is just about 0.35 mile from the kiosk. You can't go wrong here either: if you follow (or can even see) the trail sign in the star thistle, marked SOUTH FORK AMERICAN RIVER TRAIL–GERLE LOOP TRAIL, then you'll be following the hike as described. If you want to go to the river on your first loop, then you'll have to read ahead.

Pull yourself away from the shade of the glorious blue oaks and follow the trail right (southeast) across another short stretch of open hillside, until you reach a ravine that you enter heading west and exit promptly facing east. Fortunately, the track stays shaded for a while on this south-facing hillside. You'll generally maintain about a 120-foot advantage on the river.

The blue oaks, live oaks, and foothill pines continue to cool you for the next 0.6 mile or so until your next junction. With no decisions to make along the way, you can enjoy cruising in and out of the small folds. At the next junction, among a small copse of oak, the South Fork American River Trail (SFART) and the Gerle Loop take separate courses. If you look straight ahead on the Gerle Loop, you can just see the next junction, 200 feet ahead. You'll pass it soon, and you'll return to the junction you're at right now if you hike the river option as well.

For this route, though, you'll turn left to stay on the SFART. A picnic table and hitching post stand just 500 feet down toward the river. Swing northwest and turn right at the next junction, marked SFART, GERLE LOOP, and CONNECTER TRAIL. Within another 500 feet comes the junction that you could see minutes earlier, marked by a fence post and a fence line running northeast. Turn slightly left to follow the fence briefly and then the trail, as you can now see the trailhead. As you walk by, take note of the birdhouses attached to the fence. A spare moment of observation may reveal some surprising diversity.

If you want some trail diversity, either take another loop around or return and try the river trail. Simply pass the two-oak junction on the left and descend the footpath to the river. Turning left will take you to the Greenwood River Access Area, so turn right. Head south along the river and notice the unusual flood debris that has remained in bushes and trees. Also notice the healing flower, yarrow, and blackberry. Take your time here, but remember—skunks love the berries, too.

When the river curves west, take some more time at the excellent beaches along the bend. Perhaps the most unusual feature along this stretch of the river isn't really an unfamiliar sight . . . but how often do you see a two-story outhouse (or even say it without giggling?) To serve the high number of rafters and kayakers who come through, a composting outhouse was constructed just off the trail at the base of the hill. The location is signed; just be prepared to see a large structure, not a little privy. Innovations like this one have truly helped keep the rivers and surrounding areas clean and natural.

If you've worked up a bit of an appetite, stroll ahead and take a snack break in the little parklike setting with a river view, about 100 yards from the outhouse.

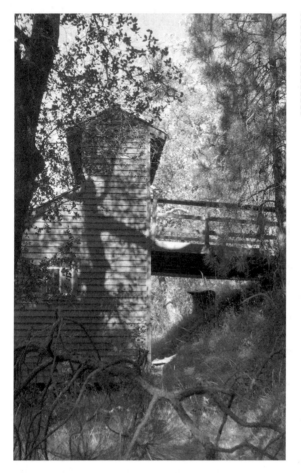

There's nothing funny about this two-story outhouse. Its state-of-the-art composting technology means river rafters, kayakers, and hikers can enjoy the South Fork of the American River minus a large ecological footprint.

From there, I observed a red fox (maybe more than one?) going back and forth to the river. After leaving the oak-and-willow-shaded rest stop, continue walking northwest and cross the stream. With 500 or 600 paces to go along the river, try counting how many times your toe hits a rock in the trail.

When you reach the old jeep trail, ascend it a few hundred feet to the junctions you stopped at earlier. Proceed to the fence line and make your way back to the trailhead.

NEARBY ACTIVITIES

There's a whole lot of nature in the diminutive Dave Moore Nature Area (see previous profile), 2.1 miles east of Magnolia Ranch on CA 49.

SOUTH FORK AMERICAN RIVER TRAIL

IN BRIEF

From the outset, your trail follows the track of the South Fork American River–Gerle Loop Trail in the previous hike. You'll pass the movie site at Cronan Ranch (see next hike), then continue on open terrain all the way to Skunk Hollow at the Salmon Falls Bridge. You trail generally stays about 120 feet above the river. From that vantage, vistas encompass the whole ecosystem throughout the hike.

You'll be in and out of shade for most of this hike, but sun becomes particularly cheap in the last 2 miles. If you start early, you'll be finishing in the heat of the day. Bring along more-than-sufficient water on this hike—sources along the way dry up early.

DESCRIPTION

This 12-mile section of hiking trail was opened in October 2010, joining a 25-mile trail system along the South Fork of the American River. Thanks are due to many volunteers, donors, and organizations, especially the American River Conservancy and the

Directions

From the junction of I-80 East and the Capital City Freeway, drive 25 miles on I-80 East toward Auburn and take Exit 119C/Elm Avenue. Turn left at the traffic light, onto Elm Avenue. At the bottom of the hill, turn left again, onto High Street. Drive under the railroad overpass before heading 2.3 miles downhill on CA 193 East/CA 49 South to the confluence and turning right. Follow CA 193 East/CA 49 South 10.7 miles through Cool and Pilot Hill to the Magnolia Ranch trailhead. Park on the west side of the lot. The trailhead is past the south end of the lot, at the information kiosk.

KEY AT-A-GLANCE INFORMATION

LENGTH: 11.6 miles

CONFIGURATION: Point-to-point

DIFFICULTY: Challenging

WATER REQUIRED: 5–6 liters

SCENERY: Foothill, riparian, and oak woodland, including all of their plants and animals

EXPOSURE: Shade is at a real premium on this long hike. A floppy hat is advisable. Sunscreen is a must.

TRAIL TRAFFIC: Light

TRAIL SURFACE: Dirt, duff, and rock

HIKING TIME: 4–5 hours

SEASON: Year-round, sunrise–sunset

ACCESS: No fees or permits

MAPS: USGS Pilot Hill, Coloma; PDFs at arconservancy.org (click "Activities," then "Hit the Trail" for a list)

WHEELCHAIR ACCESS: None

FACILITIES: Pit toilets and parking at the trailhead and destination, Skunk Hollow

DRIVING DISTANCE: 38 miles

SPECIAL COMMENTS: If you leave a car at Skunk Hollow, there's a $10 day-use parking fee.

GPS TRAILHEAD COORDINATES

Latitude   N38° 49.539´

Longitude   W120° 57.321´

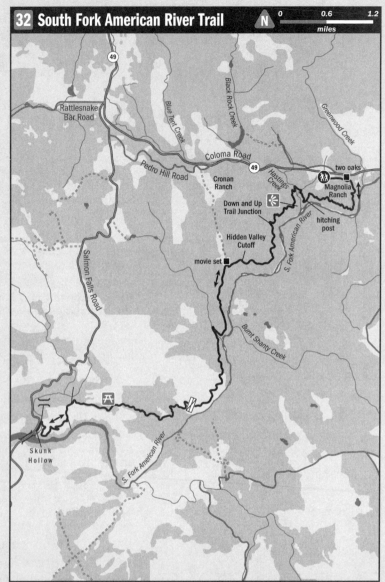

N

| 0 | 0.6 | 1.2 |

miles

49

Rattlesnake
Bar Road

Blue Tent Creek

Black Rock Creek

Greenwood Creek

Coloma Road

49

Pedro Hill Road

Cronan
Ranch

Hastings Creek

two oaks

Magnolia
Ranch

Down and Up
Trail Junction

hitching
post

Hidden Valley
Cutoff

movie set

S. Fork American River

Salmon Falls Road

Burnt Shanty Creek

Skunk
Hollow

S. Fork American River

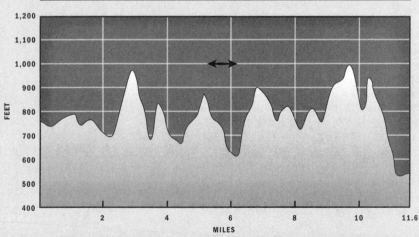

1,200						
1,100						
1,000						
900						
800						
700						
600						
500						
400						

FEET

2   4   6   8   10   11.6

MILES

Bureau of Land Management, for their efforts in securing the land to provide a protected natural area along the river.

The trailhead for this hike is officially in the Greenwood River Access Area, 0.3 mile down CA 49. But the trail signs seem to originate here at Magnolia Ranch, and the parking is free as well, so this seems to be a superior trailhead location.

Follow the previous hike description for 2.1 miles, to the junction with the Connecter Trail (that's the spelling on the sign). Just before that junction, you'll pass a picnic table with hitching posts nearby. Continue around the hill until you come to the junction with the Connecter Trail. Stay left and follow the signs for the Connecter Trail and the South Fork American River Trail (SFART) as the path heads toward a ravine.

As you descend toward Hastings Creek, notice the trail getting broader. The rock wall on the left supports a massive number of blackberry vines, and valley oak is sprinkled among the incense cedar and live oak. Daisylike madia lightly carpets the open areas. Cross Hastings Creek and ascend from its ravine on some short switchbacks. Your total elevation gain and loss favors loss by a margin of about 1,600 feet lost versus about 1,300 feet gained. (These figures are "horseback observations" and should be used for comparison purposes only. Your mileage may vary.) The point is that while you aren't going to wear yourself out on the uphills, you will get a pretty good workout.

A vista opens as you near the 2.75-mile point. In another 0.25 mile, you enter the cooling shade of blue oak, just as you're about to gain more than 300 of those 1,300 feet. Speaking of feet, alert hikers will notice the wiggly snake tracks in the soft dirt. In moments you'll have a nice view of your distant destination. Your next junction lies 0.5 mile ahead, at Cronan Ranch's Down and Up Trail.

Take the Down and Up Trail downhill to the left and follow the SFART signs. Begin ascending after you've crossed the small stream. The uphill trail crosses slopes filled with tiny white flowers and rivers of golden madia. On the distant horizon, you may notice a *casa blanca* standing on a distant hill. The sight will stick with you as you cross these open meadows.

Bypass the river-access trail and opt for the SFART, which stays about 75 feet above the river as it and you head west. Likewise, pass the Hidden Valley Cutoff in favor of a hot uphill for 0.25 mile, halted only by a copse of oak on the right, to the western-movie set that sits astride your trail. Pass between the house and the barn along the trail, walk past the Long Valley Trail junction, and take a left turn around to the southwest, as indicated by the signs for the SFART and a single sign in the grass marked TRAIL.

In a few hundred feet, the trail turns to a jeep road and you've completed 5 miles of hiking. Turn southward as the trail roughly traces the hillside. A junction with the West Ridge Trail occurs 5.6 miles along. Within 0.1 mile, you'll pass through a former gate as you head downhill a bit. Look closely for signs of some larger mammals along here. Black bear leave particularly large signs, so watch your step.

As if poking its head out to look around, this distinctive foothill pine stands above the surrounding fir-and-pine forest.

After coming out of the next big ravine, you'll gain about 200 feet of elevation on a singletrack as vista after vista opens before you. After 7 miles, your path turns west among manzanita and chamise and remains very sunny for the next mile (about 20 minutes).

Enter and exit a ravine and canyon, gaining and losing a bit of elevation in each transaction, and within 0.5 mile you'll thankfully be hiking in the shade of oak and pine. There are no navigational challenges, as evidenced by the plentiful signs along the way. Just past a dry ravine, close to 9 miles along, you'll begin ascending via a few switchbacks. A quarter-mile after that, you'll pass a small pond to your right. A left turn 250 feet after the pond is mandatory. Two picnic tables further mark this direction change.

Uphill from the tables, just 250 feet away, is the Pine Hill Preserve. To preserve the integrity of the natural area's species, visitors are asked to remove seeds from their packs, shoes, gear, and pets using the brushes attached to the convenient bench placed here for that purpose. You can then proceed to the side of the gate.

Hike alongside foothill (gray) pine and oak to your right and chaparral to your sun-baked left. Watch carefully overhead for the cones of the foothill pine—these things weigh over 6 pounds and have spikes, so a blow to the noggin wouldn't be pleasant. An uneasy feeling hits as roosting turkey vultures begin to take off.

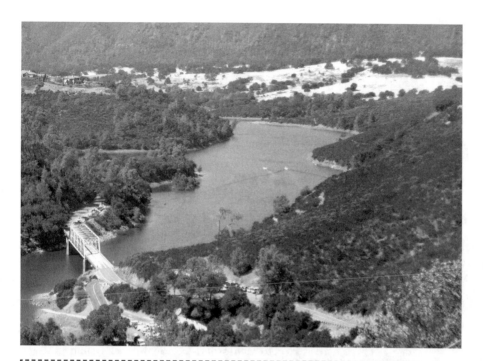

The Salmon Falls Road Bridge and the river-access point at Skunk Hollow, on the South Fork of the American River

The rock-and-manzanita trail is tantalizingly close to Skunk Hollow. Leading up to Mile 11, the trail winds slowly downhill. With Folsom Lake and your destination in sight, anxious or thirsty hikers are teased by 15 minutes of serpentine descent—all while watching their goal.

Descending the final 0.25 mile to Acorn Creek, one can appreciate the value of the newly constructed bridge spanning the stream. Another tip of the hat to the volunteers who worked on that project. Now it's just 250 yards to a nice bench under cool shade. Or perhaps a quick dip in the river.

NEARBY ACTIVITIES

For a shorter trip along the shore of Folsom Lake, check out the great vistas on the Sweetwater Trail, Hike 28 (page 153).

33 CRONAN RANCH TRAILS

KEY AT-A-GLANCE INFORMATION

LENGTH: 4.5 miles

CONFIGURATION: Balloon

DIFFICULTY: Moderate

WATER REQUIRED: 2 liters

SCENERY: Foothill woodland; views of the South Fork of the American River

EXPOSURE: Extremely sunny–pleasantly shaded

TRAIL TRAFFIC: Moderate; the trails are open to runners, bikers, hikers, and equestrians.

TRAIL SURFACE: Rock, dirt, duff

HIKING TIME: 2–3 hours

SEASON: Year-round, sunrise–sunset

ACCESS: No fees or permits

MAPS: USGS Coloma; BLM map at tinyurl.com/crtparkguide-pdf

WHEELCHAIR ACCESS: None

FACILITIES: Pit toilet in parking lot

DRIVING DISTANCE: 36 miles

SPECIAL COMMENTS: There are buildings to see at this made-for-movies ranch site. There are also mountain lions and rattlesnakes. In season, there are also hunters with bows, muzzle-loaders, and shotguns.

GPS TRAILHEAD COORDINATES

Latitude   N38° 49.560´
Longitude W120° 59.329´

IN BRIEF

In Pilot Hill's Cronan Ranch Regional Trails Park, this hike of connected trails offers a varied terrain—riparian zone along the South Fork of the American River, blue-oak savanna and foothill woodland above it. Some open-terrain trails lead to a movie-set ranch and then loop back to the trailhead.

DESCRIPTION

Thanks to the collaboration and cooperation of the American River Conservancy, the BLM, private individuals, and state agencies, the Cronan Ranch Regional Trails Park was added to California's regional-parks system in 2005 and expanded in 2006. The trailhead for this hike stands only about 5 air miles downriver from Coloma, the birthplace of the Gold Rush. Above and below the section of river that borders the ranch, streams, bars, and hillsides, gold miners sought their fortunes throughout the 1850s.

One of the forebears of the Cronan Ranch's owners settled in this area. Like many gold miners, William Bacchi arrived in 1851

Directions

From the junction of I-80 East and the Capital City Freeway, drive 25 miles on I-80 East toward Auburn and take Exit 119C/Elm Avenue. Turn left at the traffic light, onto Elm Avenue. At the bottom of the hill, turn left again, onto High Street. Drive under the railroad overpass before heading 2.3 miles downhill on CA 193 East/CA 49 South to the confluence and turning right. Follow CA 193 East/CA 49 South 8.8 miles through Cool and Pilot Hill. Turn right on Pedro Hill Road and drive to the south end of the equestrian parking lot. The trailhead is directly in front of you, past the pit toilets.

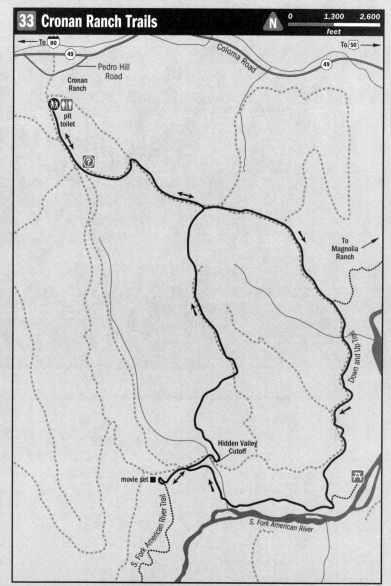

To 80

49

Pedro Hill
Road

Cronan
Ranch

Coloma Road

To 50

49

pit
toilet

?

To
Magnolia
Ranch

Down and Up Trail

Hidden Valley
Cutoff

movie set ■

S. Fork American River Trail

S. Fork American River

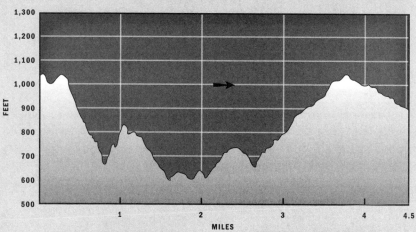

FEET				
1,300				
1,200				
1,100				
1,000		→		
900				
800				
700				
600				
500	1	2	3	4 4.5

MILES

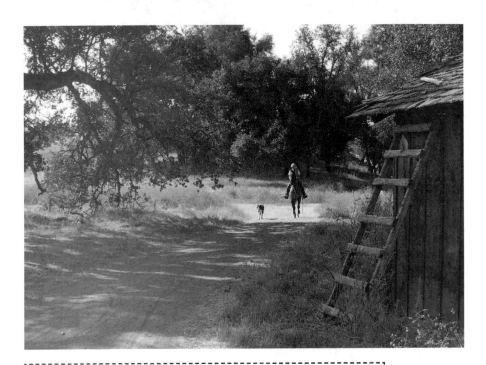

As if on cue, an equestrian and her cattle dog trot onto this former movie-ranch set.

or 1852 but by 1856 had turned from mining to ranching. This part of the Cronan Ranch was purchased by the Central Pacific Railroad in 1887 and then sold to Michael Cronan, who ran cattle on it until 1918. Descendants of William Bacchi retain some portions of the original ranch and sold other portions of it to create this park.

The ranch trails trend roughly north–south and run somewhat parallel to each other along ridges or valleys leading from CA 49 down to the South Fork of the American River. The Down and Up Trail leads through all three habitat zones on its way to the river.

So tighten your laces and make sure you've liberally applied sunscreen before you leave the parking lot on southward-heading Cronan Ranch Road. Bypass the West Ridge Trail, entering from the right and heading toward the kiosk 500 feet ahead. The displayed map of the trails and their names is helpful if you haven't already downloaded one. All of the junctions are clearly signed, and the directions are easy.

Cronan Ranch Road heads south while your track, the Down and Up Trail, bears left (resist the temptation of spring water, promised to the right). Arc across this broad, open slope and enjoy the views to the south. A solitary blue oak provides some midroute comfort. The next junction, in 0.6 mile, combines the Down and Up and East Ridge trails. Remember this junction— you'll see it again on your return.

From this junction, the track ascends a bit more, then begins descending alongside a stand of mixed oak and pine. The real show along here is in the path beneath your feet, where last night's parade of local inhabitants passed, however briefly. A good natural-history field guide is helpful at times like this, if for no other reason than to learn what was here before you wipe the memory of its presence from your sole. Some tracks may reveal a gathering of turkeys, while other signs clearly point to raccoons and others hint at an impromptu quail party.

A trail junction at about 1.5 miles along gathers the Down and Up Trail with the Connector Trail from Hastings Creek and the South Fork American River Trail. Stay on your grassy path, past the blackberries. Continue left at the upcoming stream crossing, which is followed by a brief bit of shaded uphill track.

Pleasant vistas greet you at the next junction with the East Ridge Trail (which diagonally bisects this loop route). In 0.2 mile, a junction with a river-access trail will let you turn downhill to the left if you're hiking between Labor Day and Memorial Day. Otherwise, rather than turning left, you'll continue 0.7 mile straight ahead to reach the movie set. Regardless of the date, you can always descend this trail and use the picnic area on the spur trail to the left, but you'll have to return to this spot rather than treading next to the river.

If the stars are aligned properly, movie fans may recognize the landscape along this stretch of the river as the background for scenes in *Memoirs of a Geisha*. This is a great spot for a lunch break. You'll be sitting right at the river on bedrock greenstone. A 0.6-mile hike along the bottom of this loop will lead you to another movie set: a western-ranch set (surprise!) on a hillside dotted with poppies. As you walk westward, the skyline is dominated by a *casa blanca* that you can't miss on a bright day.

Climb the hill to the northwest, where you join with the connector trail from the Hidden Valley Cutoff, and head uphill 0.1 mile to the ranch set, which consists of a two-room house, a barn and corral, a well, and a chicken coop, all under the shade of a majestic valley oak. (The picnic table isn't authentic.)

After the appropriate memory-making, you could return to the trailhead via the ranch road or the Long Valley Trail, but both are more exposed than even the sparsely treed Hidden Valley Cutoff. So turn back the way you entered this ersatz homestead and walk 0.4 mile downhill, past the huge oak now on your left, to the signed junction with the Hidden Valley Cutoff Trail. Head over the oak-dotted hillside for 0.8 mile, past a junction with the East Valley Trail (again), and you're back at a familiar landmark. Turn left at this junction and you'll be at the trailhead in less than a mile.

NEARBY ACTIVITIES

On your way home, stop for a bite to eat at the Coloma Club in nearby Lotus (530-626-6390; **colomaclub.com**).

34 OLMSTEAD LOOP TRAIL

KEY AT-A-GLANCE INFORMATION

LENGTH: 9 miles

CONFIGURATION: Loop

DIFFICULTY: Moderate

WATER REQUIRED: 3 liters

SCENERY: Open meadows full of wildflowers in spring

EXPOSURE: Rarely shaded

TRAIL TRAFFIC: Moderate; heavy on the weekend

TRAIL SURFACE: Dirt

HIKING TIME: 4 hours

SEASON: Year-round, 7 a.m.–9 p.m.

ACCESS: $10 day-use fee

MAPS: USGS Auburn, Pilot Hill; ASRA map

WHEELCHAIR ACCESS: None

FACILITIES: Parking lot, picnic table, information kiosk, pit toilet, telephone, water

DRIVING DISTANCE: 30 miles

SPECIAL COMMENTS: The trail becomes more challenging following heavy rains.

GPS TRAILHEAD COORDINATES

Latitude   N38° 53.294´
Longitude W121° 01.068´

IN BRIEF

The Olmstead Loop Trail leads hikers around and through large meadows fringed by live oaks and blackberry thickets. Songbirds, turkeys, and deer are easily observed across the fields of wildflowers.

DESCRIPTION

Facing west in front of the shaded information kiosk, hikers can study the area map and learn about the flora and fauna that can be observed on the trail. Walk into the equestrian parking lot and turn left, and 200 feet to the south you'll find the trailhead, which is clearly marked as the 0-mile point for the Olmstead Loop Trail. Walk through the pedestrian gate at the corner of the fence.

The Olmstead Loop Trail is a favorite among mountain bikers for good reason. The trail is named in memory of Dan Olmstead, a local bike-shop owner who promoted the creation of multiuse trails and stressed courtesy among trail users. When you arrive at the spacious trailhead parking lot, you will see evidence of his work in the hoofprints, bicycle tracks, and boot prints in the dirt.

- -

Directions ⎯⎯⎯⎯⎯⎯⎯⎯⎯⎯⟶

From the junction of I-80 and the Capital City Freeway, drive 24 miles on I-80 East toward Auburn and take Exit 119C/Elm Avenue. Turn left at the traffic light, onto Elm Avenue. At the bottom of the hill, turn left again, onto High Street. Drive under the railroad overpass and follow CA 49 downhill, turning right to cross the American River. Drive 5 miles to Cool. Turn right on St. Florian Court, which is the first right turn in Cool, before the flashing light and next to the fire station. The trailhead parking lot is behind the fire station. Your signed trailhead is in the southeast corner of the equestrian parking lot.

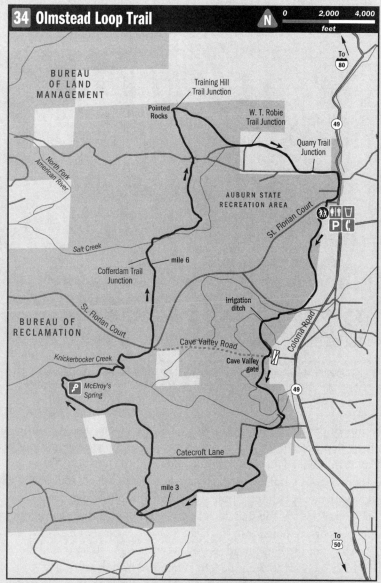

N

0   2,000   4,000
feet

BUREAU
OF LAND
MANAGEMENT

Training Hill
Trail Junction

Pointed
Rocks

W. T. Robie
Trail Junction

Quarry Trail
Junction

North Fork
American River

AUBURN STATE
RECREATION AREA

St. Florian Court

Salt Creek

mile 6

Cofferdam Trail
Junction

irrigation
ditch

Coloma Road

St. Florian Court

BUREAU OF
RECLAMATION

Cave Valley Road

Cave Valley
gate

Knickerbocker Creek

McElroy's
Spring

Catecroft Lane

mile 3

To
80

49

49

To
50
US

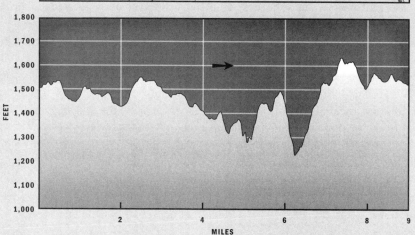

1,800

1,700

1,600

1,500

1,400

1,300

1,200

1,100

1,000

FEET

2   4   6   8   9
MILES

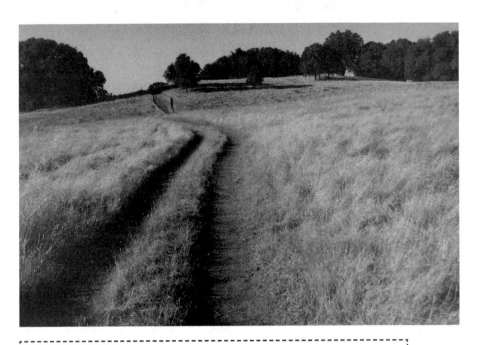

Filled with wildflowers in late spring, the hillsides turn golden brown by late summer.

Although the trail is very well signed, the placement of some of the markers can leave hikers scratching their heads. Right out of the gate, literally, is just such a trail split: the trail sign is smack in the middle of the junction. Take the left fork as the trail roughly parallels the highway, heading south. A trail sign ahead will reinforce your correct choice. Trail signs are so frequent that navigational skills are almost unnecessary. You only have to pay attention so that you don't ignore or miss a few important junctions.

Live oaks dot the huge meadow you are walking past. Your trail, bordered by a fence, passes a few houses on the left. When you near a large metal-roofed horse barn, the trail bears right. The next trail sign is conveniently located beside a blackberry patch full of ripening berries if you arrive in late summer. A second large berry thicket is on your left after you take the right fork at the next split. (Another trail goes around the berries to the left and joins your path again, so you can't go wrong here.)

Turn right, onto the doubletrack, and head up the dirt road. An irrigation ditch runs underneath it just before the 1-mile mark. Follow the trail sign up to the right. Shortly, an alternate entrance gate, marked GATE 156—CAVE VALLEY GATE, appears on the left. Continue past this point, with another trail sign on your right. You'll pass Northside Elementary School as you walk uphill. Ignore any side trails that lead to the right and walk straight ahead, toward a smaller, open gate. The trail becomes ditchlike and rock-strewn at the gate. Ahead is another trail sign to keep you on track.

Watch the slopes for wildlife, the most visible being the wild turkeys that abound here. Despite their being highly visible in contrast to the golden grasses, they can disappear in exactly the time it takes you to reach for a camera. Wally baskets, brodiaea, and popcorn flowers make these slopes pop with color in the spring and early summer. The next trail sign is at the 1.5-mile point. Again, posted right between two trails, this sign is also ambiguous. Take the fork to the left to continue on the correct route.

Your track swings west, bordered on the left by a blackberry-encrusted fence and on the right by blackberry-encrusted earth. Watch for a trail-etiquette sign on the left and a trail sign near that—turn left at this junction. Raccoons have visited these berry patches and have left plenty of evidence in the middle of the trail. Watch your step.

The long slope in front of you leads about 1,000 feet up, past milkweed and buttercup, to a copse of blue and live oak, which you'll walk through before turning southwest. The next 0.65 mile affords scant shade until you reach the stand of oaks in the distance. Your progress toward them can be measured by the radio towers and fence line to the south. Auburn comes into view about when you reach the corner of the fence. At the stand of oaks, a trail sign beneath a tall foothill pine directs you back to the northeast and 5.8 miles to Cool.

At 3 miles, you once again have some solid cover, thanks to blue and live oak. A sweeping turn to the left takes you downhill, now under the cover of tall foothill pines. When you finally encounter these long-needled trees, you'll have completed half the hike. Walk down a short, rocky stretch and watch for a sign on the right that announces MCELROY'S SPRING. This handwritten posting is attached high up in an oak tree that serves as a corner post for the fence. The spring can be easily spotted by the lush growth to the right of it.

Take a right at the end of the fence (or at the open gate just before it) and soon begin descending under the cover of foothill pine and Douglas fir until you reach Knickerbocker Creek. Enjoy the cool shade beside this stream, where a trail sign among the bushes on the opposite bank marks your fifth mile. Catch your breath here before you begin a fairly steep uphill trudge for the next 5 minutes or so. When you emerge from the trees, a grand vista of the terrain you have crossed spreads before you. The trail eases left and crosses paved St. Florian Court.

To the left, St. Florian Court leads to the site of the proposed Auburn Dam. To the right, it heads northeast, back to the fire station. Cross the road and continue north 0.5 mile across more open fields, making sure to ignore trails leading left. The foothill pine and live oak are now joined by manzanita stands, which help shade the trail. A signed junction indicates that Cofferdam Trail heads left. You should continue to the right, down to a crossing of Salt Creek, where a large, showy buttonbush crowds the narrow creek's crossing.

Take a drink of water and a deep breath here before you begin an uphill grind that takes 10 minutes or so. Travel about 0.33 mile northeast, then turn north for another 0.33 mile or so to reach flat ground among the oak and pine.

The next trail junction is signed and will direct you to the left, just west of north. Your trailhead lies southeast of this point.

The blue oaks covering this hillside are spaced exactly far enough apart for their crowns to nearly touch. If you decide to take some shade, be cautious of poison oak, which commonly appears red on these slopes. Wally baskets and blue dicks add to the color along your trail, which dead-ends at the junction with a doubletrack. According to the sign on the left, turning that way would lead you to the steep Training Hill Trail more than 1 mile away. Turning right, you have about 1.5 miles to your destination.

Your trail is fully exposed as you descend; watch for trail signs to keep on track. Your trail will swing left a bit, toward the east. As you again head uphill, the Wendell T. Robie Trail joins the Olmstead Loop Trail from the left, then exits to the left in another 100 yards. At the next junction, turn left and walk uphill on a rocky doubletrack under sparse shade.

The Quarry Trail leads north at a signed junction on your left. Continue uphill until you have a view of the backside of Cool and your original trailhead. Approaching the corner of the fence line, turn right, with the barbwire fence at your side. A few minutes more and you're back at the trailhead.

ROBIE POINT FIREBREAK TRAIL **35**

IN BRIEF

You can hike in the Auburn State Recreation Area (ASRA) today on trails that were developed by California natives and pioneers. And the reason you can hike—rather than swim over—them is that the Auburn Dam was never built. This reminder of what could have been lost *if* may increase your appetite to see what's over the next hill.

DESCRIPTION

With more than 70 miles of hiking, biking, and horse-riding trails, the Auburn State Recreation Area is a gift for outdoors enthusiasts whose interests vary from fly-fishing to gold-panning. Twenty miles of the North Fork and Middle Fork of the American River are covered by ASRA, which is governed by the California State Parks for the U.S. Bureau of Reclamation.

The Robie Point Firebreak Trail guides the hiker through an area filled with the history of what once was, what is, and what once was to be. Heading downhill from the

Directions —————————————➤

From the junction of I-80 East and Capital City Freeway, drive 25 miles on I-80 East toward Auburn and take Exit 119C/Elm Avenue. Turn left at the traffic light, onto Elm Avenue. At the bottom of the hill, turn left again, onto High Street. Pass beneath the Southern Pacific Railroad trestle as you continue downhill on CA 49. Look for the AUBURN STATE RECREATION AREA sign on the right. The trailhead is 0.2 mile after that sign, also on the right. The number of horseshoes attached to the oak distinguishes this large lot. Your trailhead is at the green gate marked GATE 130—MURPHY'S GATE TO ROBIE POINT.

(i) KEY AT-A-GLANCE
INFORMATION

LENGTH: 6 miles

CONFIGURATION: Out-and-back

DIFFICULTY: Moderate

WATER REQUIRED: 2–3 liters

SCENERY: Foothill woodland; views of the North Fork of the American River and the site of the proposed Auburn Dam

EXPOSURE: In and out of shade

TRAIL TRAFFIC: This multiuse trail is used regularly by local residents.

TRAIL SURFACE: Dirt and duff, rock

HIKING TIME: 3 hours

SEASON: Year-round

ACCESS: No fees or permits

MAPS: USGS Auburn; ASRA topo trail map

WHEELCHAIR ACCESS: None

FACILITIES: None at trailhead; picnic tables, water, pit toilets, and trash receptacles at the Auburn Equestrian Staging Area, your turn-around point

DRIVING DISTANCE: 26 miles

SPECIAL COMMENTS: Heed the mountain-lion, rattlesnake, and poison-oak warnings.

GPS TRAILHEAD COORDINATES

Latitude   N38° 54.004´
Longitude   W121° 03.543´

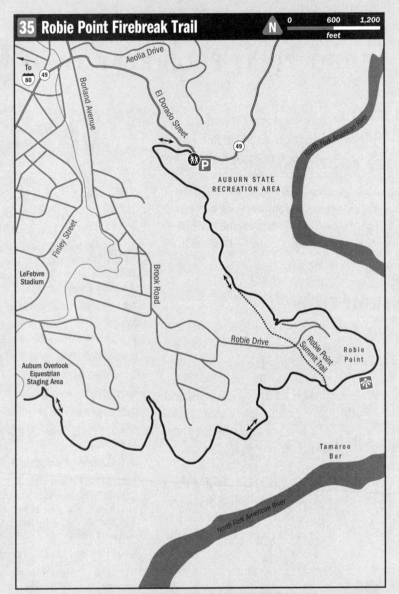

35 Robie Point Firebreak Trail

N

| 0 | 600 | 1,200 |
feet

To 80 49

Aeolia Drive

Borland Avenue

El Dorado Street

49

P

AUBURN STATE
RECREATION AREA

North Fork American River

Finley Street

LeFebvre
Stadium

Brook Road

Robie Drive

Robie Point
Summit Trail

Robie
Point

Auburn Overlook
Equestrian
Staging Area

Tamaroo
Bar

North Fork American River

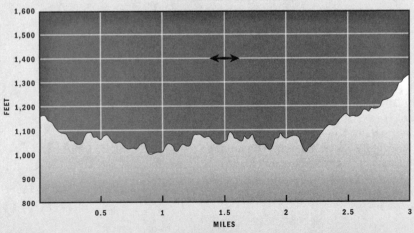

| 1,600 |
| 1,500 |
| 1,400 |
| 1,300 |
FEET
| 1,200 |
| 1,100 |
| 1,000 |
| 900 |
| 800 |

0.5   1   1.5   2   2.5   3

MILES

trailhead on broken asphalt, look left and you'll see the foundation of a hillside homestead just below the trail, which you should take to the right. Your wide path is bounded by lupine, buckeye, and rose. Ignore an old road to the right. Head past the blackberries and meander along the grassy trail. Within 0.25 mile, the sounds of the road diminish as you enter and exit a ravine.

Heading generally southeast, the wide dirt trail is occasionally shaded by oak on the hillside above. At about 0.4 mile, turn back toward the confluence for a good view of the Foresthill Bridge, the pylons of which were to be completely submerged by the Auburn Dam reservoir.

A small dirt trail leading down to No Hands Bridge enters your path from the left at 0.7 mile, where you continue heading straight uphill. A sign 100 yards uphill says AMERICAN DISCOVERY TRAIL—MILE 2, indicating an uphill track to the right—take the trail to the left. On your return, you may descend to this inter-section from Robie Point. Turn around and look down to see the old road cuts and fills braced by walls of dry-laid stone, which accommodated the track of the Mountain Quarries Railroad.

As you make your way around the hillside below Robie Point, whiteleaf manzanita will shade you and Indian paintbrush will color the trailside. The path joining yours from the right, 0.5 mile ahead, is another trail leading up to Robie Point. Yet another route over Robie Point, just 0.25 mile farther, is described on the return route. Note the WST marker and the four-by-four post adjacent to it.

Turkey vultures hang out at the vista point beneath Robie Point, waiting for the air to warm before taking the leap. From that spot, the entire Auburn Dam site comes into view to reveal the terracing, the diversion-tunnel site, and the western keyway for the dam itself.

The 0.5-mile-long diversion tunnel is no longer visible at this point in the river's reclamation process. It was originally opened to redirect the waters of the North Fork to allow construction of the dam, which began in the dry riverbed to the right of the tunnel. In 1978, extensive seismic studies revealed the risk to the dam as it was then designed. By the late 1980s, the dam project had been stalled by additional design concerns. The project was later abandoned due to funding concerns. The original riverbed has now been restored, and the reclamation pro-cess is visible on the surrounding hillsides and terraces.

Descend, stay on the WST, and ignore trails that enter or leave it. At a dis-tinct fork in the trail, the WST heads right and past a green gate. Follow that right fork past the gate.

Markers indicate that this is the WST and riders have only 1 mile to go to the finish. Wendell T. Robie was the founder of the Western States "100 Miles–One Day" Trail Ride, and it is in his memory that many trails have been named. As you enter a narrow, cooling ravine, you have less than a mile to your destination: an equestrian staging area at the eastern terminus of the Pioneer Express Trail.

As you hike this newly created tread, you have some excellent photo ops. Vistas of the restored channel of the North Fork of the American River, along with the downstream canyon, spread to the south and west. Keep a sharp eye out for foxes, which come out to investigate passersby. Continue on this easy uphill section to the Auburn Staging Area, where you can find water and a seat before you return to the trailhead.

When you reach the marked WST trail junction and the four-by-four post, take this left-hand trail uphill to reach Robie Point. The trail comes out next to Gate 135, Robie Point to Murphy's Gate–Highway 49, which is on one side of a cul-de-sac; opposite it are Gates 133, Robie Point to Marion Way, and 134, Robie Point to WST. Walk down the trail past Gate 135 to rejoin the doubletrack you traveled earlier.

Large yellow-and-black western tiger swallowtail butterflies will outpace you down the trail as they head for the big cone-shaped collection of flowers gracing branches of California buckeye. Other butterflies are also attracted to these sweet-smelling bouquets: amusingly, the little gray hairstreaks and California sisters seem to demand aerial battles before they will permit intruders to drink up the nectar.

On your way back to the trailhead, the fragrances of Chinese houses, lupine, buckeye, California rose, and larkspur waft around you. A final plunge into the ravine will cool you off before the short climb to the trailhead.

LAKE CLEMENTINE TRAIL

IN BRIEF

Lake Clementine Trail features the tallest bridge in California, Gold Rush–era bridge remains, exposed Jurassic-period geology, riparian zone and foothill flora, a rock-lined swimming hole, and a tree-lined lake. This pleasant hike along the North Fork of the American River is largely shaded. A gentle grade offers some exercise along this 2.2-mile hike on a trail shared with runners and mountain bikers. Imagine hiking in Utah's Glen Canyon *before* it was inundated by the Colorado. A similar experience awaits here at the confluence of the North and Middle forks of the American.

DESCRIPTION

The confluence of the North and Middle forks of the American River flows about 15 miles due north of the site where James Marshall first discovered gold on the South Fork of the American River. Since the time of the forty-niners, a dozen bridges have spanned these tributaries. Today, only four remain, three of which are used by motor vehicles. They are No Hands Bridge, formerly the Mountain

- -

Directions —————————➤

From Sacramento, drive 25 miles on I-80 East toward Auburn and take Exit 119C/Elm Avenue. Turn left at the traffic light, onto Elm Avenue. At the bottom of the hill, turn left again, onto High Street. Pass beneath the Southern Pacific Railroad trestle and drive 2.2 miles downhill on CA 49. Continue straight (past the CA 49 turnoff toward Cool) on Old Foresthill Road for another 0.3 mile, crossing Old Foresthill Bridge to find trail-head parking along the side of the road. If you must park far from this spot, the trail-head is on the east side of the confluence.

KEY AT-A-GLANCE INFORMATION

LENGTH: 4.4 miles

CONFIGURATION: Out-and-back

DIFFICULTY: Moderate

WATER REQUIRED: 1–2 liters, depending on season and time of day

SCENERY: River views in a widening canyon lead up to a dammed lake

EXPOSURE: Shaded except during midday hours

TRAIL TRAFFIC: Busy

TRAIL SURFACE: Sand, gravel, river rock, dirt, mud, and pavement

HIKING TIME: 2–3 hours

SEASON: Year-round, sunrise–sunset

ACCESS: No fees or permits

MAPS: USGS Auburn

WHEELCHAIR ACCESS: None

FACILITIES: Information kiosks and pit toilet, along with scant parking, are north of the trailhead on the north side of the road, at the west end of Old Foresthill Bridge. Pit toilet at North Fork Dam parking lot.

DRIVING DISTANCE: 27.5 miles

SPECIAL COMMENTS: This trail is also popular with mountain bikers. Look over your shoulder frequently.

GPS TRAILHEAD COORDINATES

Latitude   N38° 54.981´
Longitude   W121° 02.128´

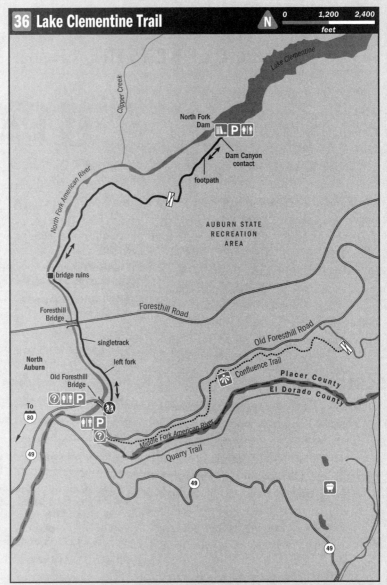

36 Lake Clementine Trail

N

0   1,200   2,400
feet

Lake Clementine

Clipper Creek

North Fork Dam

Dam Canyon contact

footpath

North Fork American River

AUBURN STATE RECREATION AREA

bridge ruins

Foresthill Road

Foresthill Bridge

singletrack

Old Foresthill Road

North Auburn

left fork

Confluence Trail

Placer County

El Dorado County

Old Foresthill Bridge

To 80

49

Middle Fork American River

Quarry Trail

49

49

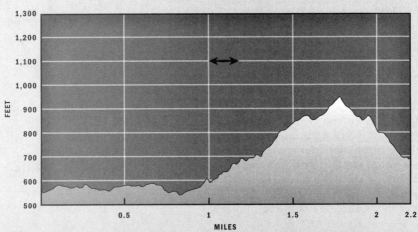

1,300
1,200
1,100
1,000
900
800
700
600
500

FEET

0.5   1   1.5   2   2.2

MILES

Quarries Railroad Bridge and famous for its proximity to the finish of the Tevis Cup Trail Ride; the CA 49 bridge to Cool; the Old Foresthill Road Bridge; and the most spectacular of all—Foresthill Bridge.

Lake Clementine Trail begins to the east of the confluence on the southeast side of Old Foresthill Road. The trailhead is marked by a gate signed TRAIL 139. Lined with boulders, this jeep trail borders the east flank of the North Fork of the American River as it flows past you toward the confluence with the Middle Fork.

Your destination lies at the end of a steady uphill amble to Lake Clementine, a reservoir created by the North Fork Dam, a debris dam built in 1939 by the U.S. Army Corps of Engineers. The flows along this fork of the American are not dam-controlled, so as summer wanes, the waters below you become slower and warmer—making for great swimming opportunities. In late spring, by contrast, the high flow over the North Fork Dam creates a spectacular mist and a thundering rumble.

Walking parallel to the river, look left, to the west side, and you will see Stagecoach Trail, which climbs to join the route of an 1852 toll road known then as Yankee Jim's Turnpike. While you're looking, glance over your shoulder often—mountain bikes can approach quickly.

At about 1,000 feet from the trailhead, descend the first left fork toward the river's edge. A hundred feet farther, a pretty stream crosses from your right. Take a moment to look left, though, to see the first of many bridge remains.

The biozones in this area—riparian and foothill woodland—are easy to tell apart, because most of the riparian zone is on your left and the river and foothill woodland are on your right, along the canyon walls.

You'll see interior live oak, canyon live oak, madrone, foothill ("digger") pine, and California bay laurel. Watch for the spiky leaves of the toyon and colorful redbuds interspersed with manzanita and poison oak.

As you look down the slope toward the river, you'll pass cottonwoods, willows, valley oaks, and bigleaf maples. If the season is right, you'll find an abundance of blackberries along here as well.

When the trail turns into a singletrack and hugs the river, you'll have walked a little more than 0.5 mile. Bikers have no place to pass you along here, so be alert. Look up to see the concrete pier and roadway of the Foresthill Bridge looming across the canyon. Walk about 500 feet and it will be directly overhead.

The bridge is a record-setting 730 feet above the river, making it the tallest bridge in California and the third-tallest in the United States. Finished in 1973, it was built to carry traffic across the reservoir that would have been created by the Auburn Dam.

In the late 1970s, before the planned construction of the Auburn Dam, seismological risks were revealed that halted those plans. Downriver from the confluence, a diversion tunnel was built that still stands. The dam's impact had it been built is most easily visualized when you look up at the Foresthill Bridge:

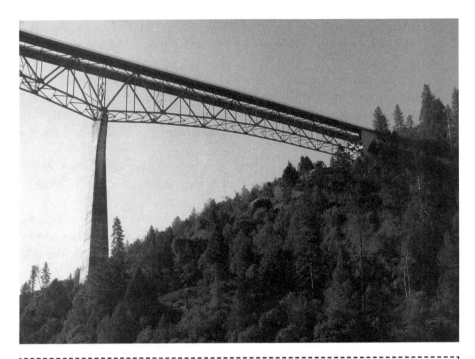

Seven hundred thirty feet above your riverside trail, the Foresthill Bridge is the tallest in California and the third tallest in the United States.

the water level would have reached just 22 feet below the top of the concrete pier above you.

After hiking 0.8 mile, look along both riverbanks for stone or concrete abutments marking original bridge sites. The concrete abutments supported the steel bridges of the early 20th century. Stone and rock abutments that supported several wooden bridges can be seen upriver within the next 0.3 mile.

Shaded by live oak and manzanita, boulder-lined pools of lazy, clear water lie within view. Stretching for almost 0.5 mile, this portion of the river is known as Clark's Hole. Placer miners made dams of stacked boulders and river cobble, which formed these connected pools. The warm, slow waters are now popular for swimming.

The midday sun at your back can be uncomfortable, and your moderately rolling trail has now turned into a fairly steady uphill exercise. To your right, the canyon wall rises sharply above you. The welcome coolness of ferns and mosses, which thrive wherever water seeps out of the manzanita-covered hillside, helps relieve the heat.

The increasingly loud sound of water signals that you're approaching the North Fork Dam. As the trail turns southeast, you will have a brief view upstream to the dam.

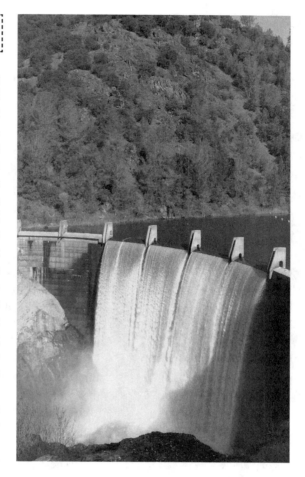

The North Fork Dam above the confluence

The gravel trail ends at 1.95 miles, at a gate signed 1.4 MILES TO FUEL BREAK ROAD AND CULVERT TRAIL. Follow the paved road as it turns left and begins to drop to the dam site and Lake Clementine. In 0.3 mile, a dirt footpath leaves the road and descends left. Those who want a very close look at the dam should take this short spur, which leads to the exact point at which the dam is anchored to the rock of the canyon wall. Along the way to this spot, notice the informal use-trail that descends to the river.

For a tamer look at the dam from a lakeside vantage point, continue along the paved road, turn left into the day-use parking lot, and descend to the lake level.

Retracing your steps gives you a chance to look for wildlife along the canyon side and flowers along the riverside. There is a long list of both, but you'll be able to spot plenty of turkey vultures, squirrels, signs of coyotes, California quails, and scrub jays, along with turkeys and red-tailed hawks. Springtime brings a riot of color to this area, with Indian paintbrush, California poppy, lupine, and larkspur among the many flowers. Your hour-long return to the car will be a relaxing walk in one of the Foothills' finest hiking regions.

NEARBY ACTIVITIES

Auburn State Recreation Area (ASRA) has more than 50 recognized trails extending hundreds of miles throughout the North and Middle forks of the American River. Whitewater rafting is very popular on both forks, and several commercial raft and kayak outfitters operate from Auburn, Colfax, Cool, and Foresthill.

37 CONFLUENCE TRAIL

KEY AT-A-GLANCE INFORMATION

LENGTH: 3.5 miles

CONFIGURATION: Out-and-back

DIFFICULTY: Easy

WATER REQUIRED: 1 liter

SCENERY: Spectacular panorama of the Middle Fork of the American River

EXPOSURE: Exposed south-facing slope, with some trailside shade

TRAIL TRAFFIC: This is a popular hiking and mountain-biking trail.

TRAIL SURFACE: Dirt and rock

HIKING TIME: 1.5–2 hours

SEASON: Year-round, sunrise–sunset

ACCESS: No fees or permits

MAPS: USGS Auburn

WHEELCHAIR ACCESS: None

FACILITIES: Pit toilet and information kiosk at the trailhead

DRIVING DISTANCE: 28 miles

SPECIAL COMMENTS: This trail follows an eastward route up-canyon and is exposed, so it becomes quite hot. A wide-brimmed hat and sunglasses are welcome gear on this hike.

GPS TRAILHEAD COORDINATES

Latitude   N38° 54.931´

Longitude   W121° 02.161´

IN BRIEF

A short, gradual climb above the Middle Fork of the American River provides more than exercise. Hikers will be treated to panoramic upriver views of the Middle Fork, overlooking placer-mining and quarrying operations as they were left more than 100 years ago.

DESCRIPTION

The shaded trailhead is below the parking area on the west side of Old Foresthill Road. To reach it, descend from the parking area to the information kiosk and pit toilet. As you walk down toward the river, imagine cooling your feet at the river's edge after your hike.

Begin by walking south along the trail, directly toward the river. The first 500 feet make a sweeping curve from south to east. As you head away from the confluence, the trail begins an easy but steady uphill climb along a singletrack.

The trail is sparsely shaded by foothill pine and cool manzanita. The pines can be recognized by their large (6- to 10-inch) globe-shaped cones, which are heavily armored with

----

Directions ⟶

From Sacramento, drive 25 miles on I-80 East toward Auburn and take Exit 119C/Elm Avenue. Turn left at the traffic light, onto Elm Avenue. At the bottom of the hill, turn left again, onto High Street. Pass beneath the Southern Pacific Railroad trestle and drive 2.2 miles downhill on CA 49. Continue straight (past the CA 49 turnoff toward Cool) on Old Foresthill Road for another 0.3 mile, crossing Old Foresthill Bridge to find trailhead parking along the side of the road. If you must park far from this spot, the trailhead is on the east side of the confluence.

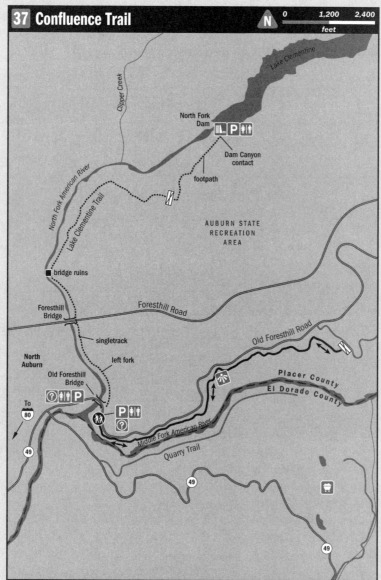

N   0   1,200   2,400
feet

Lake Clementine

Clipper Creek

North Fork
Dam

Dam Canyon
contact

footpath

North Fork American River

Lake Clementine Trail

AUBURN STATE
RECREATION
AREA

bridge ruins

Foresthill
Bridge

Foresthill Road

Old Foresthill Road

North
Auburn

singletrack

left fork

Old Foresthill
Bridge

Placer County

El Dorado County

To
80

49

Middle Fork American River

Quarry Trail

49

49

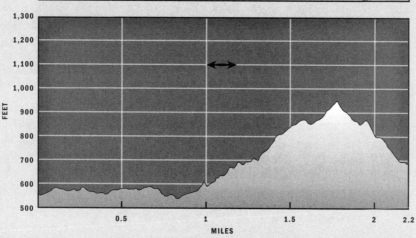

curved 1-inch hooks at the ends of their scales—oddly overprotected and showy compared with the sparse, uneven growth of the tree itself.

Look to the south side of the middle fork, where the Quarry Trail runs parallel past Louisiana Bar, Warner's Ravine, New York Bar, Murderer's Bar, Mammoth Bar, Murderer's Gulch, Texas Bar, Hoosier Bar, and on. The placer miners named these spots to remind them of home, and the names endure to this day.

Imagine looking down from this point at long wood-and-canvas sluice boxes lining the river, being worked by hundreds of gold miners. The scene is largely the same as it was in the mid–19th century. But the only thing that moves the rocks now is the river.

Keep your eyes peeled as you look across at Warner Ravine. The trail closely contours along the canyon side, and footing can be slippery at times. You might also look down at the trail and see signs of coyotes, raccoons, and dogs.

On this exposed slope, watch for rattlesnakes—an important part of this ecosystem—lazing in the afternoon sun. They are shy and will not attack unless disturbed or provoked. Respect them and walk away from them.

Depending on the time of day, sun can be an issue. Early-morning hikers will enjoy not only a cool trail but also brilliant shows of light and shadow on the opposite hills.

The vehicular Old Foresthill Road parallels this path as it rounds the mountain. Although the road is close, one has a hard time hearing any traffic. The trail surface changes from dirt and rock to old, broken pavement.

The exposed hillsides here lack the abundance of mosses seen on the North Fork trail. However, the mosses and ferns are replaced on this slope by chaparral flora, which now includes many nonnative grasses and flowers.

After about 0.75 mile, your singletrack trail becomes a four-wheel-drive trail (or fire-suppression trail) that long ago saw its last vehicle. As the path turns east, admire the view upriver from New York Bar below you to Murderer's Bar.

The Mammoth Bar area is reserved on specific days for off-highway-vehicle (OHV) users. Check with the park for the seasonal schedule by calling 530-885-4527. Established OHV trails may be hiked when not reserved for OHV users.

After 1.75 miles, the trail ends at a gate signed TRAIL #107—EAST GATE and CONFLUENCE TRAIL. Retrace your steps to the trailhead. As you approach the confluence, the refreshing sounds of water will welcome you back.

NEARBY ACTIVITIES

The Confluence Trail is well known to mountain-biking enthusiasts. ASRA has hundreds of miles of multiuse trails shared among equestrians, bikers, and hikers. Lake Clementine Trail and Quarry Road Trail in the Confluence area (Hikes 36 and 38, respectively) are well-regarded bike trails. The Olmstead Loop Trail in Cool (Hike 34), named in honor of a local bike-shop owner, is a favorite among off-road cyclists.

QUARRY ROAD TRAIL TO AMERICAN CANYON FALLS 38

IN BRIEF

Quarry Road Trail is the easiest of walks—for the first 2 miles. Just by adding an idyllic destination, you can turn this simple walk into a challenging adventure. The falls and pool hidden away on American Canyon Creek are worth every step you take along this historic mining trail.

DESCRIPTION

Your hike starts at the green gate, followed by signs indicating distances to various locations and facilities along the trail. You'll find picnic tables at 0.2, 0.6, and 1.2 miles into the hike, as well as pit toilets and trash receptacles at the first and last of these. As you wind around the first shaded curve, you'll probably notice more informative signs lining the track.

As you exit the shade of the first bend, look over your shoulder to a nice view of Foresthill Bridge. As you walk along the river toward Warner Ravine and the rapids at New York Bar, your wide trail is lined with fairy lanterns and buttercups in the spring and

KEY AT-A-GLANCE INFORMATION

LENGTH: 14.5 miles

CONFIGURATION: Out-and-back

DIFFICULTY: Challenging

WATER REQUIRED: 4–5 liters

SCENERY: Exceptional views along the Middle Fork and American Canyon Creek, with a beautiful cascade and pool at the end

EXPOSURE: Lots of shaded trail, but sunscreen is handy for the long, exposed part.

TRAIL TRAFFIC: Heavy on weekends

TRAIL SURFACE: Gravel and dirt, duff and dirt

HIKING TIME: 6 hours

SEASON: Year-round

ACCESS: $10 day-use fee

MAPS: USGS Greenwood, Auburn

WHEELCHAIR ACCESS: None

FACILITIES: Large gravel parking lot, information kiosk, picnic table, critter-proof trash receptacles, and pit toilet; pit toilets and picnic tables along first 1.2 miles

DRIVING DISTANCE: 27 miles

SPECIAL COMMENTS: If the lot is full, parking is permitted alongside the road. The trail to the cascade in American Canyon descends steeply on loose rock and dirt.

Directions ⟶

From the junction of I-80 East and the Capital City Freeway, drive 25 miles on I-80 East toward Auburn and take Exit 119C/Elm Avenue. Turn left at the traffic light, onto Elm Avenue. At the bottom of the hill, turn left again, onto High Street. Pass beneath the Southern Pacific Railroad trestle as you continue downhill on CA 49. Drive 2.3 miles down the winding highway to the confluence, where you follow the road, making a right turn at the bottom of the hill over the American River, toward Cool. The trailhead parking lot is 0.3 mile uphill on the left. There's plenty of parking in this gravel lot, which adjoins the trailhead.

GPS TRAILHEAD COORDINATES

Latitude N38° 54.697´

Longitude W121° 02.078´

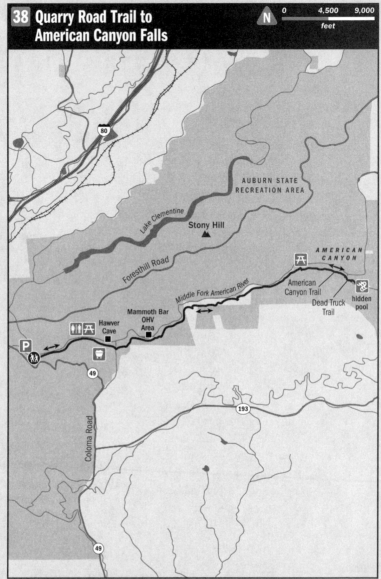

N

| 0 | 4,500 | 9,000 |

feet

AUBURN STATE
RECREATION AREA

Lake Clementine

Stony Hill

Foresthill Road

Middle Fork American River

AMERICAN
CANYON

American
Canyon Trail

Dead Truck
Trail

hidden
pool

Hawver
Cave

Mammoth Bar
OHV
Area

49

Coloma Road

193

49

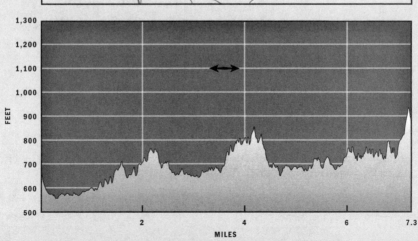

nicely shaded by live oaks and foothill pines year-round. Your trail tells of three periods of history.

Most recently, your trail was the track bed for the Mountain Quarries Railroad, which carried limestone from the quarry's loading platform near the gated entrance to Hawver Cave across the famous Mountain Quarries Railroad Bridge (a.k.a. the No Hands Bridge) on its way to Auburn. Built in the early 1900s, the railroad was abandoned and ultimately dismantled during World War II to recycle the rail's steel. You may be able to see some of the leftover ties embedded in the trail before you reach the picnic area below Hawver Cave.

An earlier incarnation of the Quarry Trail was a flume bed. The Confluence area was occupied and worked by nearly 10,000 miners during the Gold Rush years. In the late 1850s, individuals banded together to form mining companies—building and operating a 13-mile-long flume-works that was destroyed annually by spring floods. Using canvas and wood, builders literally fabricated the flume from scratch each year. Today, the riparian area and the riverbed have been almost entirely reclaimed through natural processes.

It was the process of water dripping through limestone that created the cavernous Hawver Cave. For years, curious settlers found strange animal bones in the cave. In 1906, an Auburn paleontologist named Dr. J. C. Hawver identified many species of animals from the Pleistocene Age, including the mastodon and ground sloth. A few years later, human bones were discovered, leading to the understanding that Native Americans had used the cave as a burial chamber. Quarrying destroyed the cave, which is now gated. A popular side trail—the PG&E Road Trail—leads 0.6 mile to a quarry overlook. Bypass these side trails if your goal is the falls on American Canyon Creek.

At the next trail junction, a path down to the left will lead you to a spacious picnic area. With three tables beneath pergolas, three toilets, and one enormous view, this is a terrific destination for families with small children. Above the tables stand the blackberry-shrouded remains of the limestone loading-platform foundations.

Hiking up on the right-hand trail at the junction leads you past these concrete blocks and Hawver Cave. Continue straight past the cave entrance and its running stream. You have a nice view of the river from this point. Your trail will be clearly signed at every important junction, and informative signs will pinpoint mileages and trail names.

Continue straight ahead toward Brown's Bar Trail, Maine Bar Trail, and Poverty Bar, which lie 2–5 miles ahead. You will pass above Murderer's Bar before coming opposite Mammoth Bar on the far bank. Blackberry bushes and black oaks cool and shade you, and swarms of California sister and yellow tiger swallowtail butterflies descend on pretty face, Indian pink, and larkspur as you hike on to Texas Bar, at around 2.7 miles.

The long stretches of exposure are occasionally interrupted by madrone hanging over the trail. Round the pool below the small cascades, and you will

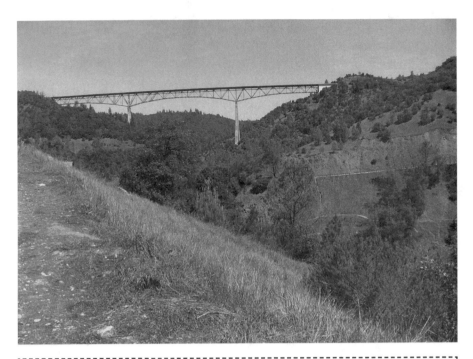

Had the Auburn Dam been completed, the water level would have been expected to rise to within 22 feet of the Foresthill Bridge deck.

come to a cool, shady glen that buzzes with activity. Butterflies, bees, and water ouzels dart around in this air-conditioned trailside rest area. A sound in the brush next to the water draws your attention to the king snake—black with striking yellow bands—as it hustles away beneath the duff. This well-timed pause above Brown's Bar offers welcome rest before you walk toward Maine Bar Trail—about 2 miles ahead with a bit of climbing.

All right, so it was hardly a grind uphill. Now the trail is graced by more flowers, the slope above and below steepens, and the dense cover of tall white firs cloaks you in deep shade as you descend into Wildcat Canyon above Hoosier Bar. Imagine, as you look through the trees, how this area would look with thousands of miners working the river and its streams. Moments after you exit the ravine at Wildcat Canyon, you'll need to make a sharp right turn before diving into the river. Your singletrack will lead you upstream alongside the rocky cobble and sand of Hoosier Bar before it climbs above the river and heads to Brushy Mountain Canyon, where you'll find a pleasant glade in which to cool your heels. Less than 500 yards away is an oak grove shading a picnic table and pit toilet.

Just about the time the picnic site comes into view, you should spot a trail sign on the left. A right turn at this sign is important so that you can take the Maine Bar Trail just 0.1 mile uphill to the American Canyon Trail, where you will again head east. This junction is easy to miss because of the distinct trail beyond the picnic table in front of you, which then leads across the exposed Philadelphia Bar on an indistinct trail to Poverty Bar. Although this can be a great alternate route, the one described here leads you away from the river into a beautiful side canyon.

Walk uphill 0.1 mile on the upended sedimentary rock to the signed junction with the Western States Trail (WST). American Canyon Trail is 0.9 mile away. This happens to be the worst section of the trail but is entirely worth it as long as you are careful. The trail—actually a soft-dirt-and-duff singletrack that feels great underfoot—is choked with poison oak for most of the way to American Canyon. Wearing gaiters or long pants or carrying trekking poles is about the only way to ward off these thick plants along here. About halfway along the trail, keep right, heading uphill on the WST at the junction with the trail that descends to Poverty Bar. As the trail steepens farther along, the WST branches to the right, going in and out of a ravine. Stay on the trail to the left.

Watch for the small cascades as they grow and slice through the greenstone, guiding you uphill into American Canyon. These beautiful pools and cascades lead to a crossing of the American Canyon Creek, just below its confluence with Hoboken Creek. A sign after the crossing identifies this as American Canyon Creek. But your destination, exceeding even this spot in beauty, is just 1,000 feet around the bend.

Head uphill on a rough trail leading to a trail sign, which marks a junction with the American Canyon Trail and Dead Truck Trail and lists distances to other locations. Look downhill behind you for a use-trail angling across the slope to the hidden creek below. As you approach the sound of rushing water, the creek and then the pool comes into range. Crossing bedrock greenstone, the water pools beneath a semicircular bowl carved into the bedrock. Only by descending to the creek and pool level can you see up into the waterfall that is the source of all of the sound.

The crystal-clear water offers overheated hikers a great place to completely dunk in and cool off—totally rejuvenating themselves for the hike out. If you don't take the time to swim in this pristine pool, you might look around for California (firebelly) newts (look but don't touch—their slippery skin coating is toxic to humans) or water ouzels as they motor around this spot. However long you happen to stay here, you'll be sure to think of this as one of the jewels of the Auburn State Recreation Area.

Your route out to the trailhead requires a slow escape from the lure of the waters; just retrace your path. All the important intersections and trail junctions are clearly signed.

NEARBY ACTIVITIES

Another excellent route to the same waterfall and pool is the American Canyon–Dead Truck Trail (see next profile).

39 AMERICAN CANYON– DEAD TRUCK TRAIL

KEY AT-A-GLANCE INFORMATION

LENGTH: 5.3 miles

CONFIGURATION: Loop

DIFFICULTY: Moderate with brief, strenuous uphills

WATER REQUIRED: 2 liters

SCENERY: Falls, streams, cascades, pools, wildflowers, foothill woodlands, birds

EXPOSURE: Mostly shaded

TRAIL TRAFFIC: Light

TRAIL SURFACE: Dirt and duff, dirt and rock

HIKING TIME: 3–4 hours

SEASON: Year-round

ACCESS: No fees or permits

MAPS: USGS Greenwood

WHEELCHAIR ACCESS: None

FACILITIES: None

DRIVING DISTANCE: 35 miles

SPECIAL COMMENTS: The trail is restricted to hikers and equestrians. There is limited parking at the trailhead. Heed the mountain-lion and poison-oak warnings. The trail to the cascade and pool descends steeply on loose soil.

GPS TRAILHEAD COORDINATES

Latitude   N38° 54.806´

Longitude   W120° 55.623´

IN BRIEF

American Canyon Trail, an easy route down to the Middle Fork of the American River, lets you explore the streams, waterfalls, and ice-cold pools on the way to Poverty Bar. This route loops back before descending to the river; you'll climb just enough to sweat hard before you walk the gentle route back to your car. The simple quarter-mile excursion on to Poverty Bar is described but not mapped.

DESCRIPTION

The trails of the Auburn State Recreation Area (ASRA) take advantage of miners' trails, pioneer roads, newly constructed trails, and some reclaimed mining ditches. This gentle descent into American Canyon takes hikers across two

----

Directions ————————————➤

From the junction of I-80 East and the Capital City Freeway, drive 25 miles on I-80 East toward Auburn and take Exit 119C/Elm Avenue. Turn left at the traffic light, onto Elm Avenue. At the bottom of the hill, turn left again, onto High Street. Pass beneath the Southern Pacific Railroad trestle as you continue downhill on CA 49. Drive 2.3 miles down the winding highway to the confluence, where you follow the highway as it turns right across the American River toward Cool, where in 6 miles you'll turn left onto CA 193 toward Georgetown. Drive 5.3 miles, then turn left onto Sweetwater Trail on the north side, which is opposite Pilgrim Court on the south. (This turn comes before you reach the village of Greenwood.) Your trailhead is on the right, just at the top of the street, before the gates to Auburn Lake Trails. Parking at the trailhead is limited, but you can park on the shoulder back down the road. The trailhead is signed AMERICAN CANYON TRAIL—THIRD GATE.

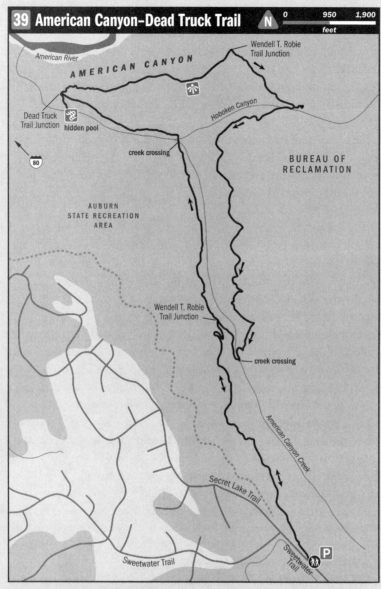

N

0   950   1,900
                  feet

American River

AMERICAN CANYON

Wendell T. Robie
Trail Junction

Dead Truck
Trail Junction

hidden pool

Hoboken Canyon

creek crossing

80

BUREAU OF
RECLAMATION

AUBURN
STATE RECREATION
AREA

Wendell T. Robie
Trail Junction

creek crossing

American Canyon Creek

Secret Lake Trail

Sweetwater Trail

Sweetwater Trail

P

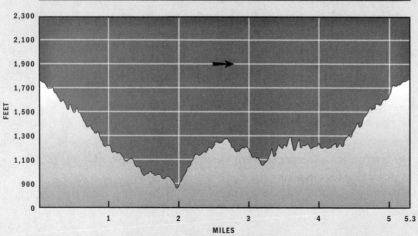

2,300
2,100
1,900
1,700
1,500
1,300
1,100
900
0

FEET

1   2   3   4   5 5.3

MILES

pleasant streams and to a secluded waterfall with a pool carved out of metamorphic bedrock.

The sign at the trailhead lists the mileages to points on this route: Wendell T. Robie Trail (0.8), Western States Trail via American Canyon (2.2), and Sliger Mine Road (3.9).

Hikers start under a canopy of foothill pine and Douglas fir among live oak, black oak, and buckeye. The trail's descent heightens the steepness of the hillside, dramatized by the tall firs and pines on both sides of the trail. The first trail that joins yours enters from above, to the left. It's just a connector leading from the community uphill.

In the spring, the scent of flowering buckeye follows you down the trail. Later in the summer, the blackberries are sure to delay your hike for a while. As you look to the right, don't be surprised if you meet the gaze of a turkey vulture playing chicken with the treetops. Along this doubletrack, you'll see trees growing horizontally from the hillside before they stretch up toward the sun.

As promised, Wendell T. Robie Trail meets your trail head-on at 0.8 mile, where you will make a U-turn to the right, heading downhill toward Sliger Mine Road. Sliger Mine is reported to have been the source of half the $5 million of gold mined in the Greenwood District. From 1848 to 1852, the creeks and canyons in Greenwood District filled with thousands of miners. Although it's difficult to tell now, your destination and areas around it were both the home and workplace of thousands of people as early as 1849. Nature has erased most of the evidence, but you can still see some of it in the form of walls, culverts, and ditches, as well as platforms and trails.

The next trail junction appears shortly—continue straight ahead as the broad trail narrows. Trail volunteers have made excellent progress in pushing back the poison oak along this next mile to the cascades. Scotch broom, ferns, mosses, and spiderwebs dominate the trail now. You're sure to see some firebellies as they make their way across the leaf litter covering the trail. These unflappable California newts are indeed slow, but no, they won't lie still while you take a picture of their bright-orange belly. Newts have toxins in their skin, so look but don't touch.

Continue heading north as these cheeky amphibians stare after you. Your next trail junction is a crossing of American Canyon Creek. Your trail will dip below abundant blackberry bushes as you approach this signed crossing. An ASRA sign will let you know your position both here and at the next crossing, of Hoboken Creek, less than 100 feet away. This area is also thick with firebellies—in the water, under rocks, and in the leaves. Watch your step.

As you walk above American Canyon Creek, the singletrack is lined with fairy lanterns and larkspur. This dirt-and-duff trail follows wherever the rock outcrops permit it. You emerge from the shade of live oak and manzanita to a hillside fragrant with bush lupine and deep purple larkspur.

A sign verifies your position at Dead Truck Trail—steeply uphill to the right. But here you have choices for a bit more adventure and exploring fun. Look to the left as you face the trail downhill: a side trail angles across the slope beneath you, leading to a real hidden treasure.

Following the trail in front of you downhill, you'll reach the lower section of this creek and then Poverty Bar on the river. Continue along the trail, and you'll soon cross to the west side of the creek. Your trail stays just above and 10 feet to the side of the creek as it descends by cascade and pool, stairstepping its way through the forest to the river. A right at the first trail junction will take you down to Poverty Bar.

If you forgo the river, then head down the trail on the slope below you, past the sedum-covered boulders, through the popcorn flowers and lupine, down to the sounds of water rushing below. When the pool first comes into view, the creek's waterfalls are still hidden to the left. Descend to the water level to get a good look up into the narrow cascades. Refresh, play, or photograph. Whenever you're ready, ascend to the trail junction above, catch your breath, and head up Dead Truck Trail, where you'll soon see the trail's namesake off to the left.

Why does the sign say STEEP? A clear example of truth in advertising. But it really isn't *that* steep, or long. No doubt you'll be glad when the brief climb is over, though. A beautiful vista point awaits as you top out along the ridge, which grants excellent views to the southeast over Hoboken Creek and up the canyon you originally descended.

The trail intersects the ubiquitous Wendell T. Robie Trail; turn right, toward Cool. Losing elevation seems unfair along here; judging from the trail's condition, the horses didn't like it either. Perhaps the mosquitoes will draw your attention away from the ruts. The path crosses one creek's washed-out footbridge before crossing the upended concrete culvert at Hoboken Creek.

Your trail is signed now with markers for the Western States Trail, which indicate that you're about 19 miles from Auburn. The annual horse race—the Western States "100 Miles–One Day" Trail Ride—was founded by Wendell T. Robie in 1955. The Wendell and Inez Robie Foundation currently helps support and maintain the trails and programs for trail users in the Tahoe and Foothills areas.

Fairy lanterns and irises line the trail as you enter and exit several small ravines without gaining or losing significant elevation. Keep to the right when you encounter any unsigned trails in the next 0.5 mile. When you come to a picturesque glade with a small cascade pooling at the trail crossing, head uphill to the right. Your homeward turn comes at an intersection about 500 feet ahead that you passed earlier. Making a left uphill will return you to the trailhead, about 1 mile away. If you're looking down as you trudge uphill, check out the pretty face all over the right bank.

NEARBY ACTIVITIES

Greenwood Pioneer Cemetery is right next to the south side of CA 193, about halfway between Cool and Georgetown. Many of the tombstones here date to the Gold Rush era.

40 WENDELL T. ROBIE TRAIL

KEY AT-A-GLANCE INFORMATION

LENGTH: 8.4 miles

CONFIGURATION: Out-and-back

DIFFICULTY: Challenging

WATER REQUIRED: 3 liters

SCENERY: Grand vistas of the Middle Fork of the American River

EXPOSURE: Nicely shaded

TRAIL TRAFFIC: Light

TRAIL SURFACE: Dirt and duff, rock

HIKING TIME: 3–4 hours

SEASON: Year-round, sunrise–sunset

ACCESS: No fees or permits

MAPS: USGS Greenwood; ASRA map

WHEELCHAIR ACCESS: None

FACILITIES: None

DRIVING DISTANCE: 50 miles

SPECIAL COMMENTS: Part race-course, part waterway; a hike for solitude

GPS TRAILHEAD COORDINATES

Latitude   N38° 57.011´

Longitude   W120° 55.845´

IN BRIEF

Wendell T. Robie Trail begins with blood-pumping switchbacks that boost hikers up above Cherokee Flat and around Summit Hill so they can contour along a historic mining flume with views overlooking the Middle Fork of the American River. Walk past some abandoned mining equipment, hardrock-mine shafts, and dry-stacked walls on this easy-to-follow trail, which leads to a cool, shaded crossing of

----

Directions ——————————————————→

From the junction of I-80 East and the Capital City Freeway, drive 25 miles on I-80 East toward Auburn and take Exit 119C/Elm Avenue. Turn left at the traffic light, onto Elm Avenue. At the bottom of the hill, turn left again, onto High Street. Drive 6 miles, traveling beneath the railroad overpass, descending the hill on CA 49, and turning right, across the CA 49 bridge toward Cool. Turn left in Cool on CA 193 toward Greenwood. Drive 6.2 miles to Sliger Mine Road, where you'll turn left. Continue left at the junction with Spanish Dry Diggins Road and bear left at the Spanish Dry Diggins Cemetery, which is surrounded by a white wire fence. In 0.3 mile, make a right where Foxglove Lane bears left. From here down, a high-clearance vehicle is advisable but not absolutely necessary. At the next flat spot, look in the bushes on the right for a sign indicating the Cherokee Flat Recreation Area. You can park here and walk or continue 0.6 mile downhill to the junction where Sliger Mine Road turns left. Some parking is available on the roadsides nearby.

The trailhead is marked with WESTERN STATES TRAIL and ROBIE TRAIL stickers on a bullet-riddled marker post that leans against a foothill pine on the right-hand side of the road. Sliger Mine Road turns left, directly away from this marker, and a four-wheel-drive road with an open gate continues downhill. Park hours are posted on a sign to the left.

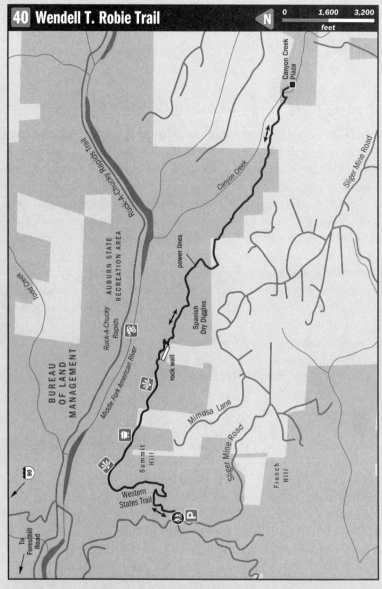

0   1,600   3,200
feet

N

Canyon Creek Plaza

Canyon Creek

Sliger Mine Road

Ruck-A-Chucky Rapids Trail

AUBURN STATE RECREATION AREA

power lines

Spanish Dry Diggins

rock wall

Todd Creek

Ruck-A-Chucky Rapids

Middle Fork American River

BUREAU OF LAND MANAGEMENT

Mimosa Lane

Sliger Mine Road

Summit Hill

French Hill

80

Western States Trail

To Foresthill Road

P

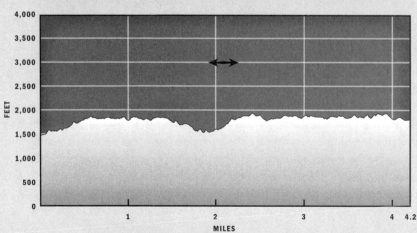

MILES

the wide, cobble-strewn Canyon Creek. Bring a picnic and insect repellent to this picturesque spot.

DESCRIPTION

From the trailhead signpost, the trail immediately climbs steeply up three serious switchbacks and continues uphill. When the dirt-and-duff trail levels out a bit, you can admire the handiwork of the trail builders whose stonework makes up the fills, walls, and culverts along here. In the early morning, deer can be seen navigating over boulders on their way uphill through thick stands of live oak and huge ponderosa pine. A few more switchbacks lead you past the 21.5-mile trail marker for the Western States Trail. You're now about 250 feet above the trail-head elevation, with a bit more to come.

Continue climbing for another 150 feet. A couple of switchbacks will get you oriented to traverse northwest around Summit Hill. Your track levels out at around 1,860 feet elevation, in the line of a former mining ditch. Now, with Douglas fir towering overhead to shade your flattened trail, get your camera ready for some fantastic vistas. Your well-worn path allows for some easy ambling, but don't ignore the pretty three-leaved plant at trailside. These red and/or green beauties may be the only color left on the trail by midsummer, but poison oak will ruin the rest of your day if you come in contact with it. Not to worry, though: squadrons of face flies will be constantly escorting you, taking your mind off the poison oak.

After rounding to the north-facing slope, you'll have hiked for perhaps 30 minutes. At 0.9 mile, upon reaching a large outcrop, the trees yield to reveal a panorama of the Middle Fork of the American River, 1,175 feet below and miles in either direction. Downstream lies the site of the Greenwood Bridge, just below Paradise Canyon's junction with the river. Across from your perch is the Ruck-A-Chucky Trail, leading from Drivers Flat Road to Slug Gulch and Fords Bar.

As you wind downhill for the next 10 or 15 minutes, you will (grudgingly) lose 300 of the feet that you gained earlier. They're relatively free of navigational obstacles, but when you're faced with trail choices on the way in, follow the track that heads left. Some of the trail markers have been imaginatively placed in trees, above your line of sight, so look around occasionally for stray signs. You've probably noticed the dry-laid rock walls above and below the trail. You may see a shallow cave or mine that was an impromptu quarry for the trail- and ditch-builders of the 1850s.

Before you reach the next vista point, you'll traverse a couple of ravines, which may be graced with water cascading across the trail. You may find other streams flowing out of seeps before they cross the path. If you linger, you may be fascinated by the flights of the water ouzel, or dipper, diving into the pools from moss-covered rocks. These water spots are, you may be sure, also visited nightly by critters galore. You can see the animal signs that line the center and margins of the trail (watch your step). Squirrel-sized tracks cross the dirt path and disappear into the uphill duff. This stretch of narrow canyon trail will stick in your memory due to the abundant and unavoidable signs of black bear and the distinctive scent of skunk.

Your descent tapers off at a vista point—a flat rock next to a madrone. Here, at about 1,560 feet elevation, you resume hiking in the line of the former ditch. As you avoid the poison oak along here, look for discarded mining and ditch-construction equipment on the left. Momentarily, you'll be directed around a large outcrop by means of a dry-laid stone wall. This wall, part of the flumeworks built to carry water from Canyon Creek, has withstood the test of time. A shaft dug into the outcrop on the right was evidently the source of the stone for this handcrafted wall. The Ruck-A-Chucky Rapids churn below here.

More switchbacks take you through some patches of blackberries, across a creek with some lovely cascades, and through some cuts in the rock. Another small stream in the ravine appears just after you pass the trail's 23.5-mile marker. The pools above Ruck-A-Chucky can be glimpsed from your trail in a few minutes. Within 5 minutes of sighting the pools, you'll pass under a trio of power lines.

The Middle Fork now changes direction, flowing down from the northeast as your trail remains on a southeast course under tall foothill pine, fragrant buckeye, and cool manzanita. Another creek, amid cool woodland shade, has pleasant cascades, and the water appears to slither across these very slippery rocks.

Another picturesque stream of water squeezes out of the greenstone, down a jumble of rocks and boulders, then into small pools—handy for cooling one's face. Scarlet monkeyflower flares alongside this small oasis of blackberries and fairy lanterns. Within 5 minutes, your trail will briefly ascend through red columbine. Watch for the path coming in from the right as yours starts to drop. Stay on the descending trail to the left. A trail marker lies just ahead on the right among the purple brodiaea.

Descend this wooded trail, zigzagging across a shallow creek atop very slippery rocks for the next hundred feet or so to the crossing at Canyon Creek. Crossing here offers no advantage to hikers. Exploring upstream on the south side takes you to some sunny, flat areas a few feet from the stream.

Take pictures along these sun-splattered wet rocks to remind yourself of this cool retreat when you get home. To beat the heat on the walk out, dip your hands in and take a faceful of cold, clear foothill refreshment. Your hike out retraces your steps.

41 RUCK-A-CHUCKY RAPIDS TRAIL

KEY AT-A-GLANCE INFORMATION

LENGTH: 6.4 miles

CONFIGURATION: Out-and-back

DIFFICULTY: Moderate

WATER REQUIRED: 3 liters

SCENERY: Middle Fork canyon and rapids

EXPOSURE: Very sunny

TRAIL TRAFFIC: Moderate

TRAIL SURFACE: Dirt and rock

HIKING TIME: 3–4 hours, depending on fishing time

SEASON: Year-round

ACCESS: $10 day-use fee. Stop at the self-pay station at the Driver's Flat staging area.

MAPS: USGS Greenwood, Georgetown

WHEELCHAIR ACCESS: None

FACILITIES: Picnic table, parking, pit toilet, and trash receptacle at both Ruck-A-Chucky Campground and trailhead

DRIVING DISTANCE: 40 miles

SPECIAL COMMENTS: High-clearance vehicles are best but not required for descending Drivers Flat Road. This trail ends at a broad, rocky beach below a lazy stretch of the Middle Fork. Slug Gulch, only 1,000 feet before the beach, makes for an easy side exploration.

GPS TRAILHEAD COORDINATES

Latitude   N38° 57.663´
Longitude   W120° 55.318´

IN BRIEF

This trail leads past the churning rapids of the Middle Fork of the American River, along the margins of a foothill-woodland forest. The trail is largely level, staying above the river until about a mile before Ford's Bar. Stop at Slug Gulch to explore, or continue along to fish or swim in the pools leading up to Ford's Bar.

DESCRIPTION

The trip really starts up on Drivers Flat Road as you crawl down the slope—hugging the inside of every curve. But assuming you arrived safely at the trailhead, you can rest easy because this hike is no sweat. There are long stretches in the sun, but you won't have to contend with lengthy hills to grind up or navigation problems to solve. There are gold-mining relics and sites along the way, so put your wandering shoes on and head upstream.

The Middle Fork plows through and over the solid bedrock about 100 feet below you as you start out. Right away you'll pass the wreckage of the Greenwood Bridge—one of the casualties of the flooding after the Hell Hole Dam failed as its reservoir was first filling in 1964—

Directions

From the junction of I-80 East and the Capital City Freeway, drive 26 miles on I-80 East toward Auburn and take Exit 121/Foresthill Road. Turn right and drive 8 miles, crossing the Foresthill Bridge, to Drivers Flat Road on the right at Eight Mile Curve. Drive slowly down this 5-mile road to the river, and ford Gas Creek just before you pass Ruck-A-Chucky Campground. Drive another 0.1 mile to the day-use parking area, which has a pit toilet and a trash receptacle. Your trailhead is 100 feet to the east, at the open gate.

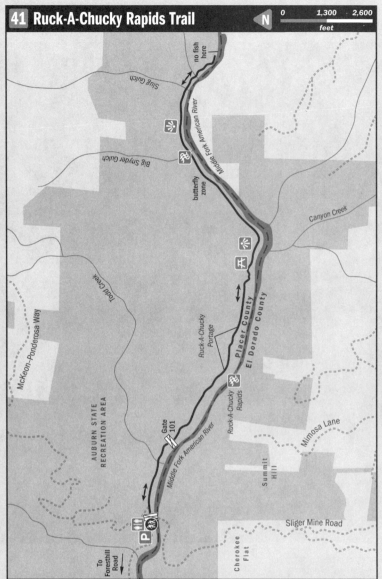

N

0   1,300   2,600
feet

no fish here

Slug Gulch

Middle Fork American River

Big Snyder Gulch

butterfly zone

Canyon Creek

Todd Creek

McKeon–Ponderosa Way

Placer County

El Dorado County

Ruck-A-Chucky Portage

Ruck-A-Chucky Rapids

Mimosa Lane

AUBURN STATE RECREATION AREA

Gate 101

Summit Hill

Middle Fork American River

Sliger Mine Road

P

Cherokee Flat

To Foresthill Road

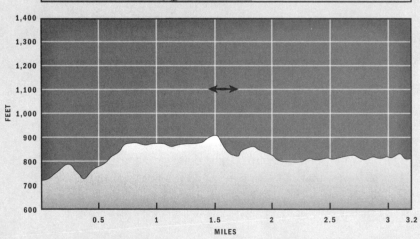

FEET							
1,400							
1,300							
1,200							
1,100							
1,000							
900							
800							
700							
600							

0.5   1   1.5   2   2.5   3   3.2

MILES

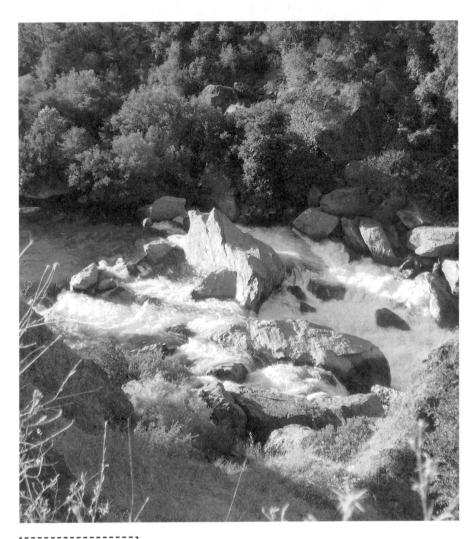

Ruck-A-Chucky Rapids

so you may have some idea of the power that water has as it sweeps downstream. Look at your trail occasionally and imagine how the sand came to be up there.

Your trail is a doubletrack that runs along the Western States Trail route from Lake Tahoe to Auburn. For the first mile, your trail ascends or maintains elevation above the river. A few Class III and IV rapids lend drama to the river scene beneath you. From a distance you can hear the roar of Ruck-A-Chucky Rapids—portaged by everyone on the river. Where a stand of live oak to your right suddenly stops, look below to see the portage trail around Ruck-A-Chucky Falls. The trail drops straight down to it—or up from it—right at the live oak.

The trail descends slightly closer to the river while a side trail drops all the way down to a conveniently located picnic table and the river just below it. Walk past the picnic table, and the trail becomes a singletrack as a beautiful pool appears in the river ahead. The air along here is filled in spring with the fragrance of the flowering buckeye, which grows among the shady, cool, smooth-barked madrone.

The oak trees along the trail are festooned with the vines of wild grapes, inviting you to dally and snack in the late summer. In the early summer, huge clusters of bush monkeyflower sweep down the slopes and crossing the trail on their way to the river. Bumblebees and California sister butterflies work over the patches fairly methodically, missing not a single blossom.

Ruck-A-Chucky Trail continues downhill a bit along a rocky patch. The river below is shallower, clearly exposing all sizes of cobble and gravel. If you haven't already filled up on grapes, sample the blackberries that are plentiful on both sides of the trail.

The trail continues to be distinct and well maintained through this second mile. Notice the copious amounts of sand on the path and the occasional cluster of debris in the trees. Imagine the power of the river that caused that debris and sand to land in the branches of trees and on the trail, some 50 feet above the water.

Still on a singletrack, drop down next to the river through this foothill-woodland community. Foothill pine, madrone, toyon, live oak, manzanita, and laurel abound on these hillsides. Sedges line the trail, and canyon or sawtooth ferns cling to moist seeps along the slope above you. Grapevines hang from moist out-croppings or manzanita bushes above you. The trail becomes a butterfly zone among the thick blackberries. You will enter and quickly exit a small ravine, with some pleasant cascades above you. Next to you, the river narrows and turns east.

The trail remains sandy and sticks close to the river, which appears to be only 2 feet deep and 100 feet wide now. Boulders the size of a small apartment line the river as you continue along the now-rocky trail. Watching the trail as it becomes chunkier is hard to do because the wildflowers are thick along here. Brodiaea, monkeyflower, penstemon, wandering daisy, and more grapes and blackberries greet you at Slug Gulch, where miners were reported to have found gold nuggets as large as slugs in the early days of the Gold Rush.

The waters in Slug Gulch spill across polished greenstone before tumbling over broken rocks on the way to the river. Climb up the side and over the bed-rock, which sits under the cascade, to reach a plateau that hundreds of miners before you have worked. To the left, hand-laid walls are clear evidence of the ter-raforming that miners undertook to move around the streambed. Walls, trails, platforms, and waterwheel pools are crammed into this tight ravine.

Climb to the upriver side of the creek, where a huge display of rockwork cov-ers the hillside. As you explore the paths, try to ascertain whether method or mad-ness governed this construction. A huge clue to this area's attraction lies in the rock, which is deeply ingrained with veins of white, ore-bearing quartz—still visible along the ravine's walls. The pools of the stream are great for cooling your heels after touring the mining operations. When you feel rested and ready for more trail or fish, descend to the path and continue another 0.5–1 mile—the choice is yours.

Broad, rocky bars line the river from here to Ford's Bar. Swimming in these calm pools is exhilarating—mostly because of the zero-degree water, and the hot sun feels great and dries anything in minutes. Make sure you're wearing a hat before lazing on these bars. The sun also *bakes* anything—heads, especially—in those few minutes. If you plan to fish, this is a superb spot to relax while you wet a line. If you plan on actually *catching* fish, there may be better spots, but that just means another hike. Ah well.

If you missed any photo opportunities on the way in, the river's orientation and changing light will give the scene an entirely different aspect as you return to the trailhead via your original route.

FORESTHILL DIVIDE LOOP TRAIL 42

IN BRIEF

Meadows with wildflowers galore and trails winding through foothill-woodland forests provide the backdrop to this pleasantly shaded hike. It's long enough that you'll break a sweat, but you won't have any difficulty staying on-route, with only minor elevation gain and loss.

DESCRIPTION

This loop's reputation as one of the best all-around hiking trails in the Auburn State Recreation Area is well deserved. Foresthill Divide Loop Trail has a number of access points along the way, so hikers can choose to take shorter versions or start from different points. You will start at the largest of four trailheads on Foresthill Road. Park near Gate 128, Eight Mile Curve, which is your trailhead.

Step over the pass-through and walk straight ahead, with the picnic table to your left, toward the pit toilet and trash receptacles. Your trail is the sand-and-dirt singletrack that heads left. It's immediately evident that your trail is shared with nonhikers. Farther along, the trail is generally smooth dirt, duff, or gravel. It does suffer from ruts in some areas, but it has been protected from ruts in other, sensitive areas.

A wildflower guide and a pair of light gaiters are excellent gear for this trail. As you

KEY AT-A-GLANCE INFORMATION

LENGTH: 10 miles

CONFIGURATION: Loop

DIFFICULTY: Challenging

WATER REQUIRED: 4 liters

SCENERY: Foothill-woodland forest; spectacular springtime wildflower displays in the open meadows and along trails

EXPOSURE: Shaded more than half the time

TRAIL TRAFFIC: Heavy on weekends

TRAIL SURFACE: Dirt and duff, rock and gravel

HIKING TIME: 5 hours

SEASON: Year-round, sunrise–sunset

ACCESS: No fees or permits

MAPS: USGS Greenwood; ASRA trail map

WHEELCHAIR ACCESS: None

FACILITIES: Picnic table and pit toilet at the trailhead

DRIVING DISTANCE: 33 miles

SPECIAL COMMENTS: The first half of this trail is bordered by poison oak, which is incredibly thick in places. Watch where you step when you sniff the wildflowers.

Directions

From the junction of I-80 East and the Capital City Freeway, drive 26 miles on I-80 East toward Auburn and take Exit 121/Foresthill Road. Drive 8.1 miles on Foresthill Road to the large parking lot on the left, just 0.2 mile after Drivers Flat Road. The trailhead is the gate marked #128—EIGHT MILE CURVE.

GPS TRAILHEAD COORDINATES

Latitude   N38° 58.440´

Longitude   W120° 57.243´

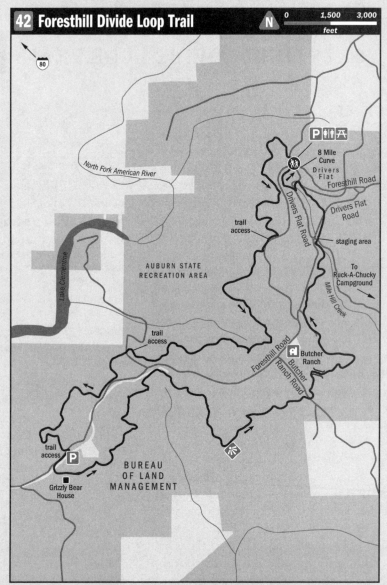

42 Foresthill Divide Loop Trail

N

0   1,500   3,000
feet

80

North Fork American River

8 Mile Curve

Drivers Flat

Drivers Flat Road

Foresthill Road

Drivers Flat Road

trail access

staging area

To Ruck-A-Chucky Campground

Mile Hill Creek

AUBURN STATE RECREATION AREA

Lake Clementine

trail access

Foresthill Road

Butcher Ranch Road

Butcher Ranch

trail access

P

Grizzly Bear House

BUREAU OF LAND MANAGEMENT

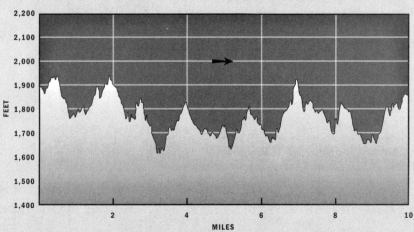

FEET

2,200
2,100
2,000
1,900
1,800
1,700
1,600
1,500
1,400

2   4   6   8   10

MILES

head into the forest cover of toyon, foothill pine, live oak, and manzanita, look down to the sides of the trail at the vast swaths of poison oak.

This is somewhat of a cruel irony in that the wildflowers—both beautiful and fragrant—are surrounded by the oily-leafed plant. Staying on the trail will pay off. The flowers you see among the madrone and buckeye—lupine, iris, globe lily, poppy, star tulip, buttercup, blue dicks, pretty face—all appear along the length of your hike.

As your trail heads generally south, you'll have occasional views of the North Fork as it flows into Lake Clementine. In midautumn, the display of colors along this trail into the North Fork is spectacular.

Throughout the ASRA, signs warn of the danger of mountain lions. This trail is no exception. About the time you read the second warning (the one with bullet holes in it, next to one that says NO SHOOTING), try to sight a couple of very large foothill pines towering above the black oak. Just after these trees, at about 2.2 miles, an open hillside displays its colorful treasures—clover, buttercup, baby lupine, and vetch.

Evidence of bike traffic is fairly noticeable, but some interesting effort has gone into prevention, including caution signs and protection in the form of "tree armor," such as the garbage-can wrapper on a live oak. The trail meanders up and down and in and out of ravines. Additions to the flora now include white fir and the white globe lily—both growing on the uphill side.

Sierra lily and whiteleaf manzanita announce an opening in the forest to reveal a view over Lake Clementine. When the trail breaks out of the trees at about 3.25 miles, the open hillside appears spotted and striped with the blue and violet of blue dicks and lupine.

Continue across the gravel road leading to Upper Lake Clementine and walk through the grove of madrone, but stay on the trail. The forest floor surrounding the madrone, and as far as you can see downhill, is poison oak. Don't be alarmed if you happen to hear gunfire from the nearby target range. At the next fork, stay to the left, pass a broad, colorful meadow, and then reach Foresthill Road, where you will cross.

Cross the road a bit to the left of your exit, then walk through the fence to the right. Your trail heads southwest to skirt the oak-covered knoll above your left shoulder. The open vista of meadows, covered with blue and white flowers waving in the wind, is a welcome change of view.

At the next junction with a trail from the right, a sign indicates that you're on the correct trail and that Drivers Flat is 5 miles straight ahead. Over the next mile, glimpse the Middle Fork of the American River 800 feet below.

A trail sign will lead you to the left and down a rocky doubletrack, which exposes vertically oriented mudstone. You'll walk across a few hundred feet of mudstone—about 500,000 years of accumulated alluvial deposits—all turned on edge and surrounded by baby lupine, which yields to larger varieties, joined by buttercups.

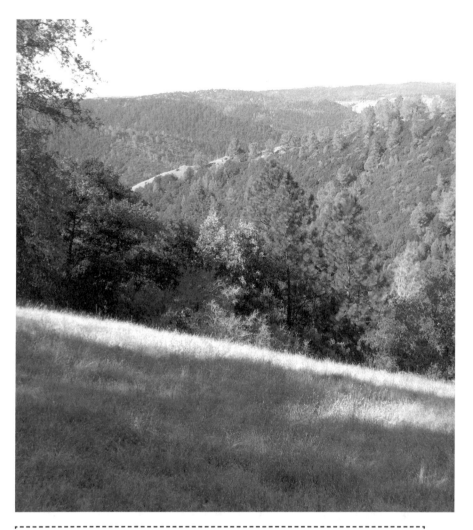

As you look west from Foresthill Divide, Auburn and the confluence are visible on the horizon.

Walking in and out of the ravines, you'll feel grateful for the wet areas that sport gatherings of sierra lily. If you lose your way along here, just follow the fragrant ceanothus. Pretty face and sierra iris abound, and a trail sign indicates that you need to abandon the level jeep road to descend to the right, through more buttercups and lupine and past an enormous black oak. As the trail turns into rocky singletrack, you'll reach Mile Marker 6.

Butterflies feast everywhere around this trail, and if you watch the trail closely, you can see caterpillars moving across it. You'll occasionally see signs of smaller mammals along the dirt-and-duff trail, where they've feasted on the cones of foothill pines—often leaving surprisingly large piles of cone scales and whittled-down stems.

Within 0.75 mile, you'll have an excellent view down into the Middle Fork. You'll soon cross some wide-open meadows, which continue to boast a colorful assortment of flowers already seen, along with a number of grasses. The trail is now a singletrack through the grass.

When you encounter a doubletrack, turn left onto it. A few hundred feet along, turn right at the trail sign. Cross the bridge in this area, cooled by the boughs of the live oak spreading across the trail. At the next split, the choice is yours. If you turn left at the next trail sign onto a dirt doubletrack, you'll head through some fire-scarred manzanita and downed trees toward Foresthill Road, visible from this vantage.

Descending 0.5 mile from this vista delivers you to a gate on the left, numbered 127 and signed BUTCHER REPEATER ROAD. This road continues within your sight for another 0.5 mile to the Drivers Flat Road staging area. Turn away from the sign and continue on your trail, mindful that in about 500 feet it will join the road for another 350 feet before oozing off to the right again, rambling loosely alongside the road. Deer prints are all over the area as you pass a ranch gate that appears to have rusted open. Before the track splits again, you'll pass through a copse of live oak. Stay on the singletrack, which delivers you to the Drivers Flat Road staging area and Gate 126, signed MILE HILL CREEK. The road to the right leads to the Ruck-A-Chucky Campground. Walk across the parking area toward the pit toilet. Your trail continues at the sign just past the recycling station.

Sierra irises decorate the flanks of your trail, which passes two interesting but dead giants. On the left of the trail and perpendicular to it is a fallen foothill pine that is just beginning its return to the soil. Compare this one with the same species 100 feet along, on the right.

Wind your way along the bike trail as it grinds and twists its way up the hill beside Drivers Flat Road. Your trailhead is at the top of the hill and across the road.

NEARBY ACTIVITIES

The Ruck-A-Chucky Rapids Trail (see previous profile) begins at the base of Drivers Flat Road and leads to picturesque Slug Gulch, where the gold that was pried out of the rocks was "as big as slugs," according to those who were first to stake their claim.

43   CODFISH FALLS TRAIL

KEY AT-A-GLANCE INFORMATION

LENGTH: 3 miles

CONFIGURATION: Out-and-back

DIFFICULTY: Easy

WATER REQUIRED: 1 liter

SCENERY: Riparian woodland

EXPOSURE: In and out of shade and sun

TRAIL TRAFFIC: Moderate

TRAIL SURFACE: Dirt and duff

HIKING TIME: 1.5–2 hours

SEASON: Year-round, sunrise–sunset

ACCESS: $10 self-registration on north side of bridge

MAPS: USGS Colfax, Greenwood; ASRA trail map

WHEELCHAIR ACCESS: None

FACILITIES: Pit toilets and trash receptacles at parking area; pit toilets also along the trail

DRIVING DISTANCE: 40.5 miles

SPECIAL COMMENTS: The interpretive trail pamphlet was written and illustrated by Heather Mehl, a graduate of Colfax High School, for a senior project in 2001.

GPS TRAILHEAD COORDINATES

Latitude   N39° 00.016´

Longitude   W120° 56.420´

IN BRIEF

This is either a great hike with a wonderful swim at the end or a fantastic swim with a sweet hike. Either way, the hike leads you to a beautiful 40-foot waterfall with lovely pools beneath smaller cascades. Codfish Falls Trail is an easy trail with interpretive signs along a scenic section of the North Fork of the American River.

DESCRIPTION

Start for the trailhead by following the wildly curvy, dust-laden Ponderosa Way. Your view to the bottom of the canyon is unimpeded by guardrails as the road hugs the slope. As you approach the river, the bridge across the North Fork comes into view. It's amazing that the bridge is still standing, but yes, you can drive across it. And it's another good story to tell.

Park next to the river as the signs direct. Your trailhead is at end of the bridge next to the gate. The trail is visible from here, skirting the base of the slope to your right as you head downriver. The broad beach to your left

----

Directions ⎯⎯⎯⎯⎯⎯⎯⎯⎯⎯⎯→

From the junction of I-80 East and the Capital City Freeway, drive 26 miles on I-80 East toward Auburn and take Exit 121/Foresthill Road. Cross the Foresthill Bridge and drive 11 miles toward Foresthill. Turn left on Ponderosa Way, then bear right at the junction with Eagle Ridge Road. The pavement ends in 0.2 mile. Drive cautiously down this dust-coated road 3.3 miles and cross the bridge to the parking area. (Ponderosa Way can also be reached via Exit 131/Weimar Cross Road off I-80 East.) High-clearance vehicles are not required, but low-clearance vehicles are not suggested.

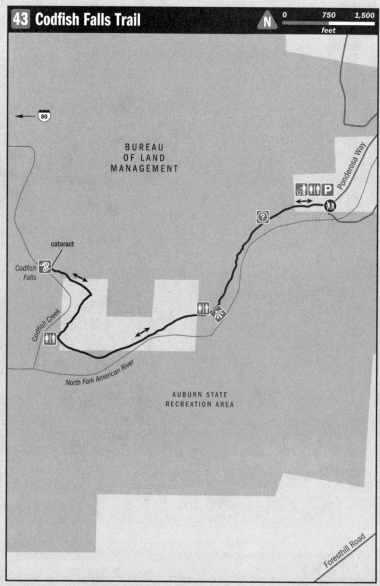

0   750   1,500
feet

80 ←

BUREAU
OF LAND
MANAGEMENT

Ponderosa Way

cataract

Codfish
Falls

Codfish Creek

North Fork American River

AUBURN STATE
RECREATION AREA

Foresthill Road

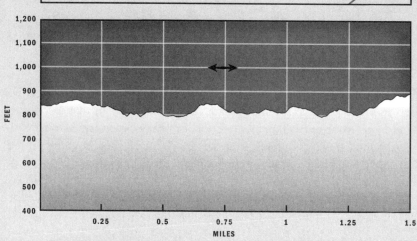

1,200
1,100
1,000
900
800
700
600
500
400

FEET

0.25   0.5   0.75   1   1.25   1.5

MILES

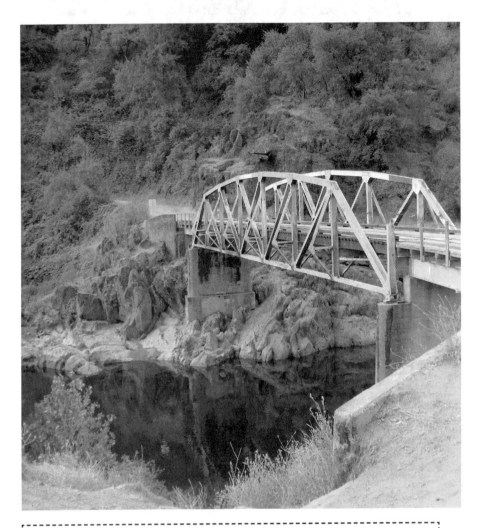

One lane, no jumping: the Ponderosa Way Bridge spans the North Fork of the American River about 4 miles below Yankee Jim's.

tempts you as you pass it on the way to the falls. If you have the will to keep walking past this great swimming spot, your sandy trail follows the beach's perimeter, then heads up to a dirt-and-duff trail.

The red-berried toyon on your left hides the view for a moment as you pass a hillside of buttercups and wally baskets on your right. In about 1,000 feet you will find a kiosk with, if your timing is right, informative leaflets that describe the flora and fauna to be seen along the trail. Codfish Falls Discovery Trail marks 14 individual points of natural interest over the next 1.2 miles. Refer to the pamphlet for descriptive text and illustrations corresponding to each marker.

Your view of the river comes and goes as the manzanita thins and thickens, alternating with clusters of foothill-pine saplings. The rock-and-dirt trail squirms around a huge shale outcropping as you look down on exposed bedrock in the river channel. Adding to the color surrounding the trail are splotches of red and green poison oak. Although the poison oak is quite pretty, don't admire it too closely. The shooting stars growing a bit farther on will better satisfy your senses.

Buckeye trees scent the trail, while tall Douglas firs shade it. Live oak and foothill pine help fill in any hot spots with their own shadows. At a wide vista point, you can look across the river to see the mounds of cobble left over from the dredging operations along here. This spot seems to be popular with animals of the riparian zone. Notice the signs of raccoon and skunk along or in the trail, including bird remains scattered among the kit-kit-dizze and poison oak. The occasional ponderosa pine breaks up the skyline as you continue walking along the river, heading southwest. You may not even notice the pit toilet concealed on the uphill side of the trail. Knock first to give critters time to slither out the side door.

Blocked by a large gravel bar, the river is pushed across to your side of the canyon. The trail, surrounded by manzanita, becomes spiderweb central for a few hundred feet. As you're flailing your arms to clear the silk, look down onto the scour zone, where trees are toppled sideways parallel to the water. Enjoy the next vista from the deep shade of the cool-skinned madrone and towering Douglas fir.

Under cover of black oak, Douglas fir, and foothill pine, your trail begins to turn away from the river and northwest for a few hundred feet. As you approach the 1-mile point, you'll see another pit toilet, well hidden among the bay laurel and poison oak, to your left on the river's side of the trail. After turning northward, you will see two fir trees—a large one on the right and a thinner one on the left. About 10 feet up in the larger tree is a white-and-blue handwritten sign that reads, DEDICATED TO RUTH MCKEE AND HELEN WAUTERS AND TO ALL OF THOSE WHO SHARE THE JOY OF NATURE, 4-19-94.

Search the ground in this area and you'll likely see some type of reptile. A ringneck snake is apt to curl up and display its fearsome red tail as a warning. These snakes are fairly slow, so you may get to see this more than once. And you can't help but hear the tree frogs as you examine this moist, shady area.

The streams may be spilling over their banks as you make your way through blackberry patches and over broken rocks. Cascades to your right make it appear that miners reworked the stream's original course. Pools, dams, and rubble piles all seem to indicate that some level of mining activity occurred here.

The stream crossings are easy, although you may get wet feet in early spring. Another stream comes from the right to join Codfish Creek. Almost immediately, a trail on the right ascends, leading you to the top of the falls. From here you can bushwhack farther up the creek to explore near the Old Vore Mine. In less than 100 feet, you'll be at the base of the 45-foot Codfish Falls.

Cascading over bedrock into pools at your feet, the water feeds an abundance of lush greenery. The Indian rhubarb hides everything but the bay laurel. Mosses and ferns cover the rocks on the periphery of the stream. Depending on the season, you may be able to hop across these refrigerator-sized boulders. Below you, a few small pools merge into one when the water is rushing. Water ouzels,

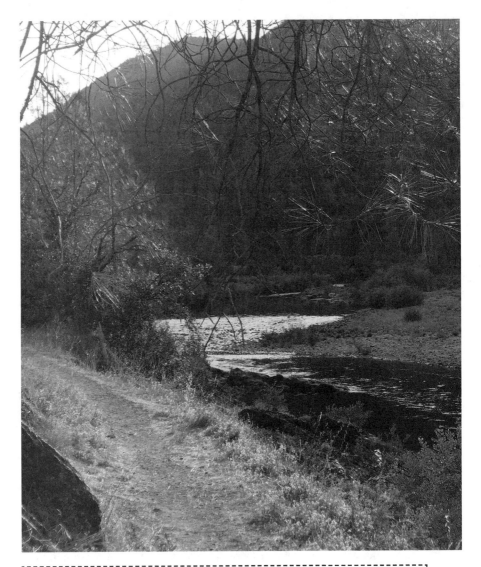

The current slows in this meandering stretch, where past gold-mining activity remains visible.

also known as dippers, peek out to grab at insects that are invisible to hikers. They must be tasty, because the robin-sized birds keep at it quite awhile.

Your trail returns via the beach you saw on the way in. After exploring the falls from top to bottom, you've earned a swim at the trailhead, if you haven't had one already.

NEARBY ACTIVITIES

Whitewater-rafting trips on the Middle Fork often originate in nearby Foresthill. Contact O.A.R.S. to arrange your own wet adventure at **oars.com**.

NORTH FORK MIDDLE FORK AMERICAN RIVER TRAIL

IN BRIEF

This trail offers easy access to a beautiful section of the American River. The gravels were worked by miners, and their imprint is faintly visible to this day. You will pass the campsites and debris of former miners and the current camps of present-day gold seekers. Aside from a few dicey spots, the trail is enjoyable all the way to the calm pools above El Dorado Canyon, where it feels like it's just you and the river.

DESCRIPTION

The Middle Fork of the American River, which flows here, above Oxbow Reservoir, has smoothed over its Gold Rush–era scars in the 150 years since the hillsides and streambeds were torn apart by hydraulic mining. The lush vegetation has regrown, and the force of the river has removed most of the waste and silts. The river itself has reclaimed the channels that were given over to sluice, flume, and water-wheel. Thousands of fortune-seekers once lived on the Middle Fork, where they worked gold claims individually or as part of a group.

Your trail begins on the east side of the road at the signed trailhead. The trail heads north, parallel to the road, as it climbs over some talus and boulders of the outcrop above you. Duck behind some manzanita, live oak,

KEY AT-A-GLANCE INFORMATION

LENGTH: 2.2 miles

CONFIGURATION: Out-and-back

DIFFICULTY: Moderate

WATER REQUIRED: 1 liter

SCENERY: Wild and Scenic River canyon, foothill woodland

EXPOSURE: Brief sun exposure

TRAIL TRAFFIC: Light

TRAIL SURFACE: Duff, dirt, and rock

HIKING TIME: 2 hours

SEASON: Year-round

ACCESS: No fees or permits

MAPS: USGS Michigan Bluff; Tahoe National Forest map at the ranger station in Foresthill

WHEELCHAIR ACCESS: None

FACILITIES: Limited roadside parking at trailhead, more across bridge

DRIVING DISTANCE: 52 miles

SPECIAL COMMENTS: The trail crosses steep hillsides on a narrow track where sure footing and balance are required. Trekking poles are particularly helpful on this hike.

Directions ⟶

From the junction of I-80 East and the Capital City Freeway, drive 26 miles on I-80 East toward Auburn and take Exit 121/Foresthill Road. Then drive 16.7 miles to Foresthill and turn right on Mosquito Ridge Road. Go 9.5 miles to the signed trailhead on the left after Circle Bridge, and park on the right.

GPS TRAILHEAD COORDINATES

Latitude   N39° 01.368´

Longitude   W120° 43.213´

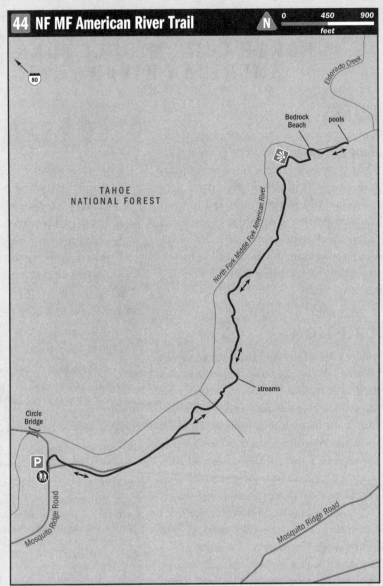

N

0   450   900
feet

80

Eldorado Creek

Bedrock Beach   pools

TAHOE
NATIONAL FOREST

North Fork Middle Fork American River

streams

Circle
Bridge

P

Mosquito Ridge Road

Mosquito Ridge Road

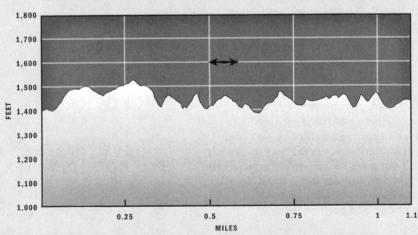

1,800
1,700
1,600
1,500
1,400
1,300
1,200
1,100
1,000

FEET

0.25   0.5   0.75   1   1.1

MILES

and Douglas fir on your way around the corner and up past a level spot offering a vista. Your trail turns east with the river, and you can see the miners' camp below on the water. The trail turns again just as you figure out the model of car that settled backward in the trees about 20 feet down the slope.

A steep slope drops to the left of your trail, which is surrounded by Douglas fir, incense cedar, live oak, and Kellogg black oak. A bay laurel crowds the trail near an imposing, fire-charred ponderosa pine as you walk along this exposed section of slippery dirt-and-pebble-covered path. You'll ascend just about 100 feet in the first 0.3 mile, then contour along to nearly the trail's end.

The hills surrounding the river are covered with glacial till, most noticeable because it forms the benches 100 feet or so above the river. This geologic characteristic was the feature that drew gold miners to the Sierra Nevada foothills in the first place. Frequent seeps or springs, often good indicators of a glacial past, are seen along this trail. Vegetation is abundant in both number and variety; the thickly forested hillsides host several types of upper-, mid-, and understory trees and plants.

The trail is often covered with the scree from outcrops of slates, granites, and quartz, which are components of the Shoo Fly Complex. Originally deposited as sediments from alluvial runoff, the rocks of the Shoo Fly Complex were pushed out from the ancient continent, buried, and transformed. Then they were pushed inland, squeezed by tectonic forces, thrust vertically upward, and finally turned 90 degrees, where we find them today. Along the way, molten quartz and granite intruded and now appear as thick gray or white bands.

After nearly 0.5 mile, your trail veers uphill on a new tread to avoid a tree wreck in the upcoming ravine. Although the walking is easy, experience is useful. Trekking poles will aid your balance on slippery spots. Cascades bounce across the trail in the rainy season but should not be difficult to cross. Just remember that the rocks are wet.

The trail is situated on soil that has slumped away from the hillside, sliding down about 6 feet. This is apparent when you look at the uphill side of the trail along the first 0.25 mile. After a particularly rainy season in the future, this trail will lower dramatically as more of the hillside slumps. You'll pass outcrops of bedrock slates and sandstones; the trail is littered with their scree and rubble. After 0.5 mile you'll walk below a scree-covered slope dotted with bay-laurel trees and bushes. Live and black oaks have shed their leaves here to form a dense mat of duff. Ponderosa pines are scattered across the slope, battling for space with Douglas fir and incense cedar. Amid the trees and bushes lies the colorful tri-leaved poison oak—ubiquitous, if not seemingly mandatory, on all foothill trails.

Along the bare dirt sections of the trail, you can easily discern the tracks of several mammals, which wander along the trail briefly, cross it momentarily, mark it as territory, or dine on it. Animal tracks and signs include black bear, fox, coyote, raccoon, deer, skunk, and squirrel.

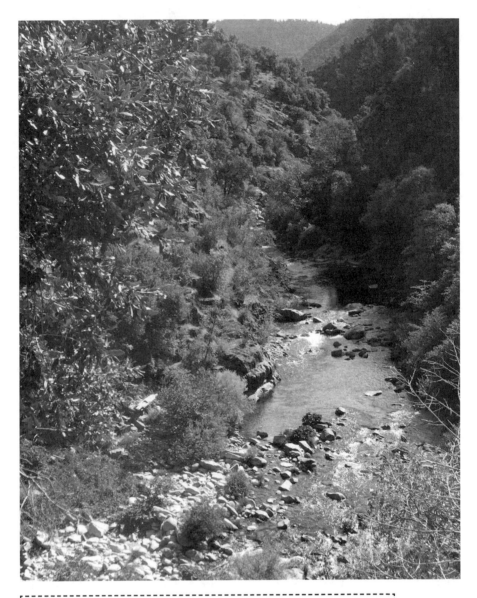

This stretch of the NFMF is about 10 miles downriver from the Deadwood mining area.

Cross a rock shelf right after the outcrop. The trail is exposed for about 5 minutes. When you reach a solitary knobcone pine at 0.9 mile, continue ahead slightly uphill to the right. The knobcone is an easily identifiable pine because it never releases its cones. They stay tucked adjacent to the trunk until the seeds are released—released by fire, which, ironically, destroys the tree, which is not fire-resistant like its Douglas-fir neighbors.

When you see a large madrone with two unusual lower limbs—one turns west, the other south—you'll be near the river overlook. A trail cuts directly through the

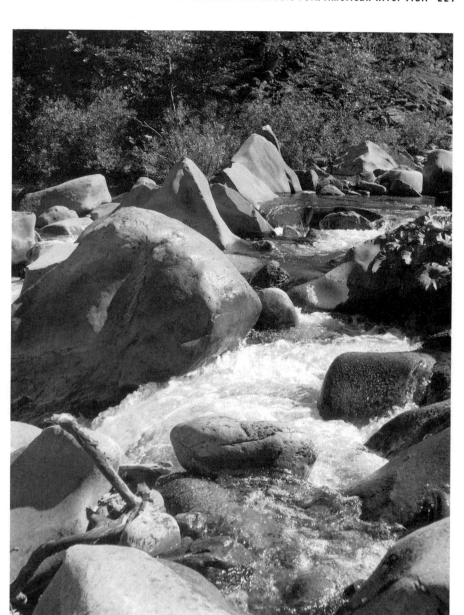

By late summer the snowmelt has abated, leaving more of these riverbound boulders exposed.

hillside on the left and leads down to the river. Keep walking another 75 feet to a prominent lookout with a great vista of the river's riffles and pools below.

You can descend to the river by walking away from the hearth area to the right, following the cliff side to the river. Steps have been cut in the rock, which makes this an easy descent, if you move cautiously. (Remember those trekking poles?) The steps are often dirt-covered and can be slippery.

As you approach the river, climb over the bedrock, back toward the cliff face. Low water levels reveal how the rock has been shaped by the water and how the water has been channeled by the rock. You can judge the river's gradient by looking across the pools upstream from here.

Calm pools await those who scramble upstream on the unmaintained trail toward El Dorado Canyon. Squeeze between the bedrock and a bigleaf maple on the left, then pass some mining debris. Pipes on the left and a sluice grate on the right, along with drill holes in the rock, testify to the past activity here. Amid boulders the size of a compact car, a rusted steel cable leads down the last 10 feet to the river.

About 200 feet shy of the mouth of El Dorado Creek, on the left at El Dorado Canyon, the large, flat rocks in the center of the river are perfect for viewing the characteristic geology of the Middle Fork. Look over to the other side of the river, where you can follow the rock forms right under your feet and on the other side of the canyon. The upturned, folded, blackened, and rotated metamorphic rock has been polished to a shine by the water. It stands like gigantic reams of paper on end—slightly flexed and bowed with quartz and granitic intrusions—making it very easy to follow across the chasm as it continues uninterrupted under the water to the south side of the river.

The pools here are slow and cool on hot late-summer afternoons. With rocks to linger on and no rafts coming from above, you may want to relax awhile before you return via the trail you came down.

NEARBY ACTIVITIES

This easy trail to the river is an introduction to the majestic beauty in the wild reaches of the Middle Fork. However, 2,000 feet above you is the Big Gun Diggings. Hydraulic mining was the man-made disaster that nearly undercut the town of Michigan City and caused it to be moved in 1859. Michigan Bluff, as it is now known, was the embarkation point for pack trains carrying supplies across the rugged canyon to the towns of Deadwood and Last Chance. To visit these sites, follow the Michigan Bluff–Deadwood Trail (Hike 45 in the first edition of this guidebook).

YANKEE JIM'S– INDIAN CREEK TRAIL

IN BRIEF

This trail leaves swimmers and boaters behind at the bridge while leading hikers on an easy walk through shaded hillsides awash in colorful wildflower displays. You'll be treated to crystal-clear pools on the river, plus secluded pools and a waterfall upstream on Indian Creek.

DESCRIPTION

Wherever you end up parking, make your way to the cables on the east end of the bridge. Some wooden-post stairs leading downhill to the north will take you in the right direction. Wander around the old mining-camp foundations and platforms. There were thousands of people working placer deposits here in the 1850s. Old photos show an alarming environmental free-for-all, but apparently nature has reclaimed and erased many of the historic scenes.

Remember that your path is north, or upriver. You need to cross Shirttail Creek right off the bat. To avoid getting bogged down in the sand and cobble on the sun-drenched river's edge, keep about 100 feet away from the river

----

Directions

From the junction of I-80 East and the Capital City Freeway, drive 38 miles on I-80 East toward Colfax. Take Exit 133/Canyon Way, turn right onto Canyon Way, and drive 0.7 mile to Yankee Jim's Road. Slowly head downhill 5 miles to the river. Alternatively, drive 26 miles on I-80 East to Exit 121/Foresthill Road in Auburn and then 17 miles to the town of Foresthill. Turn left onto Gold Street and, at the fork, take the left branch onto Yankee Jim's Road. Drive 8 miles to the bridge. Parking is available at either end of the bridge. The trailhead is at the bottom of the steps, on the east side of the bridge.

KEY AT-A-GLANCE INFORMATION

LENGTH: 3 miles

CONFIGURATION: Out-and-back

DIFFICULTY: Moderate

WATER REQUIRED: 2 liters

SCENERY: River vistas and wildflowers

EXPOSURE: Largely shaded trail, exposed on river

TRAIL TRAFFIC: Light

TRAIL SURFACE: Dirt and duff

HIKING TIME: 3 hours

SEASON: Year-round, sunrise–sunset

ACCESS: No fees or permits

MAPS: USGS Colfax

WHEELCHAIR ACCESS: None

FACILITIES: Pit toilet and trash receptacles at trailhead

DRIVING DISTANCE: 46 miles

SPECIAL COMMENTS: Plan to swim in the crystal-clear North Fork. Plan to itch like crazy if you fail to watch for poison oak. *Hint:* It's not hiding.

GPS TRAILHEAD COORDINATES

Latitude   N39° 02.423´
Longitude   W120° 54.124´

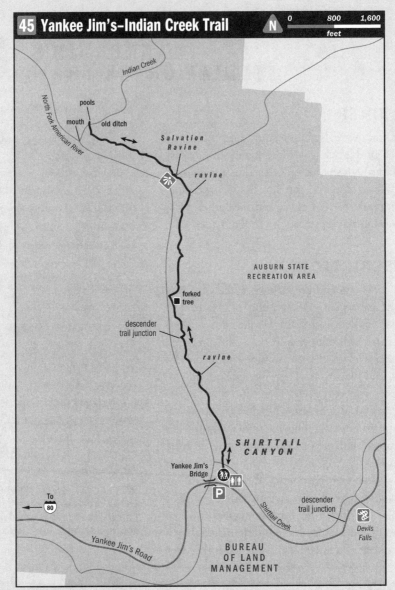

N

| 0 | 800 | 1,600 |

feet

Indian Creek

North Fork American River

pools

mouth

old ditch

Salvation Ravine

ravine

forked tree

descender trail junction

ravine

AUBURN STATE RECREATION AREA

SHIRTTAIL CANYON

Yankee Jim's Bridge

P

To
80

descender trail junction

Devils Falls

Shirttail Creek

Yankee Jim's Road

BUREAU OF LAND MANAGEMENT

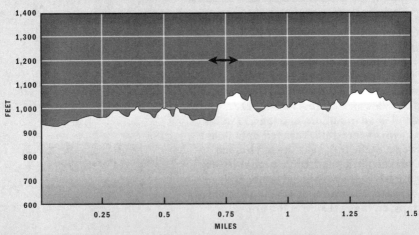

and the mouth of Shirttail Creek. If you do, your path will be fairly clear when you reach the stream. Your crossing location to get to the trail on the other side will depend somewhat on the water level. Boulder-hop carefully, without landing in the blackberry and willow, and make your way to the junction of the trail and Shirttail Creek after you cross.

Whitewater trips have originated from this crossing for several years. The evidence is seen in the small foundations (with boards covering the basement) that your track passes right after crossing. These were not for the miners. Continue on the dirt-and-duff trail northward past this bygone toilet-town and duck into the shade of the cool trail. Thistle and brodiaea cluster around the trail as it climbs about 50 feet above the river.

Silky spiderwebs pose the only impediment to travel—the creatures lie in ambush, their webs invisibly traversing the trail exactly at face-height. Apparently, wildly waving one's hands around one's head is the recommended antidote for "taking a silk hit." Press on. These adventures will just distract you from watching for rattlesnakes warming themselves on the trail. Fortunately, the slopes above and below are very steep, and the trail is very narrow in many sections, so you'll be watching your step anyway.

Enter a small, steep, rock-filled ravine and step across the slippery rocks of an unnamed stream. Keep right at any trails that descend to the river. The described route leads you right to it.

Protected from the sun by moss-covered live oak, the trail becomes little more than a singletrack, wide enough for two boots side-by-side, with fairly steep drops to the left that are somewhat exposed. Poison oak lines the trail here as you walk beneath the toyon and laurel trees. Adding nicely to the color of the forest floor, poison oak is often quite red, even in the summer. The color change, in the case of poison oak, is triggered more by heat than by any other factors. Avoid contact with any part of the plant, and wash any affected body part with lots of water as soon as possible.

The next 0.5 mile is rolling, generally heading north. The moss-covered branches of live oaks along here take on a fuzzy aura in the splattered sunlight. You can take some spectacular pictures along this section of the river. The opposite slope is bathed in light, which makes the line demarcating the scour zone and the vegetated slope above it very distinct.

Shortly, two ravines and their streams interrupt your path on the way to Indian Creek. The first is a poison-oak-bound ravine containing a jumble of rocks. Salvation Ravine appears next, with boulders the size of a small refrigerator. Walk across this ravine and climb a bit at the next jumble of boulders. The hillside you are approaching is covered with clarkia. A riot of purple, lavender, and white welcomes you into the open sun as you head down toward the river. The distinct trail narrows as it reenters tree cover.

Your trail will descend to the bedrock of the river at the mouth of Indian Creek. This is a fine spot to swim or enjoy a picnic. Upstream are a few smaller

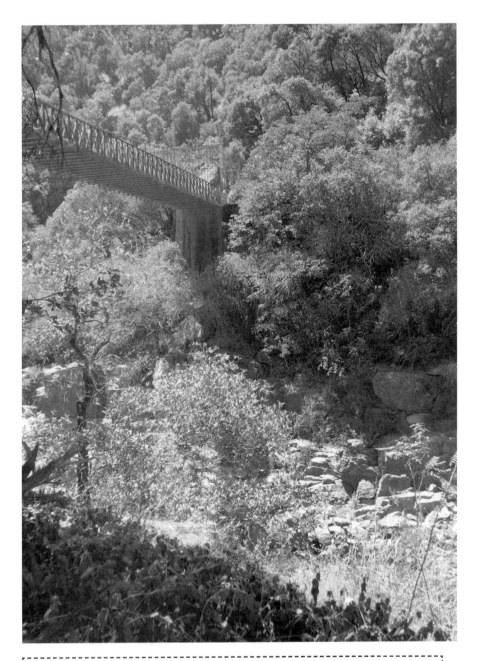

Yankee Jim's Bridge crosses the North Fork at the site where hundreds of miners lived and worked.

pools and, in wetter years, a waterfall. Bush monkeyflower and Indian paintbrush are splotched here and there at this small confluence. Bumblebees have laid claim to this patch and work it tenaciously. Above the creek on its south side are the remains of an old ditch. Hand-laid rock walls directed water around the snout of this ridge that sits north of Salvation Ravine. The ditch is difficult to follow only because it is so overgrown with poison oak, but it appears to connect to Indian Creek just above where the waterfalls would be.

Descend from that mess across a mound of talus (tailings) that is totally covered with wild grapes. Be alert for snakes here. A small king snake appeared but declined photo opportunities, preferring to slither under a rock.

Spend some time exploring upstream in the creek. Its secluded pools and many rocks make for an enjoyable adventure. The pools at the river are just right for wading and cooling off. The river is narrow enough that you can test the beaches on both sides. The trail continues for a short bit on the other side of the creek but becomes choked with overgrown-everything soon after that. At one time this trail continued upstream, where it joined with Windy Point Trail. Evidence indicates that volunteers have begun restoring and maintaining that old trail, marking it with interesting signage. It looks like a route to be explored. Otherwise, retrace your steps to Yankee Jim's Bridge.

NEARBY ACTIVITIES

Kayaks and rafts leave from the east side of Yankee Jim's Bridge. Hike 0.5 mile uphill along Yankee Jim's Road to Devils Falls. A descending trail leads to pools on Shirttail Creek. A rope hanging into the creek will help you out of the water on these slippery rocks.

46 WINDY POINT TRAIL

KEY AT-A-GLANCE INFORMATION

LENGTH: 3 miles

CONFIGURATION: Out-and-back

DIFFICULTY: Moderate

WATER REQUIRED: 2 liters

SCENERY: Spectacular vistas of the North Fork of the American River

EXPOSURE: In and out of shade and sun; southern exposure

TRAIL TRAFFIC: Light

TRAIL SURFACE: Dirt, duff, rock, scree

HIKING TIME: 3 hours

SEASON: Year-round

ACCESS: No fees or permits

MAPS: USGS Colfax; ASRA local trails map

WHEELCHAIR ACCESS: None

FACILITIES: Pit toilets at Mineral Bar campground

DRIVING DISTANCE: 50 miles

SPECIAL COMMENTS: This trail can be narrow and steep, with stretches of vertical exposure, and is often strewn with loose rock and dirt. It may not be appropriate for younger or inexperienced children. Trekking poles are very helpful on this hike.

GPS TRAILHEAD COORDINATES

Latitude   N39° 05.448´
Longitude W120° 55.259´

IN BRIEF

Breathtaking views of the North Fork begin about halfway down Iowa Hill Road, and they don't stop until you reach the river at the end of this trail. After you ascend from the crystal-clear pools below, drive up to Iowa Hill to explore the pioneer cemetery.

DESCRIPTION

Windy Point is perched more than 600 feet above the trailhead to this old miners' trail, which leads down to quartz-laden greenstone bedrock at the river. The trail begins behind the four boulders along the road, one of which has a bore hole through which you can see down the trail. The flat-topped boulders are situated perfectly for you to adjust your boots for a steep downhill hike across some dodgy sections.

Bigleaf maple and black oak shade the overgrown doubletrack at the outset, yielding to ponderosa pine and Douglas fir as you ascend a short hill. Then, at about the time that your eyes become accustomed to the

Directions

From the junction of I-80 East and the Capital City Freeway, drive 40 miles on I-80 East toward Colfax. Take Exit 133/Canyon Way, turn left onto Canyon Way, and drive 1 mile. Turn right onto Iowa Hill Road, which is paved but extremely narrow, rarely offering room for cars to pass. Iowa Hill Road is impassable to RVs or vehicles with trailers. Continue downhill about 8 miles, then uphill another 0.8 mile past the bridge at Mineral Bar Campground. The trailhead, on the right, is marked with four large boulders and a four-by-four post with no sign. There is space for a few cars to park at the trailhead.

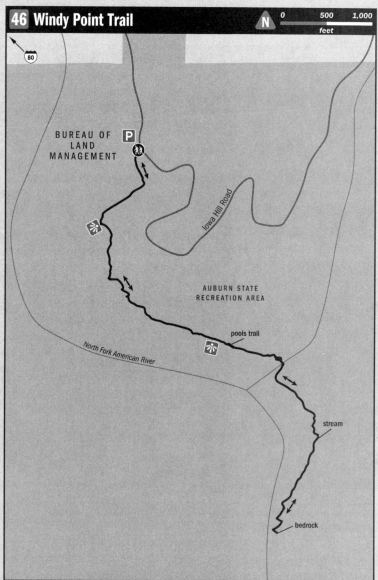

N

0   500   1,000

feet

80

BUREAU OF
LAND
MANAGEMENT

P

Iowa Hill Road

AUBURN STATE
RECREATION AREA

pools trail

North Fork American River

stream

bedrock

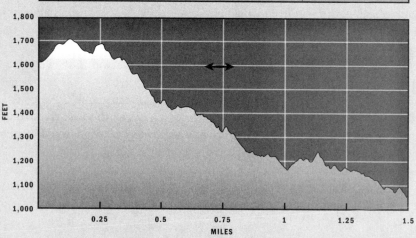

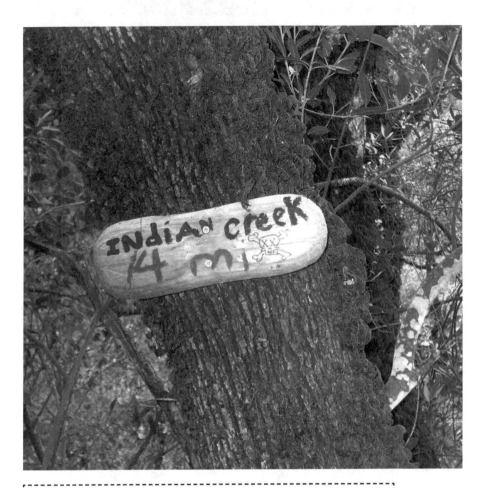

Trails from one mining camp to another have remained for us to discover. A new one appears to have been reclaimed.

darkness, the trail narrows to a tight singletrack and breaks into the sun. Just as you step into the open—at about 0.2 mile—a small rock outcrop on the right serves as a stable platform from which to frame this wide-open vista. Below, the river flows from right to left, generally north to south with some high-angle turns along the way.

In fewer than 500 feet, your trail will narrow to the width of two boots. Although the views are nonstop for 0.5 mile, watch your footing as the trail steepens and its camber tends toward the downhill side. It's very scrabbly along here, especially in the steep sections. Using your trekking poles on this trail gives you a distinct advantage as you start into a series of steep switchbacks followed by more of the same. After a couple of large outcrops, you have about 0.5 mile to hike to the creek crossing.

A nice panorama of the North Fork opens up just before you descend across a fairly open hillside on this steeply angled, narrow, scree-littered, slanted, and uneven trail with crumbly edges about 400 feet above the river. Take pictures and then descend. This is not a place where you want distractions. Stop, stand, and look around. Lupine, buttercups, popcorn flower, poppy, and brodiaea splash color over the entire hillside. From up over your shoulder down to the scour line at the river, you are treated to a blanket of blue, white, purple, orange, and yellow, accentuated with the green of live oak and foothill pine.

Continue past a side trail that descends steeply to a pair of clear pools in the North Fork. The described hike continues past the creeks ahead before descending to the river. If the first creek is impassable, take this side trail that leads to the river.

Descend some short, steep switchbacks into the darkness of a ravine's foliage, then step down a short flight of natural stairs to the creek. In high-water runoff, this crossing may be impassable. This creek emanates from a spring on Indian Knoll, 1,600 feet above and more than 2 miles to the northeast, on the other side of Race Track Hill, which towers over you. Whenever you do cross, the boulders and rocks that you must cross are always very slick when your boots are wet. Use caution here and begin your traverse from below the boulders on the right. The trail crosses the creek at a slight angle from right to left, exiting uphill through blackberries and poison oak. The latter occupies much of the trail margins from this point on.

A signed side trail uphill, which leads to a spring, is a fair warning of the upcoming creek. This second stream ahead is easily stepped over, but it's surrounded by poison oak, and the trail leading up to it is fairly crumbly. Buckeye, toyon, laurel, alder, and live oak provide cool shade along here. This stretch of trail is poorly maintained, but it remains quite distinct all the way to the river. Handwritten signs urge hikers THIS WAY to Indian Creek. With less than 0.25 mile to your destination, another sign attached to a tree pinpoints the distance to Indian Creek at 4 miles. Twenty-five feet beyond that is a trail leading uphill with signs indicating INDIAN CREEK. Judging by the loppers and choppers at the junction, this may be a work in progress that possibly offers a new and interesting adventure.

As you follow the path down, be prepared for a bit of a scramble down to the river. If it isn't already flagged, mark your exact spot so you can find it when you leave. Watch your handholds. As you hike out, keep in mind that the poison oak that was at your knees on the downhill hike in will now be at arm-level on the uphill hike out. Some water or a wet wipe can eliminate any toxic oils.

NEARBY ACTIVITIES

The Iowa Hill Cemetery has more than 100 decedents in it. Historic documents have left records of their lives, and these notes have been posted at the cemetery entrance for all to read.

47 STEVENS TRAIL WEST

KEY AT-A-GLANCE INFORMATION

LENGTH: 7.4 miles

CONFIGURATION: Out-and-back

DIFFICULTY: Moderate

WATER REQUIRED: 3 liters

SCENERY: Waterfalls, wildflowers, and panoramas of the North Fork

EXPOSURE: Some shady respites but largely exposed on a south-facing slope

TRAIL TRAFFIC: Moderate

TRAIL SURFACE: Dirt and rock

HIKING TIME: 4 hours

SEASON: Year-round

ACCESS: No fees or permits

MAPS: USGS Colfax; ASRA map

WHEELCHAIR ACCESS: None

FACILITIES: Gravel parking lot for 17 cars, pit toilet, trash container

DRIVING DISTANCE: 42 miles

SPECIAL COMMENTS: This is an easy hike down to the North Fork of the American River on a Gold Rush–era trail. Although it's not difficult, there are areas where the trail is narrow, with loose footing and steep vertical exposure.

GPS TRAILHEAD COORDINATES

Latitude   N39° 06.327´

Longitude   W120° 56.835´

IN BRIEF

Created nearly a century and a half ago as a foot- and horse-trail between Colfax and Iowa Hill, this vista-packed walk must be the easiest route down to the beautifully wild and scenic North Fork of the American River. Chinese-built railroad beds, hardrock-mine shafts, waterfalls and cascades, crystal-clear pools, and a flock of leopard lilies are all within easy reach of this historic trail.

DESCRIPTION

This descent to the North Fork is enjoyably easy. Of course, the hike in is easier—but the slope on the hike out is gentle enough for hikers of any age to enjoy. One attraction here is the wall-to-wall view of the North Fork of the American River—from above Iowa Hill Road and the bridge at Mineral Bar to the extreme close-ups of the crystal-clear water at trail's end.

The Stevens Trail descends about 1,150 feet to the North Fork of the American River. It was built in 1859 by Truman Stevens, who ran a livery stable in Colfax and a ranch in Iowa Hill. No freight was ever hauled on this foot- and stock-path, but anyone could cross the river for a toll.

Your hike begins at the parking lot set aside and marked by the Bureau of Land

Directions

From the junction of I-80 East and the Capital City Freeway, drive 40 miles on I-80 East toward Colfax and take Exit 135/CA 174– Colfax/Grass Valley. In 500 feet, keep left on South Canyon Way. In 0.5 mile, look for the signed parking lot on the left.

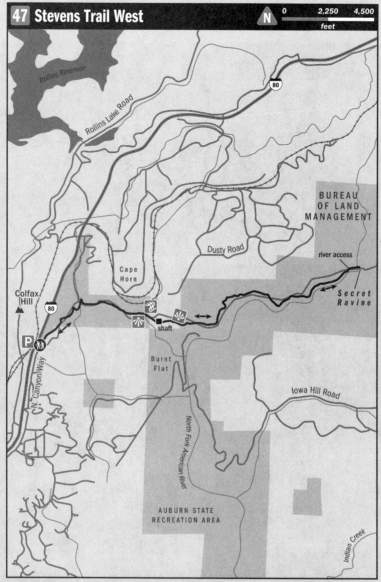

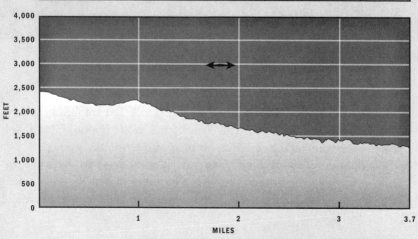

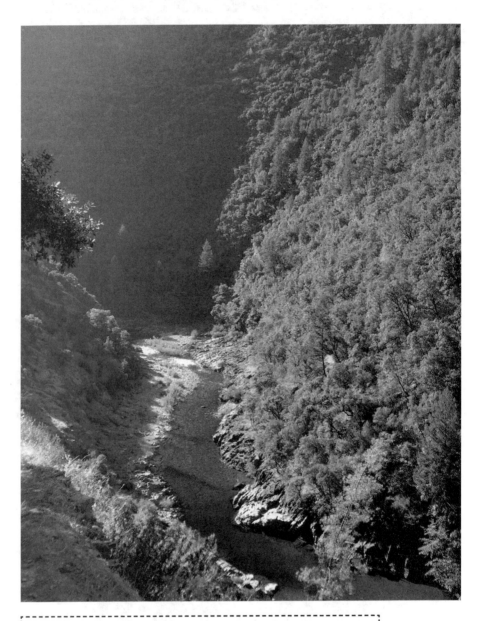

The upper canyon walls force the river through twists and turns of contorted rock.

Management on the left side of the dirt-and-gravel road. The trailhead is clearly marked at the north end of the lot. There's no water at the trailhead, but if you didn't bring your own, you'll have plenty to treat or filter on the way.

As you adjust your pack's straps, the trailhead markers—two signs and two metal posts—will guide you onto a picturesque duff trail that glides down into a cool forest. You will descend about 200 feet and weave in and out of a ravine and over two streams before the sound of the interstate fades behind you. If you're here in the right season and you stop at the massive blackberry patch, you'll hear plenty of birdcalls.

The trail is quite well defined at the outset. Shaded by fir and oak, your path is marked by signs, which seem to pop up just about everywhere you'd think one would be handy. Just after you cross a creek over a stout wooden footbridge almost 0.75 mile along, be on the watch for a trail sign directing you to the right. Head east on this uphill trail, walking 0.25 mile up the exposed four-wheel-drive road, which unfortunately leads directly into the sun on early-morning hikes.

Pass the blackberries and buckeye and head for the manzanita and oak at the top of the hill, where a very small trail sign directs you left. The doubletrack you're leaving continues ahead before veering south across Burnt Flat. (One map lists it as Stevens Trail and shows it tying into the Iowa Hill Road at Slaughter Ravine.) Another four-wheel-drive road turns right and heads uphill to the south along the ridge. Head toward Robbers Ravine to the east at the sign marked TRAIL.

Just ahead, under the shade of some midtrail foliage, is a perfect place to adjust your bootlaces and sip water. Cool manzanitas also shade this spot, which offers great seating on several large, flat boulders. After your eyes adjust to the light, you should see a profusion of bush monkeyflower all around. This spot will seem more precious for its shaded seating when you're on your hike out. So far, you've walked slightly more than 1 mile. Shortly, the trail will divide: bikers take the trail down to the right, hikers stay on the upper trail to the left.

Continue to walk southeast. As you pass beneath Cape Horn, look up and you should be able to see the dry-stacked rock walls laid by Chinese laborers, who were often suspended in baskets by their coworkers to accomplish such dangerous tasks as setting explosives in the rock. Their meticulous engineering and building skills literally supported the railroad across and through the Sierra Nevada and serve the railroad to this day. Cape Horn has two tracks: the almost-visible one skirting the edge and clinging to the cliffs above, and another that makes a tighter turn through a tunnel under the plateau above.

Look off to the right, across Burnt Flat. An outcrop of upturned shale offers a great vista point for excellent views of the hillsides downriver. You should begin to hear the sounds of cascades in Robbers Ravine. Slow down before entering the narrow slot in the rocks: every rock here is wet and slippery. The drop-off to the right would make a fall very unpleasant. But don't spend all your time watching your step. Keep your eyes open for clusters of brilliant orange leopard lilies along-side the trail in this moist area. When you find them, look to the slope above, where you will likely find even more color.

Your trail hugs the uphill slope. You have a gentle descent across a talus field, with a steep drop to the right. This rocky field is short and likely to be covered with golden poppies and Indian paintbrush. The trail along here is outfitted with the officially required number of toe-stubbing immovable rocks, so watch your step while you're watching the flowers. Delicate purple clarkia flows across the trail, revealing several minute watercourses.

Your trail is exposed to sun over the next 0.25 mile; just as it snakes along the hillside into some shade, look left and you'll see a mine shaft cut horizontally into the rock face. USGS maps do not show this shaft, a fact possibly indicating that this is more of a convenient rock quarry than a prospective gold mine. Within 100 feet, you'll need to negotiate some rock movement with care. A more spectacular vista lies ahead another 0.25 mile. From this point, you can see the Iowa Hill–Colfax Road Bridge and the Mineral Bar Campground.

The exposed sections of the trail are conveniently interrupted by the shade of foothill pine and black oak. Large seeps form at joints in the rock, feeding mosses and ferns that grow surprisingly large.

Over the next mile, you'll descend along an exposed slope. A trail to the right drops to the river, but the one described here continues left. From this vantage, it's easy to see the water below. The crystal-clear pools are lined with greenstone bedrock, reflecting green light that is seemingly unmarred by a single ripple. The scour zone reveals pickup-truck-sized boulders that channel the river back and forth across the canyon, across shallow gravel bars and through willows, straining the water before aerating it again in a rapid, then repeating the process farther downstream.

As your trail descends through thickets of blackberries, you can see through the trees that the greenstone looks bleached. The still water looks cool and inviting. The steep slopes and blackberries might be reasonable deterrents to diving into the pools right now. You have only about 0.25 mile until you reach the crossing at Secret Ravine. Just before reaching the creek, though, you'll pass an easy trail to the rocks at the river's edge below. In low-water years, the drop into the pools may be much easier than the scramble out. So plan your exit point and keep in mind that your hands will be wet and the rocks will be slippery.

The original bridge that crossed this fork has long since been washed away, leaving only pieces of foundation and sections of rusting steel cables. Look below the trail for the cables, and you can trace them as they lie buried under a century of dirt. They stick out toward the river just about 100 yards before you reach Secret Ravine. Follow the bundles of suspension cable as they lead your eye to their intended mark: the landing across the river. From there, pedestrians or riders would continue another 7 miles uphill to Iowa Hill.

The creek at Secret Ravine is very picturesque, but on a hot day you'll appreciate it for another reason. The confluence of the creek and the river is less than 100 feet to your right. Air flows over the pools above the trail and cools as it falls toward the river; at the confluence, the air is speeded up, creating a breeze as refreshing as walking into an air-conditioned room. *Voilà*— a natural swamp cooler.

Walk across the conveniently placed boulders and turn toward the river, where there is a well-established campsite and fire ring. The campsite, like others along Secret Ravine, may be used by miners routinely working upriver. A trail shown on the USGS map continues upriver for another 4,000 feet along the water's rocky margin. Secret Ravine's name seems enough to warrant an exploration upstream from the trail crossing.

An almost-distinct trail ascends the creek on the east side of the ravine. Miners' camps, both historic and current, can be found here among the laurel and cottonwood overlooking some convenient rockbound pools of crystal-clear water. Tarps and logs provide scant cover for the equipment being used today, and rust covers the equipment used in earlier days.

More leopard lilies cluster on the hillside here, above the moss-and-leaf-covered rocks below the trail. Other clusters grow about 200 feet upriver along the margin of the trees. These wonderful fragrant flowers, picturesque in early summer, are vividly orange when other spring flowers have already faded to paler colors.

The pools and shallows of the river east of the creek make great places to cool off. Your level of attire here might take into account whether miners are working or the trail is very busy—the area sees the most traffic after noon. However you do it, cool off before heading back uphill. This trail has about 2,800 feet of total elevation gain and loss. The gradual uphill grade rarely requires too much effort, but the shade is always appreciated.

NEARBY ACTIVITIES

Colfax–Iowa Hill Road winds 9 miles up to a Gold Rush–era town and a historic cemetery with informative notes regarding each of the deceased. While you can no longer cross the North Fork on Stevens's footbridge, the trail does continue on the south side of the river and leads to its original destination, Iowa Hill. The trailhead for the Stevens Trail East (see next profile) is next to the Iowa Hill Store.

48 STEVENS TRAIL EAST

KEY AT-A-GLANCE INFORMATION

LENGTH: 7.24 miles

CONFIGURATION: Out-and-back

DIFFICULTY: Moderate

WATER REQUIRED: 2–3 liters

SCENERY: Foothill woodland, Wild and Scenic River

EXPOSURE: Few patches of sun

TRAIL TRAFFIC: Light

TRAIL SURFACE: Duff, dirt, and rock

HIKING TIME: 3–4 hours

SEASON: Year-round

ACCESS: No fees or permits

MAPS: USGS Colfax, Foresthill

WHEELCHAIR ACCESS: None

FACILITIES: Parking on Iowa Hill Road opposite the store

DRIVING DISTANCE: 49 miles

SPECIAL COMMENTS: If you need a guide on this hike, tell Lyneá Daniels, the proprietor of the Iowa Hill Store, and she'll fix you up with a pro: Shorty, the affable pit-bull trail hound.

GPS TRAILHEAD COORDINATES

Latitude   N39° 06.438´

Longitude   W120° 51.615´

IN BRIEF

This is a wonderful hike to the Wild and Scenic North Fork of the American River. When T. A. Stevens built this trail in the 1860s, his plan was to move people and livestock easily between Colfax and Iowa Hill. Now you can mosey down and up with the same ease on this historic thoroughfare.

DESCRIPTION

This is the forgotten side of the Stevens Trail. In the 1860s, travelers descending from Colfax would have crossed the suspension bridge that Stevens built at Secret Ravine, then would have continued to the gold fields at Iowa Hill, which was a town of more than 10,000 people. The suspension bridge has long since carried its last toll-paying horse and rider, but at the end of this hike you can still see the cables that attached the bridge to the bedrock.

Start at the signed trailhead to the right of the store. Be aware that the trail is adjacent to private property for the next 500 feet. Walk 25 feet straight downhill to the next trail sign, and you're now on a line for the break in the

----

Directions

From the junction of I-80 East and the Capital City Freeway, drive 40.1 miles on I-80 East toward Colfax. Take Exit 133/Canyon Way to the right and turn left on Canyon Way. In 1.1 miles, turn right onto Iowa Hill Road. Drive 9.1 miles to Iowa Hill and park across from the store. *Warning:* Iowa Hill Road is a narrow mountain road, often with no place to pass. Curves are tight, with no guardrails to protect cars from the steep drop-offs. Large vehicles and trailers should stay off this road. The marked trailhead is to the right of the Iowa Hill Store.

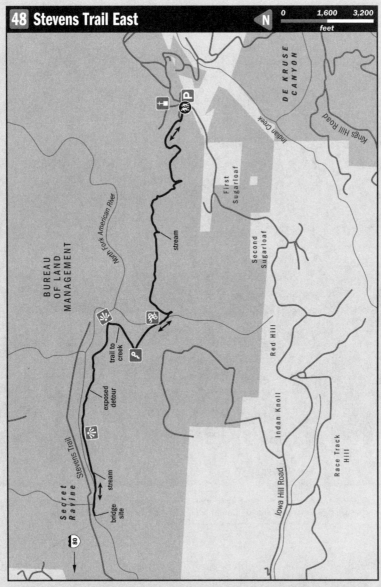

N

0   1,600   3,200
feet

DE KRUSE CANYON

Kings Hill Road

Indian Creek

First Sugarloaf

Second Sugarloaf

Red Hill

Indian Knoll

Race Track Hill

Iowa Hill Road

stream

North Fork American River

BUREAU OF LAND MANAGEMENT

trail to creek

exposed detour

Stevens Trail

Secret Ravine

stream

bridge site

80

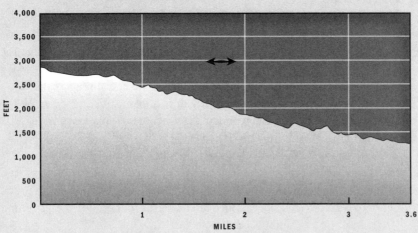

4,000
3,500
3,000
2,500
2,000
1,500
1,000
500
0

FEET

1   2   3   3.6

MILES

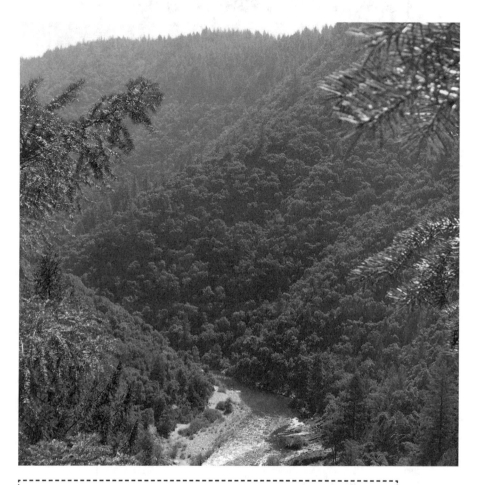

The North Fork flows around hard metamorphic rock where two geologic terranes meet.

trees ahead, where the trail enters the forest. Just follow the fence past the trail signs and blackberries.

Zigzag down among the Douglas firs and ponderosa pines as you notice old riveted iron pipes—part of the legacy of hydraulic mining that will soon become more evident. The well-signed trail leads you northwest and then around the debris field, even occupying its outlet stream for a bit. Next you head southwest, where you'll begin descending along a ravine. At 0.5 mile, a line of rocks and a new BLM trail sign direct you to the right if you're a hiker, rider, or biker. When you turn right, the bullet-riddled, wooden STEVENS TRAIL marker verifies that you're heading the right way (northwest).

The ravine to the right, now choking with shade-tolerant Douglas-fir seedlings, was once used as a runoff. The trail is bordered by kit-kit-dizze, poison oak, and manzanita. Some red-skinned madrones shade the path. As you admire them, be careful not to trip on a sugar-pine cone, and be on the lookout for the 12-pound squirrels that eat the seeds in one sitting! No small feat, that: sugar-pine cones weigh up to 4 pounds and yield about 2,100 corn-sized seeds per pound. When you walk down into the crux of the next ravine, you will run into a fallen Douglas fir that straddles the gap from trailside to trailside. Another trail sign marks the other side of the ravine just after the treetop.

Your gentle descent takes you past some surprisingly huge black oaks on the slopes above the trail, a huge ponderosa pine next to the trail, and skyscraping Douglas firs below it. A toppled bigleaf maple lives on despite being bent sideways by a fallen black oak.

When wet, this next stream crossing—steep to both sides—would be a tumultuous cascade, with slippery, moss-covered rocks covering the trail. When dry, it offers a skunk shelter in the deep rock crevices below the path. As you walk along, notice the moss, nearly half an inch thick, growing over the rocks above and below the trail. A century and a half ago, those rocks were exposed and bare. You may look behind the moss and be surprised to see stacked rocks forming a wall: Stevens built one long-lasting trail. In fact, a large boulder broke off of the outcrop next to the path ahead and landed on a section of trail supported by a wall that Stevens built. The wall held, and the boulder rests in place.

Continue your gentle descent, roughly paralleling the river below until you turn away from it and enter a ravine descending from Red Hill. This beautiful copse of dogwood, bigleaf maple, bracken ferns, and mosses is wonderfully cool on a hot day. The steep slope above the trail channels the water over large, slick blocks of blackened bedrock so that it cascades down to trail-level, pooling before falling over a similarly steep and rocky descent. Large blocks of rock on either side may provide some dry footing.

The pools below you to the right slip away as the creek plummets and you move northwest again. When you can see back through the trees to the opposite side of the ravine, it's apparent that the bigleaf maple, live oak, black oak, and even dogwood and laurel all share a very shallow vertical space on the hillside. The Douglas fir, however, starts beneath and ascends far above all other trees on the slope.

The ravine some 600 feet down the trail also hosts plunging cascades in the spring. Fifty feet after crossing the creek, you can see the water run off the hill. The next ravine, 0.2 mile farther, is the site of a spring that flows year-round. As the trail approaches it, ferns become so thick that the trail is obscured. This small yet picturesque seep is a nice place to wet your kerchief on a hot climb out.

In another 5 minutes, you'll see a small trail (not mapped in this book) descending sharply to your right that appears to lead to the creek in the ravine below. Hiking 3 minutes more on your trail takes you to an excellent vista point at the 2.2-mile point. The view upstream from here, about 450 feet above the river, looks down on the gravel and cobble arrayed on the river's bedrock channel. That little silver strand gleaming in the sun is framed by the diagonal walls of the canyons towering above it.

Another fine example of Stevens's wall-building lies about 10 minutes down the trail. At this same spot is an example of trail-failing. Look for a detour up to the left that goes above and behind the outcrop, or use the oft-employed rope to scramble carefully up the face of the rock to follow the trail. Aside from a bit of exposure here, this is an easy maneuver because there are lots of natural rock steps, and the detour is very brief. The river is now only about 200 feet below your position.

Look on the opposite slope for signs of trail-*building*. This portion of the Stevens Trail extends past Secret Ravine to enable miners to reach upstream bars. Cross another small stream as you draw within about 75 feet of the river, then cross a jumble of rocks as you continue descending to the junction of the trail and the river.

Stevens built his suspension bridge here, and you can see the cables at your feet in the duff and brush. Although they may not be the Golden Gate variety, they stood long enough for Mr. Stevens to collect a toll of 25 cents from walkers and 50 cents from riders, allowing him to retire and live in Colfax until he was 80. He was buried in the historic Colfax Cemetery, just 0.5 mile from the Colfax threshold of his historic trail.

Thanks to a partnership between the U.S. Bureau of Land Management and the Trust for Public Lands, the private property around the trail was purchased and protected for hikers and other outdoors enthusiasts to enjoy.

There are two different worlds at this point on the river. One is calming, the other raucous. If you walk west past the cables, you'll find easy access to the bed-rock-lined pools in front of you and farther downstream. You can slip into the crystal-clear water by descending to the boulder the size of an SUV—right in front of the garage-sized one. Here you can walk across bedrock into the water.

If you turn back to the right of the cables, you can descend fairly easily to the rocks leading over to the cobble-covered bars. At this spot, riffles rather than rapids churn the water into a noisy frenzy. Colorful, mineral-laden rocks line the river bottom, creating beautiful images in the sunlight. A small, sandy beach lies upstream about 100 feet, but it can't be accessed easily and, judging by the debris discarded there, isn't worth the effort.

Swim, wade, explore, and generally lounge until you're rejuvenated and inspired to hike back up to the trailhead. Wave to any fellow hikers on the opposite slope, and wave so-long to Secret Ravine on your ascent. You'll find that it's as gentle going up as it was coming down.

NEARBY ACTIVITIES

Gold Rush–era history is vividly portrayed in the display at the Iowa Hill Cemetery, on the left and about 500 feet north of the Iowa Hill Store, just before you leave the north end of town. There you can read how the deceased lived their lives, how they died, and how their peers remembered them.

GREEN VALLEY TRAIL 49

IN BRIEF

This is one of the most challenging trails in this book, yet it offers so much for so many interests. Naturalists can delve into this very active biozone, which is rich with flora and fauna from small to large. What photographer wants to miss shots of Lovers Leap in Giants Gap? Gold Rush enthusiasts can explore until the day runs out and not cover half the mining undertakings to see here. And stop me now if a geology buff wouldn't want to wander from one end of this valley to the other, exploring from slope to slope.

This trail is steep to the river—about 1,800 feet of elevation loss in only 2.5 miles—and is, for much of the route, one big vista point. Dense foothill forest near the river, combined with old trails, makes for some confusing terrain. Prepare for this hike by poring over the available maps in advance. A GPS unit, while

- -

Directions ⟶

From the junction of I-80 East and the Capital City Freeway, drive 51.5 miles on I-80 East to Exit 146/Alta. Turn right on Morton Road and turn immediately left onto Casa Loma Road. Drive 0.9 mile, then bear right to stay on Casa Loma Road. Drive 0.3 mile to the junction with Moody Ridge Road, which bears right. Drive 0.4 mile on Moody Ridge Road, past the junction with Aquilla Road, to the parking area on the left, officially signed GREEN VALLEY STAGING AREA, with another homemade marker visible high in a corner of the lot. Your trailhead is in the northeast corner of the lot, where a line of boulders leads the way to the actual trail. Follow the narrow path as it leads to Aquilla Road. There, an abundance of signs will lead you to this historic trail, where you can see that the Placer Legacy has secured a conservation easement for access. As the legacy requests, please respect private property.

KEY AT-A-GLANCE INFORMATION

LENGTH: 6 miles

CONFIGURATION: Out-and-back

DIFFICULTY: Hard

WATER REQUIRED: 2–3 liters

SCENERY: Lush foothill woodland with vistas of remote foothill canyons and snowcapped Sierra Nevada mountains

EXPOSURE: Partially or fully shaded most often; some brief periods of full sun

TRAIL TRAFFIC: Light

TRAIL SURFACE: Dirt, duff, rock

HIKING TIME: 3–5 hours

SEASON: Year-round, weather permitting

ACCESS: No fees or permits

MAPS: USGS Dutch Flat; Tahoe National Forest map

WHEELCHAIR ACCESS: None

FACILITIES: None

DRIVING DISTANCE: 63.5 miles

SPECIAL COMMENTS: Green Valley can be accessed from three trailhead locations: from this one, on Moody Ridge; from the Euchre Bar Trail, at Iron Point; and from the Foresthill side of the North Fork, near Sugar Pine Reservoir (see Hike 46, *60 Hikes within 60 Miles: Sacramento,* first edition).

GPS TRAILHEAD COORDINATES

Latitude   N39° 11.718´
Longitude   W120° 47.848´

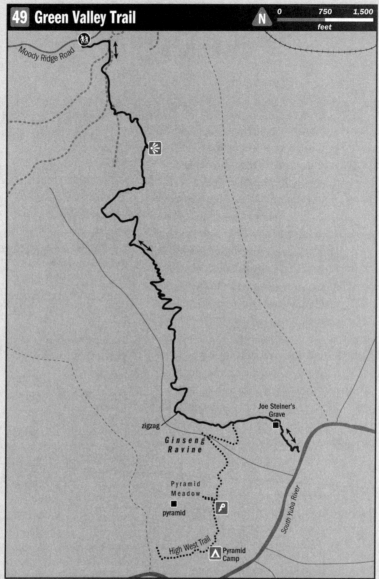

N

0   750   1,500

feet

Moody Ridge Road

Joe Steiner's Grave

zigzag

Ginseng Ravine

Pyramid Meadow

pyramid

South Yuba River

High West Trail

Pyramid Camp

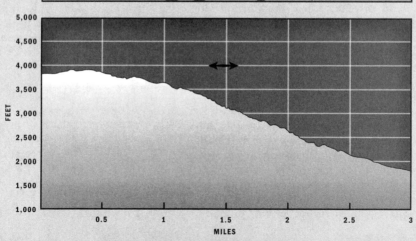

FEET

MILES

certainly not necessary, can be a real asset as you explore. If the hike up and down doesn't deter you, then this is an area you'll want to return to again.

DESCRIPTION

If you followed the signs and arrows to the final locked gate and the PLACER LEGACY sign, then you should be ready to check your bootlaces for a vista-filled downhill-switchback festival. The dirt-and-duff trail can be difficult to follow right out of the gate, as the leaf matter filling the well-worn path obscures the tight switchbacks. Under cover of black oak and manzanita, plus ponderosa and foothill pine, you hike just shy of 300 yards, whereupon you won't be able to resist your first vista of the North Fork's upriver canyon and beyond to the Sierra Nevada. There will be plenty more of these vistas, so this is the last time I'll mention them. (By the way: they're awesome.)

As your track momentarily angles southwest, your views through the manzanita become blocked by a dense stand of oak and cedar that cools the air instantly—a phenomenon you may want to recall on your return. As the tread beneath your feet narrows, you might notice other trails joining from uphill. You will continue to see them from both sides, so attention to your map and compass is important. But be sure to keep looking around at your terrain. Because there are a number of unmarked trail junctions, and because the route is densely forested at points, looking back uphill at your trail out can be a valuable task that you'll appreciate on the route home. Your track remains distinct for the next mile.

Green Valley was inhabited by some 2,000 people in 1852. It and other mining camps like it were served by mule trains, which brought in equipment, supplies, mail, and the news of the day. This was their trail into the widest valley of the North Fork, bustling with activity. Imagine the comings and goings along the trail as newcomers arrived, as mining inspectors and surveyors performed their duties, as vendors and tradesmen of all sorts moved up and down hillside and canyon. You may notice flat spots to the side of the trail at a few points—passing spots, perhaps.

At just about 1 mile from the trailhead, a seasonal runoff stream cascades across the trail. Soon you'll think that if only you could get a running start, you could practically slalom down these tight switchbacks. (I know you're going to remember these on the way up.) Watch these compact turns closely.

Essentially descending southeast along the nose of Moody Ridge, you'll face directly into the midmorning sun. As you serpentine downhill, with the larger boulders thankfully to the side of the trail, be aware that many critters have staked their claim to this trail and they renew that claim daily. The trail is narrow here, so watch for claim markers.

At around 2,300 feet elevation, you're presented with a fork in the trail. The trail to the left is a shortcut—it's fine to take, but it's steep, and if you take it you chance missing a turn. The right-hand fork, straight ahead of you, winds through

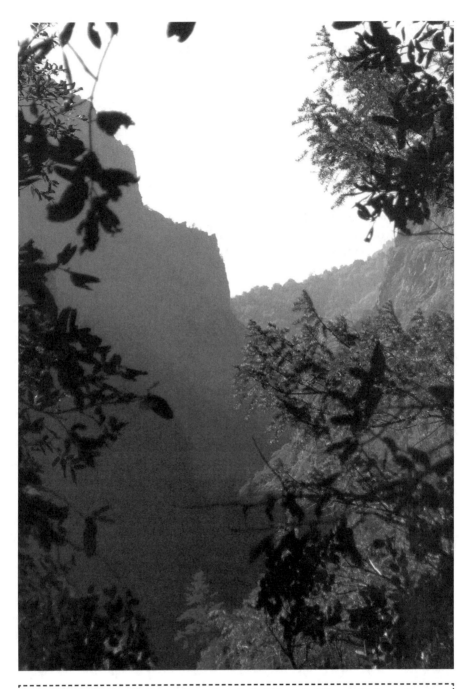

Giant's Gap, camouflaged by haze and live oak, sits in the Melones Fault Zone and is the meeting place of the Calaveras Complex and the Shoo Fly Complex.

the copse of trees visible ahead. The track then swings widely through this ponderosa-pine, Douglas-fir, and incense-cedar park before encountering the steep shortcut trail. Turn right onto it, then take ten paces downhill and turn left.

Follow the track as it leads southeast toward the river you hear. Manzanita and live oak define the trail well for the next 350 yards. More ponderosa pine, Douglas fir, and incense cedar surrounds you, and the walking is almost leisurely. At around 2,080 feet elevation, look for a mining ditch that crosses your path. This was probably what's now known as the High West Trail. This is an excellent ditch trail to begin exploring. As you're thinking about that, in a scant 500 downhill feet, you encounter the grave of prospector, miner, and caretaker Joe Steiner, a Swiss immigrant. Mining gear and debris from the hydraulic-mining era are scattered in the forest litter.

Within steps of that memorial, you enter blackberry city, where you may linger for several minutes before moving on into a grassy area beneath California bay laurel, Douglas fir, and gray pine (also known as foothill or, derogatorily, digger pine). Several trails intersect yours—explore them as time allows.

At about 1,880 feet elevation, a stream drops the final 40 feet to the river, and mining camps are situated wherever they fit. Another advance toward the river, now just 20 feet above, reveals a couple of excellent places to camp with excellent east-facing views. Unfortunately, they're perpetually strewn with the debris and junk common to miners from the 19th to the 21st century. About 100 feet upstream from this spot, it would be possible to ford the river and take a dip in the pool just beyond.

If you have the time, energy, and curiosity, you can strike out south on the ditch trail you noted on the way in. It proceeds at an easy pace and maintains its elevation. But don't get lulled into carelessness in watching your trail—it does diminish at times and entirely disappears at others. At a side trail in your now-grassy path, you can step into a pleasant round meadow, bounded by a battalion of incense cedars. From the center, you have a view of The Pyramid, just to the west. The rusted pipe in the ground, plus the soggy ground underfoot as you leave the meadow, gives some evidence of the number of cedars in the area.

Ahead lies Pyramid Camp, another picturesque miners' campsite overlooking the river. Critters have rearranged the site's gear, but one can see possibilities.

Continuing along the edge of the cliff for another 250 yards will deliver you, frustratingly, to the edge of another chasm, with Giant Gap and Lovers Leap temptingly close, even visible through the trees. Perhaps next trip. The historic trails are here for a while. The noble part of exploring is, alas, the willingness—or good sense—to retreat until another day, or another trail.

NEARBY ACTIVITIES

Green Valley can be reached from the trailhead at Euchre Bar (see next profile). There are many other trails to explore in the upper North Fork area. For maps and lists of trails, visit **northforktrails.com**. For trail notes, including in-depth historical and geological information, visit **northforktrails.blogspot.com**.

50 EUCHRE BAR TRAIL TO HUMBUG CANYON

KEY AT-A-GLANCE INFORMATION

LENGTH: 8.8 miles

CONFIGURATION: Out-and-back

DIFFICULTY: Hard

WATER REQUIRED: 4–5 liters

SCENERY: Foothill woodland and river canyon

EXPOSURE: Well shaded

TRAIL TRAFFIC: Light

TRAIL SURFACE: Duff, dirt, and rock that are slippery almost all the time

HIKING TIME: 3–4 hours

SEASON: Year-round

ACCESS: No fees or permits

MAPS: USGS Dutch Flat, Westville; Tahoe National Forest map

WHEELCHAIR ACCESS: None

FACILITIES: Pit toilet but no water at trailhead parking area

DRIVING DISTANCE: 55 miles

SPECIAL COMMENTS: Be aware and respectful of private property.

GPS TRAILHEAD COORDINATES

Latitude   N39° 11.613´

Longitude   W120° 46.186´

IN BRIEF

If you're looking for an easy way down to the North Fork of the American River, this one is a sweetheart. The word *switchback* has a good name on this well-graded trail. Descend to the river and cross it on the only suspension footbridge across the wild and scenic North Fork. You can discover mining relics and campsites when you continue upriver to Humbug Canyon.

DESCRIPTION

The sign at the parking area points you in the right direction for the trailhead—just 500 feet east. A side trail on the left, just after the hairpin turn, is a shortcut through the trees to the trailhead. Otherwise, continue on the road and look to the right for a baby-blue sedan parked backward on the right side of the road. Just beyond that on the right is the welded-metal sign for the Euchre Bar Trail. Your route to the river descends 1,525 feet in just 1.5 miles. So turn right and begin descending the dirt-and-leaf-covered trail. Watch your footing: the duff is slippery along the entire route.

A trail sign 75 feet down on your left confirms that you have the right route. Rocks line the dirt track, which is covered here with live-oak and black-oak leaves. The rocks intrude on the trail in earnest when the bay

----

Directions ————————————————→

From the junction of I-80 East and the Capital City Freeway, drive 51.5 miles on I-80 East to Exit 146/Alta. Turn right on Morton Road and turn immediately left on Casa Loma Road. Drive 2.7 miles to the second railroad crossing. Continue across the tracks. The trailhead is 0.75 mile down the dirt road. A pit toilet marks the parking area, which fits about six cars.

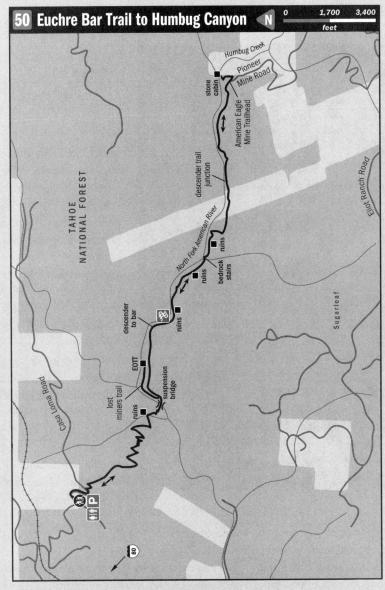

50 Euchre Bar Trail to Humbug Canyon

N

0   1,700   3,400
feet

Humbug Creek

Pioneer Mine Road

stone cabin

American Eagle Mine Trailhead

descender trail junction

North Fork American River

ruins

ruins

bedrock stairs

descender to bar

ruins

EOTT

suspension bridge

lost miners trail

ruins

Casa Loma Road

TAHOE NATIONAL FOREST

Sugarloaf

Eliot Ranch Road

80

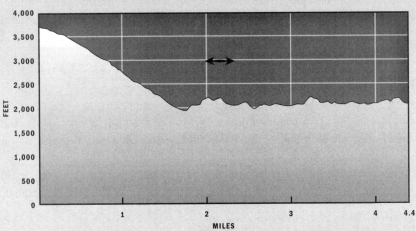

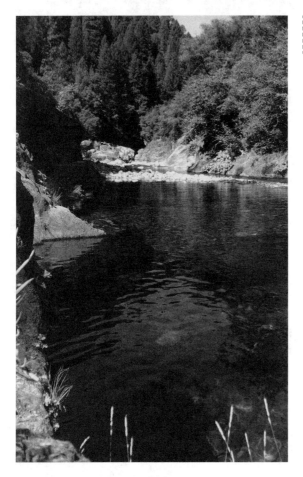

Crystal-clear water at
Humbug Bar

laurel and foothill pines begin to appear. When the rocks thin out, the oaks thicken on the slopes. Face flies and gnats swarm around you all along the trail, so it would be a good idea to apply repellent by the first switchback. The trail pretends to flatten a bit after 20 minutes of hiking.

You can see Sugarloaf Mountain and Sawtooth Ridge to the south and east when the trees cooperate. The eastbound train to Reno passes directly overhead as it rounds the point at Casa Loma. Walls built by Chinese railroad workers still support the tracks as they bend around points and span ravines. You can just hear the sound of the whistle fade through the trees as you continue to descend past the first mile.

By 1.25 miles, the trail has enough bare dirt to enable you to follow the tracks of raccoon and squirrel. Switchbacks help your downward journey under Douglas fir, black oak, and foothill pine. In 45 minutes, you'll see the first remains of gold-mining camps. Concrete pads and bed frames hint at what used to be a busy endeavor here.

Some rock steps help you over a sizable outcrop surrounded by large river cobble. It's hard to tell mining rubble from alluvial deposits around this heavily mined site. Still above the river, you'll see the bridge come into view below, where it spans the river just past some random campsites to the right of the trail. Poison oak stands sentry at each end of the bridge and persists alongside the trail as you head upstream.

When you cross the bridge, built in 1965, turn left and follow the trail uphill a few paces around to the right. Stop at the split in the trail. Note that the round, squatty boulder to your left has a rattlesnake den under the corner closest to you. Have your camera ready. If you're feeling adventurous, you can take the lost miners' trail to its end above Euchre Bar by following the left-hand track as it closely parallels the river. This trail is narrow, with steep drops to the river. Many footsteps and no maintenance have caused the tread to deteriorate dangerously. I advise extreme caution if you intend to peer down onto Euchre Bar. The route described and shown on the map takes the trail uphill to the right, leading you to Humbug Canyon.

The miners' trail involves 20 minutes of hiking on an unmaintained and somewhat overgrown trail that ends unceremoniously at a sheer drop 0.3 mile upstream, where a spike remains driven into the rock above a glistening pool at Euchre Bar. A memorable point on the trail is the site of a memorial sign, placed with care on a foothill pine growing horizontally from the slope, declaring the young deceased miner to have been "a good miner, but a better friend."

From the junction of the miners' trail, head uphill on the Euchre Bar Trail and ascend through fern, laurel, live oak, and dogwood. You can view the Wild and Scenic River down the steep slope on the side of this rocky trail. Thick moss and ferns coat the rocks and boulders at trailside. A faint path leads steeply downhill to the river, but you continue straight, as your trail—occupying tracks perhaps built only for mining crews—almost levels.

When you're hiking at about 40 feet above the river, you can spot cabin sites and campsites all along the trail. Crystal-clear water glides through the pools below you. Look to the left to spot the old mining ditch to the left of the trail. In a moment, the ditch crosses the trail and continues on the right for some distance. A number of platform sites where cabins or equipment once stood perch above the trail.

You can mentally sort among the debris, ruins, and remains to assemble a picture of life and industry here. Very little of personal life remains—the area's vegetation has regrown, and occasional floods have washed away light materials and objects. Discarded or abandoned heavy equipment yields the best idea of the sights and sounds in this canyon during the 1850s.

The remains of someone's porch and retaining walls, now holding back the laurel and scrub oak, sit on the right. Springtime has brought the color of Sierra iris, brodiaea, clarkia, and penstemon to these front yards that sit 30 feet above the water. Cross the creek and mount the steps in the bedrock as you leave Euchre Bar behind and head to Humbug Canyon.

Bedsprings, frames, stove parts, broken mugs and plates, and bits of glass compose the remnants of a formerly tidy camp to the left. A platform of rocks may have supported a pulley and a wide belt as it passed up-slope, then returned down to the equipment directly below on the bar. As you look at the wheels and pulleys, the compressors and pipes, the tramway parts, and the scoop buckets, you can only guess which piece performed which operation. More gear and cabin sites dot the trail on both sides as you continue.

Step up over bedrock to cross another creek, then walk through a forest of Douglas-fir saplings. The whipping branches are slightly less annoying than the spiderwebs strung across the crowded path. Use your trekking poles to clear the way.

The trail leads east, past vertical slopes that drop from the left side of the trail to the sun-drenched emerald pools. A large seep on the right is cloaked in oversized ferns. Now cross a narrow cascade that bounces over the trail and begins to descend to the river as the canyon walls widen. A large, round metal sheet is attached to a Douglas fir on the left—no writing, no drawing, just a blank white sheet of round metal.

The trail widens to road-width as you approach the Dorer Ranch. Uphill to the right is the ranch; avoid it, as it's private property. Follow any homemade signs leading down any of the roads or trails toward the river. Here, at Humbug Creek and the North Fork, you can rest before the return trip.

The ranch owner has made some improvements at the river's confluence with Humbug Creek. Respect this private property as you enjoy the pools and slides. Refresh yourself for the hike back to the bridge, then prepare for an uphill hike to the trailhead.

NEARBY ACTIVITIES

The American Eagle Mine Trail (see next profile) begins where this hike ends. If you have the energy, it's an exciting trail that leads to interesting mining sites.

AMERICAN EAGLE MINE TRAIL

IN BRIEF

American Eagle Mine Trail starts where Euchre Bar Trail (see previous profile) leaves off. Hiking east on this section of Wild and Scenic River offers hikers choices of relaxing in the river's pools, exploring century-and-a-half-old mining operations, and observing the plentiful flora and fauna along the trail.

DESCRIPTION

If you followed the Euchre Bar Trail to its end at the pools of Humbug Bar, you've had a taste of the river, the flora, and some of the antique mining contraptions. The trailhead for the American Eagle Mine Trail sits at the junction of Humbug Creek and the North Fork of the American River, just 30 feet from the end of your hike on the Euchre Bar Trail. Pack up your gear from the picnic table, and clear any trash. Out of concern for nearby property owners, please respect the area and its primitive amenities. Descend to the creek on the obvious path and look for your track among the streamside foliage, about 20 feet up from the river. Three steps and you're on the other side, ascending a sandy path that curves uphill to the right.

- -

Directions ⟶

The best way to reach the trailhead is from the end of Euchre Bar Trail. From the junction of I-80 and the Capital City Freeway, drive 51.5 miles on I-80 East to Exit 146/Alta. Turn right on Morton Road and make an immediate left on Casa Loma Road. Drive 2.7 miles to the second railroad crossing. Continue across the tracks. The trailhead is 0.75 mile down the dirt road. A pit toilet marks the parking area, which fits about six cars.

KEY AT-A-GLANCE INFORMATION

LENGTH: 1.8 miles

CONFIGURATION: Out-and-back

DIFFICULTY: Moderate

WATER REQUIRED: 1 liter

SCENERY: Wild and Scenic River, Gold Rush–era remains

EXPOSURE: Shaded with some sunny patches

TRAIL TRAFFIC: Light

TRAIL SURFACE: Duff, dirt, and rock

HIKING TIME: 2 hours

SEASON: Year-round

ACCESS: No fees or permits

MAPS: USGS Westville; Tahoe National Forest map

WHEELCHAIR ACCESS: None

FACILITIES: None

DRIVING DISTANCE: 55 miles

SPECIAL COMMENTS: Mining equipment and cabin sites with artifacts can be seen along the trail. This trailhead, on private property at Humbug Bar, can be reached only by completing the previous hike, Euchre Bar Trail to Humbug Canyon.

GPS TRAILHEAD COORDINATES

Latitude   N39° 10.747´

Longitude   W120° 43.636´

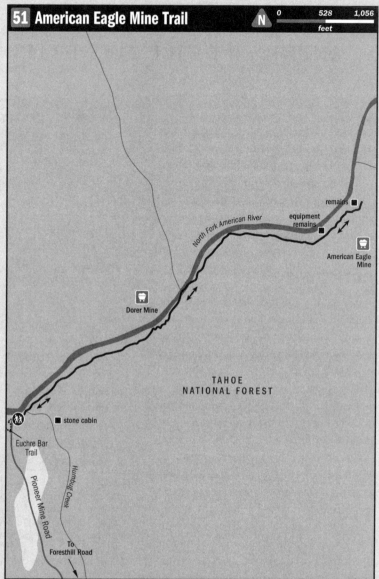

51 American Eagle Mine Trail

N 0   528   1,056
feet

North Fork American River

remains

equipment
remains

American Eagle
Mine

Dorer Mine

TAHOE
NATIONAL FOREST

stone cabin

Euchre Bar
Trail

Humbug Creek

Pioneer Mine Road

To
Foresthill Road

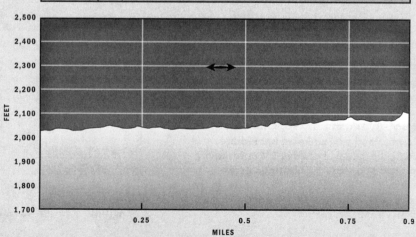

FEET

2,500
2,400
2,300
2,200
2,100
2,000
1,900
1,800
1,700

0.25   0.5   0.75   0.9

MILES

Within a hundred paces, look for a faint path leading back to the right into some patchy bushes. Push on through, and within 50 feet you'll see a roofless stone cabin on the bank above Humbug Creek.

Square on the inside, with doors, windows, and a hearth, this cabin is solid, if not windproof. It appears as if someone was trying to make a nice appearance here—perhaps for an understanding partner—by building a comfortable, albeit temporary, home. The most treasured and missed accoutrement of the gold camps was a wife, or a woman of any sort, actually. Trails lead to the creek and river, which was probably the builder's workplace.

Return to the trail and head east past some scrawny blackberries, where the trail broadens considerably. The path is clear for a few minutes, making for easy hiking as it contours alongside the river. Then, just like that, the trail becomes overgrown with bushes, seedlings, poison oak, face flies, and mosquitoes. Cross some logs, and the trail once again widens. California sister butterflies linger trail-side, lending color above the tree-shaded, duff-covered forest floor.

Rock walls, built to support the fills that the trail crosses, still hold their position. These improvements on the local trails—the miners' sidewalks and thoroughfares—enabled the workers to move around the diggings efficiently.

The river is about 15 feet below the trail now as you travel east. Wider and much calmer in this flat section, the pools look very inviting. Side trails will take you down for a brief dip. After that, keep following the old iron pipe that runs at least 500 feet alongside the trail, on the right. It looks to have been hastily sunk into the slope, then laid on top of the ground to bring spring water to those living near their claims along the river.

Climb a bit and barge forward when the trail closes in on you. The river canyon's walls are vertical now, and you pass above them on the narrow trail. Mining remains lie mostly above the trail. A large fremontia, with its softball-mitt-sized leaves, crowds the trail on the right. Pass this bush, then pass a seep emerging from above the trail. Continue east for another 10 minutes. The apparatus you see now is from the American Eagle Mine, which is technically about 200 feet above you.

Equipment, strange and primitive, rusting and overturned, is scattered about beneath the mine site. Well above the trail is a very large steel pipe, purpose unknown, held in place by laurel and oak. Adjacent to the trail, on the riverside, is another mysterious mechanism. "A steel octopus" may best describe this possible exhaust manifold cowering beneath a bigleaf maple. Another interesting piece of gear lies on the uphill side of the trail. Possibly an air compressor, it looks as if it was once housed beneath a roofed enclosure and ran a belt of some kind on each side. Similar devices and wheels are also seen down-slope.

As you head farther up the trail, the route east becomes crowded with underbrush and dissolves into the forest in another 10 minutes. You may consider the trail to have ended when you discover another piece of overturned gear. An air compressor, manufactured in 1911 by Gardner Governor Company, sits idle and rusting. Nearby, some iron spikes have been pounded into the rock, and then the forest closes off further travel.

On your return to the trailhead at Euchre Bar, look around for more remains. You'll find tramway equipment manufactured in San Francisco, steel cables, flywheels, shovels and buckets, stove parts, and rockworks. The trek down was pretty easy. The trip up is not much more difficult since you have discoveries to talk about while you slowly ascend to your car.

NEARBY ACTIVITIES

The Green Valley Trail (Hike 49, page 249) takes hikers down a ridgeline, from the trailhead on the Foresthill Divide to the Wild and Scenic River downstream from the Euchre Bar footbridge and just upstream of Giant Gap, with spectacular views of Lovers Leap.

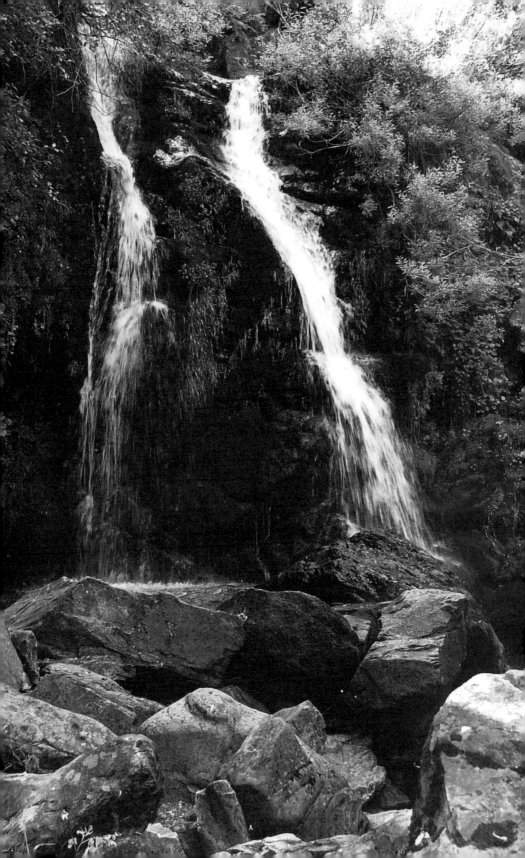

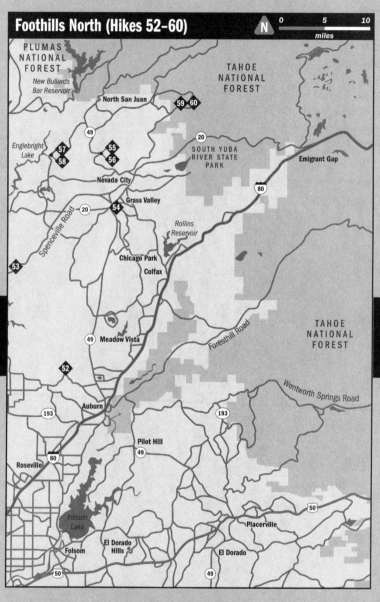

Foothills North (Hikes 52–60)

PLUMAS NATIONAL FOREST

New Bullards Bar Reservoir

TAHOE NATIONAL FOREST

North San Juan

59 60

49

20

Englebright Lake

57
58

55
56

SOUTH YUBA RIVER STATE PARK

Emigrant Gap

Nevada City

80

Spenceville Road

Grass Valley

20   54

Rollins Reservoir

53

Chicago Park

Colfax

Foresthill Road

TAHOE NATIONAL FOREST

49   Meadow Vista

52

Wentworth Springs Road

193   Auburn

80

193

Pilot Hill

Roseville

49

Folsom Lake

50

El Dorado Hills

Placerville

Folsom

El Dorado

49

50

FOOTHILLS NORTH

52 HIDDEN FALLS TRAILS

KEY AT-A-GLANCE INFORMATION

LENGTH: 5.5 miles

CONFIGURATION: Connected loops

DIFFICULTY: Moderate

WATER REQUIRED: 2 liters

SCENERY: Foothill woodland

EXPOSURE: Well shaded most of the way

TRAIL TRAFFIC: Moderate

TRAIL SURFACE: Sand and rock, dirt and duff

HIKING TIME: 2–3 hours

SEASON: Year-round, 30 minutes before sunrise–30 minutes after sunset

ACCESS: No fees or permits

MAPS: USGS Gold Hill. An excellent color map of all the trails is posted at tinyurl.com/hiddenfallstrails.

WHEELCHAIR ACCESS: Yes—the accessible Hidden Gateway Trail begins just 10 feet past the trailhead for this hike.

FACILITIES: Restrooms, water fountain, and pay phone

DRIVING DISTANCE: 32 miles

SPECIAL COMMENTS: Hidden Falls Overlook offers a view of the falls that would be unobtainable without this naturally architected platform.

GPS TRAILHEAD COORDINATES

Latitude   N38° 57.544´

Longitude   W121° 09.839´

IN BRIEF

Hidden Falls Regional Park, the crown jewel of Placer County's Placer Legacy program, is a model for suburban open-space design and use. The park's 7 miles of trails are available to hikers, bikers, runners, and horseback riders. An accessible trail—the Hidden Gateway Trail—offers excellent views of the 221-acre site. The other paths consist of either loops or out-and-back trails that range from moderate to difficult. The hike described here combines portions of each trail to give the hiker a good workout rewarded by excellent scenery. These trails are well marked, and the intersections are somewhat frequent, so becoming temporarily disoriented should not be a concern on this hike.

DESCRIPTION

Your trail, which starts out near the top of the ridge, descends to Deadman Creek, then ascends the next ridge to the north before arriving at the pools of Coon Creek. The nicely shaded path takes you along Coon Creek as you make your way west toward Deadman's Falls.

Directions _____

From the junction of I-80 East and the Capital City Freeway, drive 24 miles on I-80 East toward Auburn and take Exit 119B/Grass Valley. Drive north on CA 49 for 2.7 miles and turn left onto Atwood Road, which becomes Mount Vernon Road after 1.7 miles. Follow Mount Vernon Road 2.6 miles and turn right on Mears Road. The Hidden Valley Regional Park entrance, at 7587 Mears Road, is up the hill, on the right. Turn into the parking lot. The trailhead is to the right of the restrooms.

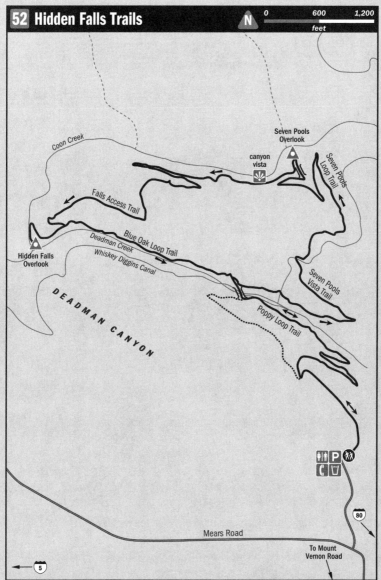

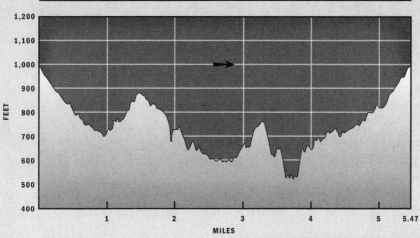

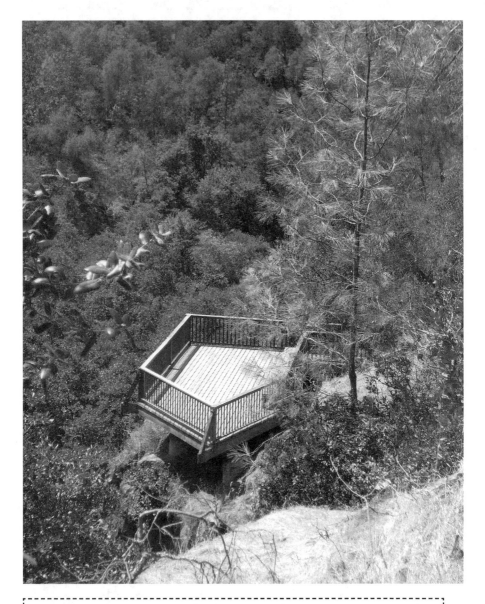

The new observation platform affords hikers views of the falls that were never before attainable.

Your trail starts at the information kiosk at the end of the parking lot, where you'll see a map of the complete trail system. The restrooms and pay phone are to your left; walk about 5 feet down the sidewalk, turn right, and descend a few concrete steps to the dirt path of Poppy Trail. Then turn left and begin walking north.

As you walk down Poppy Trail, the view to your east is of fenced cattle ranches ringed by foothill-woodland forests. This old four-wheel-drive road is rather exposed as you descend to the first U-turn. A couple of lazy switchbacks ease you down about 150 feet to Deadman Creek.

On the way down, you'll feel a nice cooling as you enter the shade of live oak and foothill pine. Within moments you'll begin to hear Deadman Creek. A restful bench has been placed here from which you can watch the sometimes-turbulent stream. Another, more appetizing sign of the upcoming creek is the appearance of miner's lettuce on the left side of your trail. Resist the temptation to pick—it's prohibited—as you head toward the bridge ahead of you.

Cross the bridge to reach Pond Turtle Trail. Take this connector 300 feet to its junction with Blue Oak Loop Trail. A sharp right uphill puts you on the side of the hill under the shade of the foothill-woodland understory: toyon and manzanita. This trail will quickly gain elevation, then level off. To your left you can see the contours of the hills in the trail cut. Notice the gentle folds of the rock strata as you pass.

After you cross a footbridge at a seasonal runoff ravine, you may begin to notice more blue oak—much of it speckled with oakmoss lichen. On the right, a rather large—and horizontal—foothill pine stretches from its roots at the canyon center to its crown tip at the trailside. Signs indicate that this tree fell during the winter of 2006. Your trail continues to gain elevation after it swings back to the northwest. As you walk in the shade, watch for weasel signs, which are usually plumb in the middle of the trail.

As you level out after 1.4 miles, you'll see a signpost (labeled #10) at the junction where you now leave the Blue Oak Loop when it turns left. Continue straight onto the Seven Pools Vista Trail.

Descend a bit to the northeast, toward the Seven Pools area. You won't actually reach the pools on this trail—the next junction will get you there. On the way, you'll find a great perch from which to use your camera. For now, the dirt-and-leaf-covered trail seems to be the easy part of the hike: gently descending, continuously shaded, quiet enough to hear birds and the stream.

Among the toyon, manzanita, and live oak, the trail will make a U-turn before reaching the Seven Pools area, then wrap around the hillside, gently descending in and out of a ravine before reaching a well-signed intersection with Seven Pools Loop. Your route turns sharply right, onto Seven Pools Loop, at Signpost #11.

Head east, descending just below the previous trail section and getting ever closer to Coon Creek. To help keep your feet dry, use the small bridge that crosses the ravine you walked around earlier. Now head north about 100 yards to a spur trail, which leads to a rock outcrop looking over the cascades and into one of the pools.

Return to the Seven Pools Loop, heading west. Notice the bits and chunks of quartz along this section of trail. Quartz-bearing gravels attracted miners' attention, as the mining ditch along Deadman Creek reminds us. The large blocks in the creek bottom testify to the general geological makeup of this region: highly fractured blocks and faults, squeezed, uplifted, folded, coated with lava and mud-flows, washed, scrubbed, bleached, and left as you find them today. To see a good example just before you reach the vista ahead on the right, look at the outcrop of rock running from the left on the hill above you—visible as it continues immediately under your feet and out to your right at the boulder-littered canyon floor.

Shortly after the vista spot, just as the trail turns away from the creek, your path crosses Pond Turtle Trail. This junction is simple: keep walking straight. But if you want a pleasant spot at which to sit and have a moment, you've gone about 2.7 miles—halfway—and the creek is right there after all.

Continuing west on Seven Pools Loop, the trail varies from 5 to 50 feet above the creek bed. Walk past any blocked trails that are marked for trail restoration. The 960-acre ranch to the west is currently being surveyed for additional trails, but vegetation recovery is needed in some areas first.

The Seven Pools Loop will switchback, ascending to the east for 0.2 mile. Turning right at the intersection with Quail Run will lead you toward Turkey Ridge Road, through a tunnel of manzanita, black oak, and toyon, for one of the real highlights of this hike.

At the junction with Turkey Ridge Road (#15), turn west through the closed gate to follow the shaded fuel-break up and over the knoll and down to Hidden Falls Trail. Head for the picnic table in the shaded cul-de-sac. A break in the rail fence, marked by a handcrafted sign, beckons you to the Falls Overlook.

Hike east 100 yards as you listen to the growing rush of the as-yet-unseen Deadman Creek. A dozen stone stairs lead you down toward tempting blackberries, but your trail is to the right. Begin a brief traverse of the hillside above the creek. Descend the rocky, fence-lined track right up to another stream, Coon Creek, then swing south with the trail. A west-facing bench overlooks Coon Creek at a well-engineered trail that descends to its bank. Your destination is a mere 150 feet ahead, as the roaring cascades foretell.

The views of these 35-foot year-round falls were limited and somewhat precipitous before this observation platform was constructed. Now visitors can view, photograph, linger, and contemplate in comfort as never before.

Return on this trail to ascend the stone steps, where you turn right and continue to the junction with Blue Oak Loop. This flat, shaded trail turns right to follow the Pond Turtle Connector across the bridge. Turn left onto Poppy Trail to walk along Deadman Creek, past another blackberry patch.

Three easy switchbacks lie between the creek and the ridge. Even though you leave the shade of foothill pines and California buckeyes for an open, dry slope, you can't help but stop and admire the massive mistletoe-blotched valley oak that towers over the trail. Walk another 500 feet to the trailhead, with this giant to your right.

FAIRY FALLS TRAIL 53

IN BRIEF

This pleasant hike to Fairy Falls takes you along a route through an area of intense geologic history to a set of waterfalls—all of which will be flooded if the proposed Waldo Dam is constructed. Fairy Falls (also known as Shingle Falls on topos) sits astride the ill-named Dry Creek and drops some 70 feet to the pool before tumbling over Lower Fairy Falls.

DESCRIPTION

This hike includes something for a wide variety of interests. Following Old Spenceville Road, where the lone oak stands, you'll walk past what was once Spenceville, founded in the 1850s and abandoned in 1915. Copper mines dot the lower trail, and gold fields can be found in the hillsides. Mines are especially dangerous and should never be entered.

Surrounded by the Spenceville Wildlife Area, the trail is visited by a vast number of migratory birds. If you're interested in rocks,

KEY AT-A-GLANCE INFORMATION

LENGTH: 5.1 miles

CONFIGURATION: Out-and-back

DIFFICULTY: Moderate

WATER REQUIRED: 2 liters

SCENERY: River, pools, cascades, 2 waterfalls, and foothill woodlands

EXPOSURE: Lots of exposure to sun; the route in provides some shade

TRAIL TRAFFIC: Moderate

TRAIL SURFACE: Dirt and gravel, dirt and duff

HIKING TIME: 2–4 hours depending on lunch, photos, and wading time

SEASON: Year-round

ACCESS: No fees or permits

MAPS: USGS Camp Far West, Wolf

WHEELCHAIR ACCESS: None

FACILITIES: None

DRIVING DISTANCE: 63 miles

SPECIAL COMMENTS: The large, clear pools below the lower falls make this an ideal destination on a hot summer day.

Directions

From the junction of I-5 North and CA 99 North after Arco Arena, take CA 99 North—which turns into CA 70—35 miles. In Marysville, turn right onto CA 20 and drive 0.2 mile, then turn left to continue on CA 20 for 0.2 mile. Make another right turn to continue on CA 20 for 18.5 miles. Turn right on Smartville Road at the Beale AFB sign and go 5.5 miles, staying to the left, to reach Waldo Road. Turn left onto this gravel road and drive 1.8 miles to Spenceville Road. Be careful when crossing the wooden-decked Waldo Bridge. Stay on Spenceville Road 2.3 miles until you reach the large dirt parking area on the left, 500 feet before the road ends. Your trailhead is at the yellow gate blocking the bridge.

GPS TRAILHEAD COORDINATES

Latitude   N39° 06.837´

Longitude   W121° 16.251´

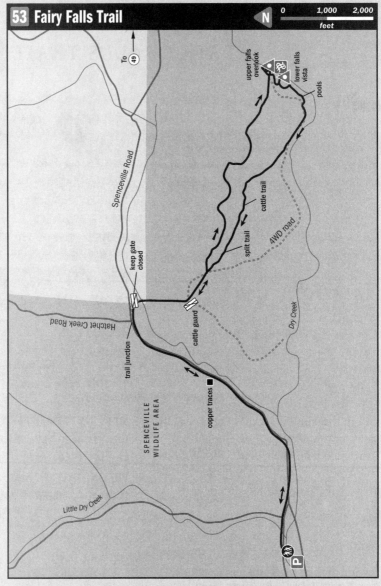

N

| 0 | 1,000 | 2,000 |

feet

To **49**

Spenceville Road

Hatchet Creek Road

keep gate closed

trail junction

cattle guard

SPENCEVILLE WILDLIFE AREA

copper traces

Little Dry Creek

split trail

cattle trail

4WD road

Dry Creek

upper falls overlook

lower falls vista

pools

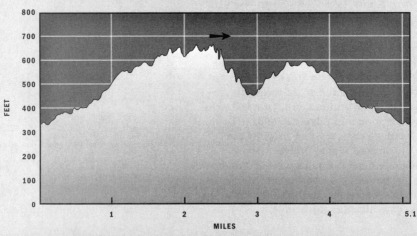

Fairy Falls and Dry Creek's canyon expose geologic features that are within easy reach. You'll find typical flora of the foothill woodlands, but the blossoming flowers alone are worth a springtime hike here. They're at their peak from March through May.

In such a broad, open space, one would expect to see large animals from a distance. Instead, they choose the cool evenings and mornings for their business. But that doesn't mean you won't see some local fauna. Within 50 feet of the bridge, I almost stepped on a medium-sized northern alligator lizard as it sat motionless in a sunny patch in the trail. Before traveling 0.5 mile, you might also spot a two-toned green Pacific tree frog as this little fellow bellows from a seep on the left side of the trail.

Look across Dry Creek at the exposed rock; the result of the heating and melting of several minerals metamorphosed this rock into what we know as serpentine, California's state rock. This greasy-looking, dark-green rock is very common in the western Foothills, largely due to the geologic forces that also created the gold here.

In fact, as you drove just south of the town of Smartville, you entered a geologic area that was formed just about 200 million years ago and is now known as California. An island 600 miles out in the Pacific Ocean began moving east at the same time that the North American continent began moving west. When they inevitably met, the resulting faulting created favorable conditions for gold and other metals to be formed and exposed.

Geologists call that arc-shaped island, which stretches from Oroville to Auburn and extends about 25 miles west into the Central Valley, the Smartville Block. This formation is largely responsible for California's legacy of gold.

This area was settled not only for its rich gold veins but also for its copper-bearing ore. Copper is so concentrated in the Smartville Block that Native Americans were able to dig it directly out of the earth. After about 0.75 mile, look for an opening in the road cut that appears to be covered by stacked blocks. That is one of the sealed copper mines, further evidenced by the red-stained clays in the path.

Walk generally northeast along Old Spenceville Road, bypassing a trail that enters from the north and leads to private property. You'll soon come upon a gate blocking your road, so turn to the south and walk toward the gate you see there. Now you have a brief but unrelenting south-facing uphill climb. Lift your spirits by turning around to look at the scenery of the surrounding hills.

When you reach the top of the hill after 1.4 miles, you'll see a cattle guard standing as lonely as the tollbooth in *Blazing Saddles*. You can ignore the road that goes southwest. Turn southeast and angle across this open slope for 250 yards to a junction of the two Fairy Falls approach trails. The choice is yours—the distances are equal, and neither involves tedious climbing. I went left on the Upper Falls Trail on my way in and returned via the right-hand trail after exploring the lower falls and pools.

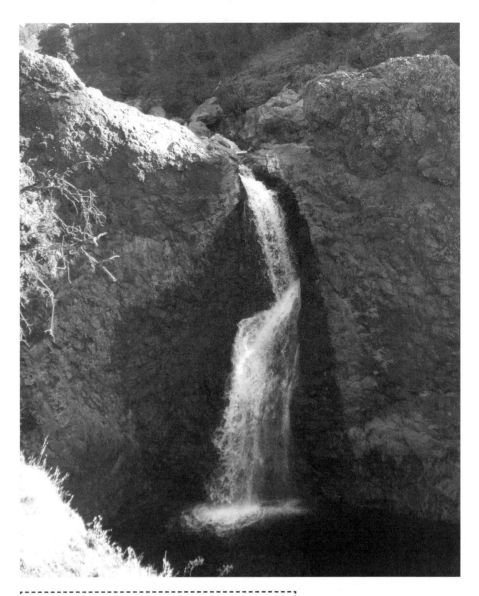

Fairy Falls, on Dry Creek, is called Shingle Falls on some maps.

Evenly dotted with blue oak, the hillsides also boast foothill pine, manzanita, toyon, and live oak. And where there is sun and space, there are flowers. On my hike, California poppies and popcorn flowers colored most open slopes, and the blue oak glowed when backlit by the sun.

The Upper Falls Trail ascends the hillside for a few moments, then begins to contour around the hills. You'll cross a jeep road about 150 yards from the falls.

Fairy Falls, Shingle Falls, Beale Falls, Dry Creek Falls—regardless of what it's called, the falls are impressive, plunging some 70 feet in the upper cascade. The chain-link fence appears to be a poor deterrent to closer viewing, but it is a reminder of the danger at the edge of the overlook.

While standing here, one *must* wonder about the bottom half of a bulldozer planted in the ground on the edge of this precipice. There are so many questions that these things bring to mind . . . but first, there's a canyon to explore.

Thin, narrow trails creep down the edge of the canyon to afford better views, different views, more views—whatever the motivation, there's a little winding trail to get you there around this brilliant cascade. You can leave the security of the fence farther downstream and, without too much difficulty, have fun exploring down to the lower falls and then to the placid pools at the creek level.

From the lower falls or the lower pools areas, begin your return on the jeep road that parallels the creek just uphill from it. After 500 feet of walking northwest, take the footpath to the right that angles slightly uphill. You'll stay on this trail until you reach the junction that you encountered on the entry route. From that point, your return track to the trailhead is a familiar one.

NEARBY ACTIVITIES

About 15 miles north, South Yuba River State Park offers miles of river recreation as well as hiking, biking, and equestrian trails. Buttermilk Bend Trail (Hike 57, page 288) and Point Defiance Trail (Hike 58, page 292) highlight pioneer engineering along a scenic river.

54 HARDROCK TRAIL

KEY AT-A-GLANCE INFORMATION

LENGTH: 4.4 miles

CONFIGURATION: Connected loops

DIFFICULTY: Moderate

WATER REQUIRED: 1 liter

SCENERY: Foothill woodland, historic mining relics and buildings

EXPOSURE: Mostly shaded

TRAIL TRAFFIC: Moderate

TRAIL SURFACE: Sand, chipped gravel, dirt and duff

HIKING TIME: 2 hours

SEASON: Year-round, sunrise–sunset

ACCESS: $7 day-use fee at visitor center; free parking at Penn Gate

MAPS: USGS Grass Valley; local trail map at visitor center and at parks .ca.gov/?page_id=26345; PDF at tinyurl.com/empire-pdf

WHEELCHAIR ACCESS: None

FACILITIES: Information kiosk at trailhead; restrooms at visitor center

DRIVING DISTANCE: 48 miles

SPECIAL COMMENTS: Hazardous-waste cleanup has temporarily closed some portions of the trails. Other trails have reopened since the area was fully restored. New and old trails are being resurfaced with gravel, making them comfortable, durable, and easy to follow.

GPS TRAILHEAD COORDINATES

Latitude   N39° 12.561´
Longitude   W121° 03.423´

IN BRIEF

The Hardrock Trail is the largest of the three loops connected for this hike. The Hardrock Trail joins the Osborn Hill Loop at a well-signed junction, and the Conlon Mine Loop swings you by a hardrock-mine site. All three reconnect to make one large but wasp-waisted sightseeing trip. Set in the 800-acre Empire Mine State Historic Park, these loops will lead you past the relics and buildings of the region's richest gold-mining area.

DESCRIPTION

Hardrock mining came to Nevada County in 1850, when George Knight discovered gold—literally a mountain of it. The Mother Lode he unearthed was not only one of the richest gold deposits in the world but also became the descriptive name for the entire region. More than half of California's gold production came from the mines in this area, with the Empire Mine and the North Star Mine yielding the greatest share of riches.

The Hardrock Trail begins at Penn Gate, which is close to the old Pennsylvania Mine site. The Pennsylvania Mine was one of many dotting the park grounds. In the 1850s, mine shafts were blasted, drilled, and dug in every direction to extract gold-bearing ore for

----

Directions _____→

From the junction of I-80 East and the Capital City Freeway, drive 24 miles on I-80 East toward Auburn and take Exit 119B/Grass Valley. Drive about 22 miles on CA 49 North to the Empire Street exit and turn right, onto West Empire Street. Cross South Auburn Street and continue 0.3 mile on East Empire Street to the Penn Gate trailhead parking area, on the right.

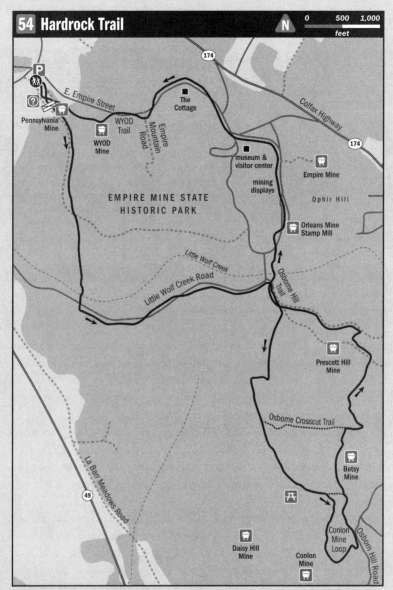

N

0   500   1,000
feet

E. Empire Street

174

Colfax Highway

174

The Cottage

Pennsylvania Mine

WYOD Trail

WYOD Mine

Empire Mountain Road

museum & visitor center

mining displays

Empire Mine

Ophir Hill

Orleans Mine Stamp Mill

EMPIRE MINE STATE HISTORIC PARK

Little Wolf Creek

Little Wolf Creek Road

Osborne Hill Trail

Prescott Hill Mine

Osborne Crosscut Trail

Betsy Mine

La Barr Meadows Road

49

Daisy Hill Mine

Conlon Mine

Conlon Mine Loop

Osborn Hill Road

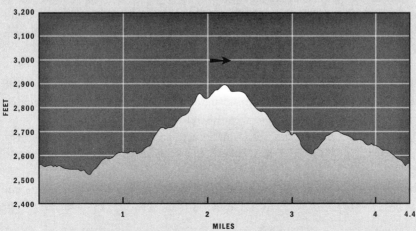

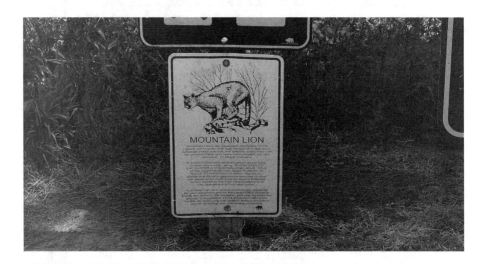

Mountain lions are a very real threat, even in urbanized areas.

further processing. Ore was crushed to sand by the numerous and noisy stamp mills. The resulting ore dust was treated with chemicals—the most hazardous of which were mercury and cyanide—to capture the gold. Your trail passes the stamp mills, tailings piles, and slurry ponds, which are currently being cleaned up so they can be reclaimed by nature.

An information kiosk at the trailhead displays a map giving an overview of the trails. It also houses a very active colony of carpenter bees, which encourages speed-reading. Better, then, to pick up a current trails guide from the visitor center. Heed the warnings about both rattlesnakes and mountain lions: they're very real threats here.

Hikers, runners, bicyclists, and horseback riders share these trails as they tour this foothill woodland in the shade of Douglas fir, ponderosa pine, foothill pine, sugar pine, live oak, black oak, bigleaf maple, and incense cedar.

Interpretive signs along the trail help visitors appreciate the area's history. What at first glance looks like a pile of useless rock turns out to be, well, a pile of useless rock that was placed there on purpose by individual miners toiling in the Work Your Own Diggins Mine. Operated somewhat like a time-share scheme, the mine was finally abandoned in 1912.

A fence on your left borders the trail as you walk south toward Little Wolf Creek. Cross a small footbridge over the creek before turning east on Little Wolf Creek Road. Under shade of ponderosa pine and a huge stand of bigleaf maple, walk at a leisurely uphill pace just above the creek flowing to your left.

After walking east for 0.5 mile, you'll encounter a well-signed junction with the Osborn Loop Trail. Spurred by the promise of several abandoned mines— Daisy Hill, Conlon, Betsy, and Prescott Hill—turn right, and then at the next junction follow the right-hand fork uphill. This is the apex of the Osborn Hill

Loop. Hazardous-waste cleanup is ongoing, and trails may be rerouted from time to time. Generous and distinct signage will guide you when it's necessary.

The next south-bearing section of trail is partially exposed, gaining about 200 feet in elevation over the next 0.6 mile. On your way, you'll reach a T under the power lines; turn right, walk 200 feet, and resume walking south on the new track. Continue your gentle ascent for another 0.4 mile to the Conlon Mine Loop Trail. On the south side of the trail, this 0.7-mile loop of fresh gravel tread ushers you through the manzanita-covered hillside surrounding this hardrock-mining site. On your way uphill to the Conlon Mine, look for the trail to the Daisy Hill Mine near a picnic table. Depending on restoration efforts, you may be able to explore that path as well.

When you complete the Conlon Mine Loop, head north on the Osborn Loop Trail in the direction of the Prescott Hill Mine and the Hardrock Trail. A spur trail to the southeast leads to a pedestrian-entry gate on Osborn Hill Road. On the way, you'll pass the trail to the Betsy Mine on your right. A fence at Osborn Hill Road will turn you around if you explore this side trail.

In about 0.2 mile, you'll be able to take a tour around the Betsy Mine site on fresh tread. No more than 600 feet north of that, you'll traverse under the power lines and begin a swing to the northwest. Only 200 yards ahead is the junction with the Prescott Hill Mine Trail. Keeping left on the Osborn Hill Loop will reconnect you with the Hardrock Trail. Continue your gentle downhill as you come to another junction with the Prescott Mine Trail. Keep left again.

At the next two familiar junctions, follow the signs that lead you to the right and downhill, where you can easily ford Little Wolf Creek. At the top of the brief uphill, the trail turns left to pass the foundations of the Orleans Stamp Mill. Signs will direct you to the left to stay on the Hardrock Trail or direct you right to reach the Union Hill trails. The return route to the trailhead continues to the left. You will soon pass some of the mining museum's outdoor displays. Walk through the parking area toward the visitor center. The Hardrock Trail continues on East Empire Street, along the stone wall in front of the Bourne Mansion. Penn Gate is only 0.5 mile ahead.

Before you reach your destination, you'll veer off into the Work Your Own Diggins (WYOD) area and soon pass the Mule Corral; here mules awaited their descent into the mines, where they worked out their lives and birthed generations of new stock. You'll again walk through the Pennsylvania Mine remains as the trailhead comes into view.

NEARBY ACTIVITIES

Explore more trails from the Gold Hill trailhead in the Union Hill area.

55 INDEPENDENCE TRAIL: EAST BRANCH

KEY AT-A-GLANCE INFORMATION

LENGTH: 4.5 miles

CONFIGURATION: Out-and-back

DIFFICULTY: Easy

WATER REQUIRED: 1–2 liters

SCENERY: Foothill woodland, river canyon

EXPOSURE: Shaded

TRAIL TRAFFIC: Moderate

TRAIL SURFACE: Dirt and duff, rock and gravel

HIKING TIME: 2–3 hours

SEASON: Year-round

ACCESS: No fees or permits

MAPS: USGS Nevada City; local trail map at Tahoe National Forest Ranger Station on CA 49

WHEELCHAIR ACCESS: None; the West Branch (see next hike) is superior in this respect.

FACILITIES: Pit toilets at trailhead

DRIVING DISTANCE: 57 miles

SPECIAL COMMENTS: Some of the flumes on this trail are in less-than-prime shape, so exercise caution when crossing them.

GPS TRAILHEAD COORDINATES

Latitude   N39° 17.499´

Longitude   W121° 05.827´

IN BRIEF

From the trailhead to a perch overlooking Hoyt Crossing in 2.3 canyon miles, including 11 flumes, this short trail in the former Excelsior Ditch offers a glimpse into the engineering methods and challenges of 19th-century gold miners. The beautiful canyon views in a foothill-woodland habitat zone are worth the trip as well.

DESCRIPTION

The Excelsior Mining and Canal Company, formed in 1854, sought to provide increasing supplies of water to hydraulic mines operating as far away as Smartville. Construction of the 17-mile Excelsior Ditch began in 1859 with the intent of delivering water from the South Yuba River to the existing China Ditch. The connection was made four years later. Following the Sawyer Decision in 1884, hydraulic mining was rendered impractical and the ditch was converted for agricultural-irrigation purposes. The Excelsior Ditch, its paths for ditch tenders, and its flumes were operated for these purposes until 1963, when it was finally abandoned.

Directions

From the junction of I-80 and the Capital City Freeway, drive 24 miles on I-80 East toward Auburn. Take Exit 119B/Grass Valley and drive 27 miles on CA 49 North to Nevada City; then turn left—following CA 49—at the split with CA 20. Immediately to your right is the Tahoe National Forest Ranger Station, where you can obtain additional trail information and a simple map. The trailhead is 6.2 miles past the ranger station. A parking area with enough room for a dozen cars is on the right side of CA 49, in front of the trailhead and restrooms. Additional parking is at the turnout just around the curve.

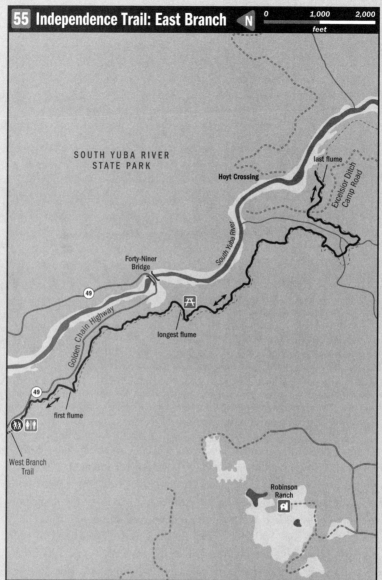

SOUTH YUBA RIVER
STATE PARK

Hoyt Crossing

last flume

Excelsior Ditch Camp Road

South Yuba River

Forty-Niner
Bridge

49

Golden Chain Highway

longest flume

49

first flume

West Branch
Trail

Robinson
Ranch

0   1,000   2,000
feet

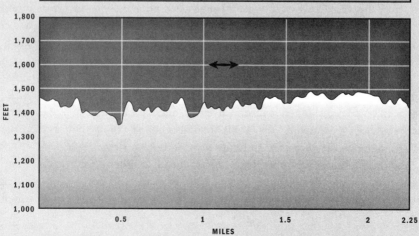

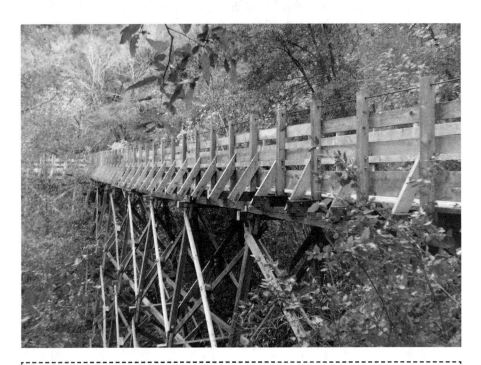

Each flume was employed so that the water ditch could shortcut ravines or skirt rock outcrops. The ditch became a three-sided box that sat on the trestle below—together they made up the flume.

So now you can take off on this easy trail. It's easy to navigate; don't turn off the path except for picnic tables. It's easy to walk; over the next 2.3 miles, the trail gains only 35 feet in elevation. It's easy for walking beside your companions—especially small ones, as this is a great trail for children. And it's easy for snagging photo ops: vistas and features are everywhere, so keep your camera handy.

Pass the stairs just 200 feet along the path, unless you need to go down to your car at the turnout. To span a ravine or bypass a rock outcrop, ditch-builders constructed a trestle—the framework beneath whatever was put on top for it to support. In this case, a wooden water trough with no ends was the ersatz ditch. The flume is the sum total of both engineered structures, trestle and trough. More importantly, the first flume you'll cross on this trail is a mere 250 yards ahead.

Hugging the hillside tightly as it rounds an outcrop, the next flume provides a stable platform from which to look out over the river and road below. Well-placed benches making a convenient spot for taking pictures. The background foliage of incense cedar and red-skinned madrone, live oak, and bigleaf maple makes for great shots throughout the canyon. Vistas will open occasionally along the way, and the trailside granite construction and outcrops are also noteworthy.

About 15 minutes (0.6 mile) from the trailhead, another photo op comes up at an impressive boulder display. Views of the new and old Forty-Niner Bridge come up as well if you look back to the west. If you dawdle around here, watch for the pretty plant at trailside with three red or green leaves together—don't touch, as it's poison oak. Surrounded by the fragrant kit-kit-dizze, equally fragrant incense cedar provides the scent of fall in place of springtime's buckeye extravaganza. The blackberries here at trailside are just nature's cherry on top.

The longest flume on this trail spans the next ravine, which brims with live oak, madrone, bigleaf maple, and willow. Just past the next flume, about 1 mile along, stands a California torreya—also known as the California nutmeg (although it is definitely not a nutmeg). This single-needle conifer is rare throughout the Sierra Nevada, their foothills, and the Coast Range. And thank goodness for that: its needles are anything but friendly—as sharp as cactus needles.

The first of two picnic sites is just beyond the next flume, and the second comes three flumes after that. Each flume has its own peculiarity: some are slippery, some have rotted a bit, and one at 2 miles in has holes in its deck to avoid. But if the explorer in you says "go on," then on you can go.

When the ditch looks completely blocked, you can continue forward on the ditch tender's trail. Below you, the Excelsior Ditch Camp Road is visible. Just ahead, in fact, the trail runs out again at a washout on this dirt road. Scramble around that to regain the trail without too much effort, and proceed.

Believe it or not, there's one more flume to deal with, and it's the funkiest so far. But just 0.1 mile beyond it is the actual end of the trail. With manzanita and chamise crowding in and live oak all around, this perch stands right over the South Yuba River. And from that point, one can point a camera lens straight into the miners' tunnel at Hoyt Crossing.

The walk back is even easier. After all, it's 35 feet downhill now.

NEARBY ACTIVITIES

Grass Valley and Nevada City are replete with Gold Rush–era historic sites. Each downtown area is easy to walk, making for a pleasant time on any day. Nevada City's Victorian Christmas displays are special.

Having seen the water-delivery process, visit Malakoff Diggins State Historic Park (Hike 60, page 300) and see what happened in step two of that process. And you can witness an entirely different type of gold hunting at Empire Mine State Historic Park (see previous profile), where hardrock mining really paid off.

56 INDEPENDENCE TRAIL: WEST BRANCH

KEY AT-A-GLANCE INFORMATION

LENGTH: 4.8 miles

CONFIGURATION: Out-and-back

DIFFICULTY: Easy

WATER REQUIRED: 1–2 liters

SCENERY: Foothill forest, canyon overlooks

EXPOSURE: Always shaded

TRAIL TRAFFIC: Moderate

TRAIL SURFACE: Leaf-covered duff and dirt

HIKING TIME: 2–3 hours

SEASON: Year-round

ACCESS: No fees or permits

MAPS: USGS Nevada City; local trail map at Tahoe National Forest Ranger Station on CA 49

WHEELCHAIR ACCESS: Yes— all facilities are accessible.

FACILITIES: Restrooms at trailhead and 2 spots along the trail; no water available

DRIVING DISTANCE: 57 miles

SPECIAL COMMENTS: This is the nation's first wheelchair-accessible wilderness trail. Groups may take a docent-guided tour by calling 530-272-0298.

GPS TRAILHEAD COORDINATES

Latitude   N39° 17.491´
Longitude   W121° 05.831´

IN BRIEF

Just 10 minutes from Nevada City, this pleasant hike makes use of the first wheelchair-accessible wilderness trail in the United States. The builders created the path from the remains of an abandoned mining and irrigation canal originally built in 1854. The level grade makes it ideal for hikers of all ages and abilities. Interpretive and identifying signs highlight the diversity of flora along the trail. A sharp eye will spot a California newt among the trail duff (and the sharp hiker won't touch it—the amphibian's slimy coating is toxic). The cascades at Rush Creek, which has a superior ramp-access system, is the glamour spot on this route.

DESCRIPTION

Gold Country trails certainly offer foothill hikers some diverse and lush flora. The trail itself runs along a mining relic: in 1854 the Excelsior Mining and Canal Company constructed the Excelsior Ditch to transport water from the South Yuba River 17 miles to join

Directions

From the junction of I-80 and the Capital City Freeway, drive 24 miles on I-80 East toward Auburn. Take Exit 119B/Grass Valley and drive 27 miles on CA 49 North to Nevada City; then turn left—following CA 49—at the split with CA 20. Immediately to your right is the Tahoe National Forest Ranger Station, where you can obtain additional trail information and a simple map. The trailhead is 6.2 miles past the ranger station. A parking area with enough room for a dozen cars is on the right side of CA 49, in front of the trailhead and restrooms. There's additional parking at the turnout just around the curve.

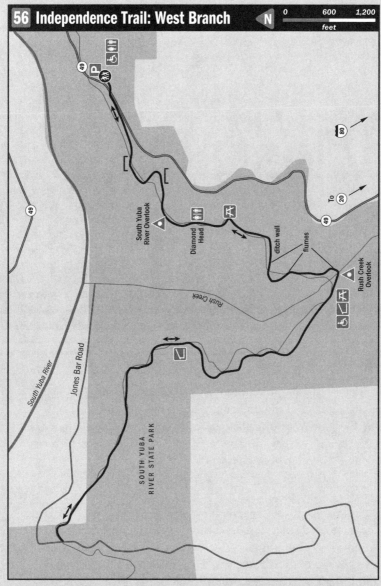

0   600   1,200
feet

N

49
P

49

80

To
20

49

South Yuba
River Overlook

Diamond
Head

ditch wall

flumes

Rush Creek
Overlook

Rush Creek

South Yuba River

Jones Bar Road

SOUTH YUBA
RIVER STATE PARK

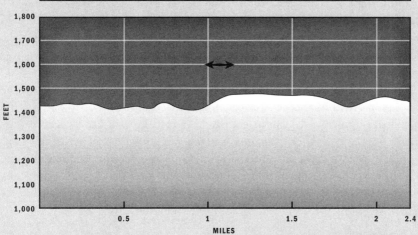

FEET				
1,800				
1,700				
1,600				
1,500				
1,400				
1,300				
1,200				
1,100				
1,000				

0.5   1   1.5   2   2.4

MILES

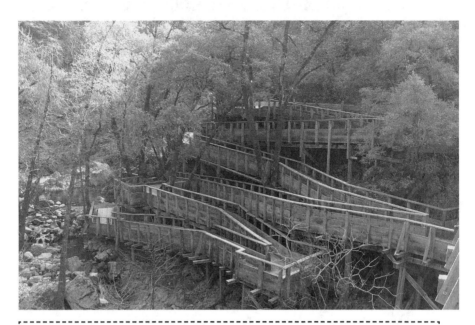

A ramp built in the style of a trestle and ditch flume allows all hikers to access the stream and enjoy the cascades of Rush Creek.

another canal near the present-day Lake Wildwood dam. This nearly level ditch and the maintenance trail beside it are now your route.

The East and West branches share a common trailhead. Your trail, the West Branch, is the more scenic of the two. Signs on the information board will direct you if you've forgotten your compass.

You almost immediately enter a short tunnel to pass safely underneath CA 49. Signs there inform hikers that leashed dogs are permitted on the trail, but bicycles, motorcycles, camping, and fires are not. And beware of the poison oak.

The reinforced fence borders this initial stretch, separating hikers from steep, exposed hillsides. The trail has three distinct segments, which you'll notice from the outset. In the first 0.1 mile, you'll see the stone wall (probably covered with moss and lichen), which is the original wall of the ditch. Adjacent to and slightly above the ditch path is the maintenance trail for the ditch tenders, who monitored the water flow and made repairs. The most unusual features along the path are the flumes—wooden troughs standing on trestles, which carried the water across ravines and other streams.

A bench fashioned from a large tree trunk sits next to the first bridge at the 0.2-mile point. Within another 50 feet, Jones Bar Trail leads north. Stay left on Independence Trail. Notice the incense cedar mixed in with Pacific madrone as you make your way down to the next bridge and another log bench.

Look closely for the interpretive signs for the towering ponderosa pine, canyon live oak, and Kellogg black oak that surround the scenic South Yuba River Overlook, which you'll reach after 0.4 mile. Here is a nice shelter in case of sudden showers.

As you walk 500 feet on, notice the deerbrush and manzanita bushes shading you from even the low morning sun. A series of ramps lead you to Diamond Head—a Class A outhouse at the 0.5-mile point in your hike.

You'll have the sensation of descending into the canyon, but it's an illusion caused by CA 49 climbing the hill as the trail stays level. As the sound of cars falls away, you'll notice more and more ferns, mosses, and lichens along the rock walls. Amble 500 feet more and you'll come upon ramps leading to a nice picnic table. So far you've traveled 0.6 mile.

Look up at the Douglas fir now towering over you and the bigleaf maple shading you when its leaves are full. In the next few hundred feet you'll notice the air becoming cooler where moist, moss-covered rocks surround you. These rocks remain as they were when laid more than 150 years ago. Although reconstructed, Flumes 26 and 27 are identical in design to the water-carrying structures of the Gold Rush days. By the time you reach Flume 27, you'll have walked just about 1 mile.

Your south-facing trail still gets plenty of shade from the surrounding manzanita and may be muddy in some spots along here. If you look carefully, you'll probably spot a California newt. The male newt may puff himself up, showing his reddish abdomen, but his defense is in his skin, whose coating is toxic to humans. Take a photo and leave him alone.

California buckeyes line the path here as you come upon another small shelter, which provides a shaded overlook to the South Yuba River below.

The best site, Flume 28, is still ahead about 500 feet. Its horseshoe shape illustrates exactly how the ditch builders shortcut most ravines by building a trestle with a flume atop it. This flume is special in that it allows easy access to the pool at the base of the cascades of Rush Creek. This is truly an idyllic spot for everyone. In winter, the ice clings to the rocks surrounding the pond, and in spring, water shoots with a roar across the rocks that these ramps overlook. Benches; a shelter; wide, shallow ramps; and a tree-shaded pool—spectacular. Here's where you're sure to linger, where children will run and splash, and where everyone can reach the stream below the cascades.

As you leave Rush Creek the trail turns north, contouring along the opposite side of the ravine. If you're ready for a snack, picnic tables are about 200 steps ahead. Ramps lead to the tables and to an outhouse at the end of the platform.

The trail ends at Jones Bar Road, an obvious turnaround spot. Retrace your steps to the trailhead, or drop down to Jones Bar and the beaches along the river.

NEARBY ACTIVITIES

Empire Mine State Park in Grass Valley features a museum and visitor center displaying a complete mining history for the Mother Lode and specifically the Empire Mine. The Hardrock Trail (Hike 54, page 276) explores the Empire Mine and several others that were operated in the same area.

57 BUTTERMILK BEND TRAIL

KEY AT-A-GLANCE INFORMATION

LENGTH: 2.5 miles

CONFIGURATION: Out-and-back

DIFFICULTY: Easy

WATER REQUIRED: 1 liter

SCENERY: Spectacular views of the South Yuba River

EXPOSURE: Partially shaded trail with exposed areas

TRAIL TRAFFIC: Moderate

TRAIL SURFACE: Dirt, sand, and rock

HIKING TIME: 1.5 hours

SEASON: Year-round, sunrise–sunset

ACCESS: No fees or permits

MAPS: USGS French Corral

WHEELCHAIR ACCESS: None

FACILITIES: Toilets in parking area and at nearby visitor center

DRIVING DISTANCE: 62.5 miles

SPECIAL COMMENTS: If you want more exercise and a different view of the river, take the Point Defiance Trail (see next profile) 1 mile to Englebright Lake and return. It begins across the road and about 100 yards down at a signed trailhead adjacent to the covered bridge.

GPS TRAILHEAD COORDINATES

Latitude   N39° 17.593´

Longitude   W121° 11.550´

IN BRIEF

Prepare for extraordinary views of the South Yuba River from rock benches along this easy trail. Here, the riparian zone holds somewhat closely to the river's edge, quickly transitioning to a foothill-woodland zone upslope. The result is a transition zone that boasts the best of both zones. The abundance of flowers and trees along this short, friendly trail makes this a favorite foothill hike for all ages.

DESCRIPTION

Starting your trip from the second parking lot is easier, but whether you park here or back across the river next to the bridge, take time to cross the Bridgeport Bridge—the longest single-span covered bridge in America. Built in 1862, it's one of only ten covered bridges left in California. Made from Douglas fir and covered with sugar-pine shingles, the bridge's double-truss-and-hoop construction is unique. The only other bridge of its design was built in New York State. Information in the visitor center explains how this bridge's architecture is responsible for its strength, durability, and beauty.

Directions ⟶

From the junction of I-80 East and the Capital City Freeway, drive 24 miles on I-80 East toward Auburn and take Exit 119B/Grass Valley. Take CA 49 North about 23 miles toward Marysville and exit on CA 20 East. Take CA 20 East 7.5 miles to Pleasant Valley Road, then bear right and drive 7.7 miles, passing Lake Wildwood, to the Bridgeport Visitor Center. Park in the lot on your left just past the large barn, or continue across the bridge and park in the lot on your right, on the road, or directly in front of the trailhead, next to the toilets.

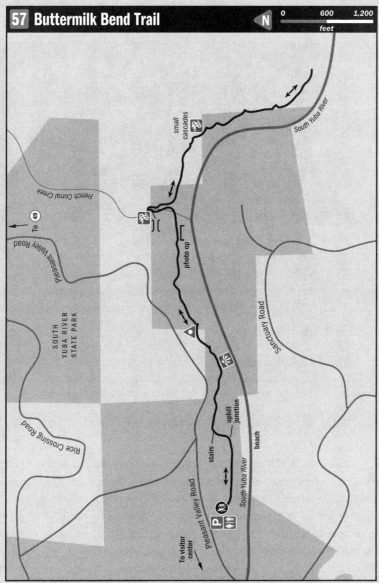

N

0   600   1,200
feet

South Yuba River

small
cascades

French Corral Creek

To 49

Pleasant Valley Road

SOUTH
YUBA
RIVER
STATE
PARK

photo op

Sanctuary Road

Rice Crossing Road

uphill junction

stairs

beach

South Yuba River

Pleasant Valley Road

To visitor
center

P

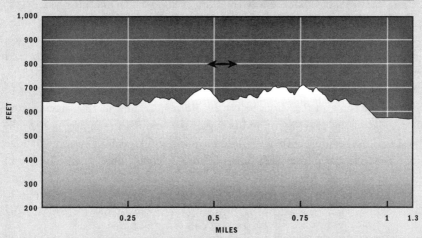

1,000
900
800
700
600
500
400
300
200

FEET

0.25   0.5   0.75   1   1.3

MILES

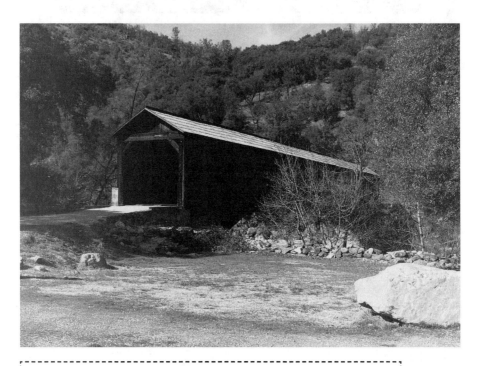

The Bridgeport Bridge is the longest wooden single-span covered bridge in America.

Your trailhead is near the toilets in the north parking lot. If you parked here, the trail is obvious. If, however, you parked next to the visitor center, traverse the bridge and turn right onto the path leading past the picnic table and information sign; then walk through the gate and cross the road to the north lot.

Signs warn of rattlesnakes and mountain lions along this trail. These are sensible warnings for the area, despite this being such an easy trail. Colorful poison oak is particularly common along spots of this trail as well.

The trail initially rises above the river so gradually that you might miss some of the interpretive signs that identify the flora along the trail and hillsides. Beginning in March, California poppies, popcorn flowers, larkspurs, shooting stars, fiddlenecks, and blue dicks are splashed across the slopes above and below you and at every seep and spring coming in from your left. Stop frequently to read about them. Smell them endlessly. But leave them to grow, as the park requests. The more seeds that fall, the more flowers that spring.

Your trail is about 75 yards below an alternate trailhead that starts at the northeast end of the parking lot and occupies the original flume dug in the hillside in 1877. You can use either route to begin or end your hike. Looking above the trail to the left, you may see some of those original flume works. Your trail will join with that leg shortly.

The trail runs above the river along an abrupt precipice—the smooth wire fence to your right is there to steady your nerves. As you begin to notice the enormous cobble littering the river in front of you, the trail will ascend a short hill. At the top of this rise, a side trail to the right descends to the river.

Follow the trail uphill to the left, past the miner's lettuce and flowering redbud. Directly after this junction, you should be able to see some stairs ahead of you. Get ready for a quick elevation gain—these 35 stairs carry you up to some switchbacks on an exposed slope. The dirt path, quite well defined now, will soon be joined from the left by the upper trail. You're now in the original flume, and the trail will remain level to its end.

When you can distinctly hear the river, just as the trail turns northeast, you'll have a great view of the pools and beach below. In another 20 steps, you'll come to a bench cut into the rock. Purple spring vetch, orange California poppy, and white canyon nemophila grow around you at this up-canyon viewpoint.

Another side trail, with stairs at the top, leads down to the river. Your path continues northeast, and you'll find a stone bench right at the bend in the trail marked by the large foothill pine. The view overlooking the cascades is fantastic.

Continue eastward, with miniature lupine and bird's-foot fern lining the trail. A small ravine has been strengthened by some recent rockwork above and below the trail. Another vantage point—allowing you to see around Buttermilk Bend—is outfitted with another stone bench. The cascades below make for a great picture.

After walking north for a few minutes, you'll cross a bridge over the ravine at French Corral Creek. The bridge is wide, and you can linger to watch the water cascading above and below. You can also head left after crossing the bridge to sit on the rocks and observe the streamside insect activity.

After crossing the bridge, make a U-turn to exit the ravine. Look back to the obvious stonework on the opposite side of the bridge, and now look on your side for similar formations. These are the abutments for the original flume that crossed the ravine.

As you leave the ravine, look for zigzag larkspur, popcorn flower, and blue dick around the rock outcropping. The toyon has been trimmed back but still shades much of the trail. Blue oak and foothill pine also ensure a cool hike.

Depending on the season, you may see relics of the gold-mining era other than your trail. The stone fireplace, about 50 feet below the trail, may indicate a dwelling more permanent than a tent—a home or a boarding house. The large metal pieces that look like monitor pipes are said to be sections of a hoist for moving rocks.

Just 1.25 miles on, South Yuba River State Park abruptly ends. You can descend one of two trails that angle toward boulders as big as midsize cars. After exploring at the river, retrace your steps to the trailhead.

NEARBY ACTIVITIES

The Kneebone Family Cemetery and the Bridgeport Barn are on the grounds of the nearby Bridgeport Visitor Center.

58 POINT DEFIANCE TRAIL

KEY AT-A-GLANCE INFORMATION

LENGTH: 2 miles

CONFIGURATION: Out-and-back

DIFFICULTY: Moderate

WATER REQUIRED: 1 liter

SCENERY: Riparian woodland and close-up river views

EXPOSURE: Well shaded

TRAIL TRAFFIC: Busy

TRAIL SURFACE: Sand, dirt, and rock

HIKING TIME: 1 hour

SEASON: Year-round; parking sunrise–sunset

ACCESS: No fees or permits

MAPS: USGS French Corral

WHEELCHAIR ACCESS: None

FACILITIES: Toilets at visitor center; picnic area and toilet at destination

DRIVING DISTANCE: 62.5 miles

SPECIAL COMMENTS: Combine this hike with the Buttermilk Bend Trail (see previous profile) for spectacular up-canyon views. The trailhead lies at the end of the longest wooden single-span covered bridge in America.

GPS TRAILHEAD COORDINATES

Latitude   N39° 17.592´

Longitude   W121° 11.692´

IN BRIEF

Point Defiance Trail is a cool riverside adventure with side trips to pebble-covered beaches. Watch the South Yuba River as it swings from bank to bank toward Harry L. Englebright Lake.

DESCRIPTION

The Point Defiance Trail is a straight, short shot downriver and back. A mere 1 mile long one-way, this trail takes you by beaches, rapids, and quiet riffles as you hike over river cobble, through rockslide debris, and under a pleasant riparian-woodland canopy.

Finding your trailhead is rarely this straightforward—as long as you can park anywhere within sight of both the barn and the covered bridge, it's a cinch. With the barn to your back, walk through the bridge to the opposite side of the river. The trailhead is uphill to your left.

This trail is also known as the Englebright Lake Trail because Point Defiance is actually a point on the South Yuba where the lake reaches farthest upriver. The dam itself was

----

Directions ⟶

From the junction of I-80 East and the Capital City Freeway, drive 24 miles on I-80 East toward Auburn and take Exit 119B/Grass Valley. Take CA 49 North about 23 miles toward Marysville and exit on CA 20 East. Take CA 20 East 7.5 miles to Pleasant Valley Road, then bear right and drive 7.7 miles, passing Lake Wildwood, to the Bridgeport Visitor Center. Park in the lot on the left, just past the large barn, or continue across the bridge and park in either the lot on your right or on the road. Your trailhead is through the bridge, on the left as you emerge on the opposite bank.

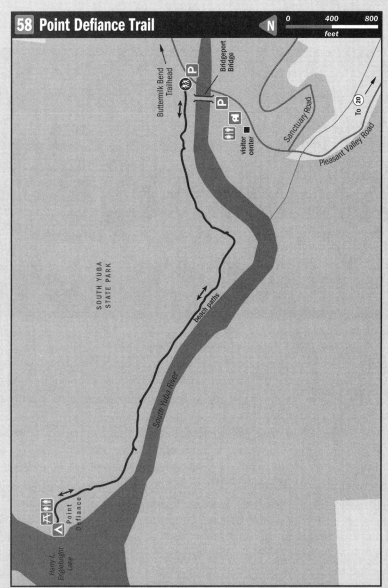

58 Point Defiance Trail

N

0   400   800
feet

Buttermilk Bend Trailhead

Bridgeport Bridge

Sanctuary Road

To 20

Pleasant Valley Road

P

P

visitor center

SOUTH YUBA STATE PARK

South Yuba River

beach paths

Point Defiance

Harry L. Englebright Lake

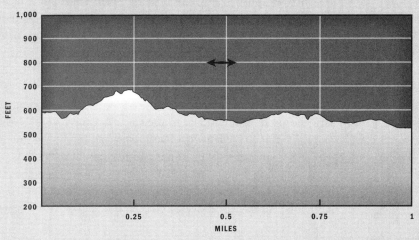

FEET

1,000
900
800
700
600
500
400
300
200

0.25   0.5   0.75   1

MILES

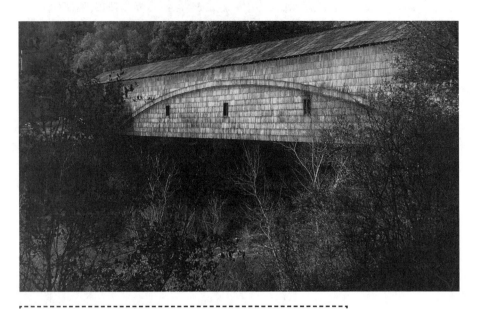

Sugar-pine shingles cover the Bridgeport Bridge's hoop-and-truss frame.

built in 1941 to catch the debris from mining operations in the South Yuba drainage. Your hike takes in the last portion of the South Yuba before the river joins the Middle Fork of the Yuba and slows as it enters the lake.

Your dirt-and-rock trail will wind along within 30 feet of the river among manzanita, toyon, and foothill pine. There really is no way to wander off-course unless you take one of the many side trails down to the beaches. Some easy access points are noted here. The first access point you'll will come to is within 100 feet of the trailhead. Note that dogs are generally unwelcome on the beaches.

After you spot the initial warning about mountain lions and rattlesnakes in the area, look across to the opposite shore through the live oak and madrone. Your trail may be damp in places because the ravines entering from the right fill each spring.

As you come upon the rapids, the trail will follow the river. Enjoy some nice views of the bar as the river turns southwest. As you overlook the bar after the riffles, you can see another beach that would be quite pleasant after a spring runoff. Watch your footing on the loose rock in this area as you gain elevation. When you cross the jumble of rocks and boulders around 0.25 mile, you're crossing the result of rockslides rather than flooding.

Just after the river and the trail turn northwest (after about 0.4 mile), you may notice a singletrack footpath leading down to the river. Another, easier path is ahead. The beach is a nice strand of coarse sand and river cobble.

As the river approaches your trail to within about 15 feet, you'll see boulders the size of compact cars, signaling a quiet area. Flood debris can be seen above your head in the oak and madrone branches. When the trail gains height on the river, notice how the channel narrows between your bank and the bar—water

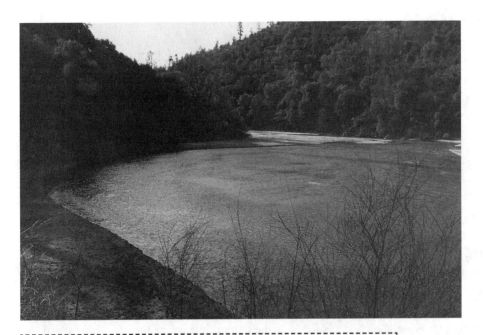

The current slows noticeably as it hits the waters of the upper end of Englebright Lake..

squeezing into such a small gap causes it to accelerate and shoot out downstream. That's the basic theory of the hydraulic-mining technique that uses a monitor: large intake pipes upstream and successively smaller diameter pipes farther and farther downstream build pressure, which is released at the monitor at a very high speed and pressure capable of decimating the hillsides.

As you near the end of the trail, the river becomes noticeably broader and calmer. You'll also catch sight of a broad patch of blackberry bushes just before you cross another jumble of boulders. A junction with a path angling left signals the picnic area. Enjoy the beach just past the composting toilet. Your return is the way you came in. If you desire some different vistas, you can continue as this track becomes a fire road and turns, climbing northeast to continue 1.7 more miles in a loop back to the bridge.

NEARBY ACTIVITIES

For a much different view of the South Yuba River, hike the Buttermilk Bend Trail, which starts from the parking lot across the road. See the previous profile for details on this view of the river.

Take a walk through the historic remains around the Bridgeport Visitor Center. A forty-niner with a very colorful story—but one not uncommon at the time—founded Bridgeport: in 1849 William Thompson, a ship's captain, abandoned his vessel in San Francisco Bay to go with his wife to the gold fields. They settled here, and their descendants live nearby and maintain the cemetery to the southwest of the visitor center.

59 HUMBUG TRAIL

KEY AT-A-GLANCE INFORMATION

LENGTH: 5.6 miles

CONFIGURATION: Out-and-back

DIFFICULTY: Moderate

WATER REQUIRED: 1–2 liters

SCENERY: Foothill woodland

EXPOSURE: Sun and shade

TRAIL TRAFFIC: Moderate

TRAIL SURFACE: Dirt, duff, rock

HIKING TIME: 2–3 hours

SEASON: Year-round, sunrise–sunset

ACCESS: $8 day-use fee

MAPS: USGS North Bloomfield; local trail map at the museum

WHEELCHAIR ACCESS: None

FACILITIES: Limited parking at the trailhead; restrooms, picnic tables, telephone, water in North Bloomfield

DRIVING DISTANCE: 77 miles

SPECIAL COMMENTS: Dogs are prohibited on California State Park trails.

GPS TRAILHEAD COORDINATES

Latitude   N39° 21.920′

Longitude   W120° 55.409′

IN BRIEF

Humbug Trail generally follows the course of Humbug Creek and often the path of the North Bloomfield Tunnel as well. You will pass close to one of the 200-foot shafts leading down to the tunnel, and you can dally along the creek, where the gold-separation flume used to be. This steadily descending trail winds along a wooded canyon and leads to a pleasant bench overlooking the South Yuba River.

DESCRIPTION

Whether you've come for the mining history, the natural history, or the plain old lure of the South Yuba on a hot day, hiking this trail is one of the most pleasant ways to justify descending 800-plus feet in 2.8 miles. This path has a fairly constant grade as it descends, with a slight steepening about halfway along.

Directions

From the junction of I-80 and the Capital City Freeway, drive 24 miles on I-80 East toward Auburn and take Exit 119C/Elm Avenue. Turn left at the light, onto Elm Avenue, and take CA 49 North 26 miles toward Nevada City. Continue on CA 49 by turning left toward Downieville. Drive 11 miles, then turn right onto Tyler–Foote Road, where you'll see a sign for Malakoff Diggins State Historic Park. Continue on Tyler–Foote Road 17 miles to the park. The name of the road will change to Cruzon Grade Road and then to Backbone Road. Turn right on Durbec Road into the park. Signs will lead you to the North Bloomfield town site. From the hotel in the center of town, drive west on North Bloomfield Road 1.25 miles to the information sign on the right, where you can learn about the famous tunnel. The trailhead is another 0.15 mile ahead, on the south side of the road. Some parking is available on the right, next to the hiker sign.

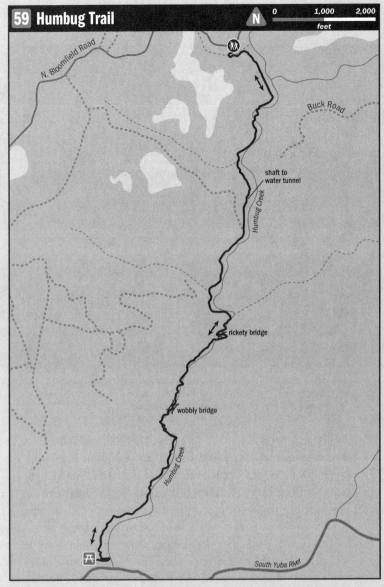

N

0   1,000   2,000
feet

N. Bloomfield Road

Buck Road

shaft to
water tunnel

Humbug Creek

rickety bridge

wobbly bridge

Humbug Creek

South Yuba River

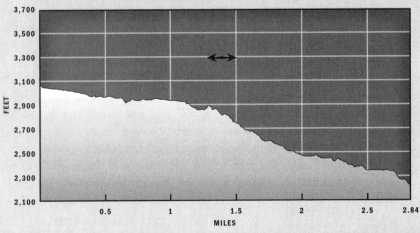

FEET							
3,700							
3,500							
3,300							
3,100							
2,900							
2,700							
2,500							
2,300							
2,100							

0.5   1   1.5   2   2.5   2.84

MILES

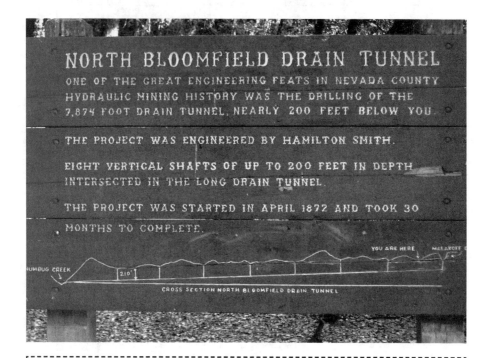

NORTH BLOOMFIELD DRAIN TUNNEL
ONE OF THE GREAT ENGINEERING FEATS IN NEVADA COUNTY
HYDRAULIC MINING HISTORY WAS THE DRILLING OF THE
7,874 FOOT DRAIN TUNNEL, NEARLY 200 FEET BELOW YOU.

THE PROJECT WAS ENGINEERED BY HAMILTON SMITH.

EIGHT VERTICAL SHAFTS OF UP TO 200 FEET IN DEPTH
INTERSECTED IN THE LONG DRAIN TUNNEL.

THE PROJECT WAS STARTED IN APRIL 1872 AND TOOK 30
MONTHS TO COMPLETE.

CROSS SECTION NORTH BLOOMFIELD DRAIN TUNNEL

An engineering marvel in its day, the North Bloomfield Drain Tunnel made it profitable to clog rivers, canyons, and farmland with rocks and mud while digging for gold.

Your track starts on the south side of North Bloomfield Road, as the sign indicates. Drop off the road into a lush foothill woodland of Ponderosa pine, bay laurel, black oak, Douglas fir, incense cedar, and dozens of understory trees and shrubs. Traverse southwest initially, cross a small stream, and then swing east back toward the creek before you settle into a generally southerly course along it.

If you had a moment to stop at the kiosk illustrating the North Bloomfield Drain Tunnel, you have a good idea of this simple plan: basically, keep the bathtub tap always on and keep the drain always open. The gaping maw of a drain hole below Diggins Pond sends water, mud, and rock into the tunnel and down to the South Yuba River. Within 5 minutes of walking, you'll cross a causeway that allows you to stay out of the horrid-looking liquid (which I suppose is water) as it exits the Diggins. Imagine tons of this stuff flowing into the Yuba daily.

As you roughly follow the creek along its steep descent, the canyon broadens after the first 0.5 mile, providing more picturesque vistas. The track has some minor ups and downs, but they're minimal since the trail doesn't have to traverse many ravines. At about 0.65 mile along, you do cross a seasonal stream; just 0.1 mile after that, keep an eye out for some shabby fencing on the left, meant to keep people away from the 200-foot-deep shaft it surrounds (or once did).

Over the next 0.5 mile, generally hiking under cover of shade, you'll climb and descend a bit, coming in and out of a runoff stream. Your views of Humbug Creek change—from "Where is it?" to "Look at that bedrock!"—until you drop right down to it. After that runoff stream, cross some boulders, thickly coated with moss, and then take a few simple switchbacks down to the creek, now just 1.3 miles along. Here at the halfway point, you have some excellent down-canyon views.

Over the next 0.2 mile, depending on the time of year and the amount of snowmelt, your views of the creek and its cascades are stunning. The trail climbs away from the creek, and as you gain about 75 feet on the creek, look back to see the changing face of the cascades. As the canyon narrows and runs out of turf, a convenient, albeit rickety bridge lets you wobble your way around rock outcrops as they bulge into the canyon. In less than 0.25 mile, you'll come to another wooden vista point that similarly wiggles beneath you as you traverse it.

In 0.1 mile, you can visit the creek at the point where the gold-collection flume was once situated. You can still see spikes driven into the bedrock to anchor the flumeworks.

Past those magnificent sights and fun bridge crossings, it's just like falling in slow motion down to a leaf-littered bench perched about 40 feet above the South Yuba River. From this point—actually on the South Yuba River Trail—the vistas range from slightly upriver to well downriver. A trail leads to the rocky beaches below, at which point the river narrows and you can reach the opposite bank before your feet freeze. You can stay in the sun at the river's edge or retreat to this spot where two picnic tables sit under constant shade, thanks to the ponderosa pine and live oak.

NEARBY ACTIVITIES

If you haven't done so already, take a walk through the North Bloomfield town site and over to the cemetery via the Church Trail. For more information on the Diggins Loop Trail and the Slaughterhouse Trail–Town Trail loop, see the next profile.

60 DIGGINS LOOP TRAIL

KEY AT-A-GLANCE INFORMATION

LENGTH: 5.4 miles

CONFIGURATION: Connected loops

DIFFICULTY: Moderate

WATER REQUIRED: 2 liters

SCENERY: Views of hillsides removed by mining operations

EXPOSURE: Very sunny

TRAIL TRAFFIC: Light

TRAIL SURFACE: Gravel, dirt and duff, sand

HIKING TIME: 2–3 hours

SEASON: Year-round, sunrise–sunset

ACCESS: $8 day-use fee

MAPS: USGS North Bloomfield, Pike. A local trail map and brochure are available at the museum.

WHEELCHAIR ACCESS: None

FACILITIES: Restrooms, picnic tables, telephone, bear-proof garbage bins, and snacks at town site

DRIVING DISTANCE: 77 miles

SPECIAL COMMENTS: Pay parking fee or self-register at the museum. Dogs are prohibited on California State Park trails. Malakoff Diggins State Historic Park will close in 2012 or 2013 for budgetary reasons. However, the hiking trails will remain open and the gates will be unlocked.

GPS TRAILHEAD COORDINATES

Latitude   N39° 22.075´

Longitude   W120° 54.053´

IN BRIEF

Your hike begins at the historic town of North Bloomfield, then passes the old school, church, and cemetery on the way to a loop through Diggins Pond, the scene of intense hydraulic mining. The route then climbs to the rim overlook before returning to the town site and your original trailhead.

DESCRIPTION

Gold was first plucked by hand from the rivers; then it was drilled for and dug from hard rock. Here's the best example of how the hills were blown apart and washed away by water to reach the gold-bearing gravels. Your trail loops through the floor of the diggings and then heads up to the rim to give you a bird's-eye view of the area, its devastation, and its recovery.

Gold was discovered in the creeks and hills in the surrounding area, but its extraction from the ore-bearing gravels was inefficient and uneconomical. When three mining partners devised a method to deliver water to their diggings to process the gravels, a new and

----

Directions

From the junction of I-80 and the Capital City Freeway, drive 24 miles on I-80 East toward Auburn and take Exit 119C/Elm Avenue. Turn left at the light, onto Elm Avenue, and take CA 49 North 26 miles toward Nevada City. Continue on CA 49 by turning left toward Downieville. Drive 11 miles, then turn right onto Tyler–Foote Road, where you will see a sign for Malakoff Diggins State Historic Park. Continue on Tyler–Foote Road 17 miles to the park. The name of the road will change to Cruzon Grade Road and then to Backbone Road. Turn right on Durbec Road into the park. Signs will lead you to the North Bloomfield town site.

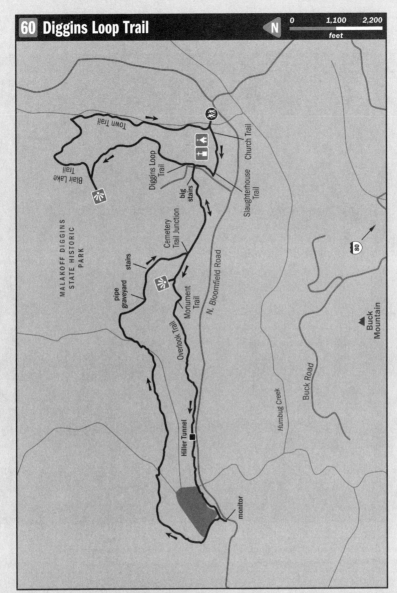

0   1,100   2,200
feet

N

MALAKOFF DIGGINS
STATE HISTORIC
PARK

Town Trail

Blair Lake Trail

Diggins Loop Trail

big stairs

Cemetery Trail Junction

stairs

pipe graveyard

Overlook Trail

Monument Trail

N. Bloomfield Road

Slaughterhouse Church Trail

Hiller Tunnel

monitor

Humbug Creek

Buck Road

Buck Mountain

80

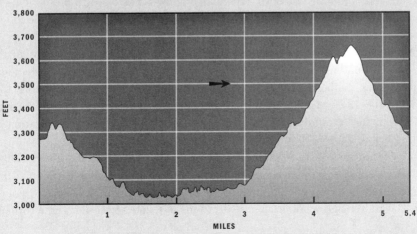

FEET

3,800
3,700
3,600
3,500
3,400
3,300
3,200
3,100
3,000

1   2   3   4   5.4

MILES

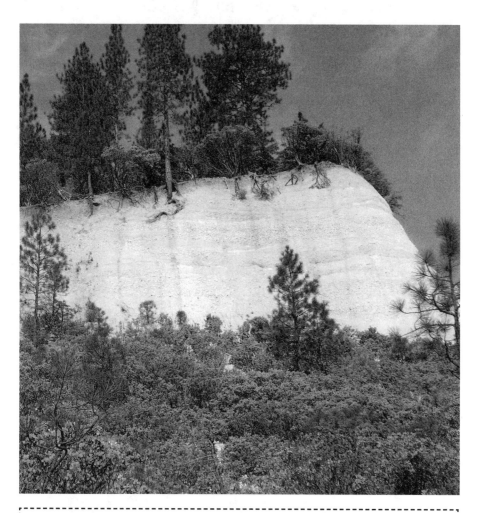

These trees were moments away from being washed away by a monitor's spray when operations ceased a century-and-a-quarter ago.

cheap method of mining was born. Hydraulic mining came to North Bloomfield—originally called Humbug because of its poor production—and the landscape soon changed forever.

Walk around the town of North Bloomfield, which boasts several original and restored buildings along with displays of the huge water cannons known as monitors. Your trailhead sits across the street from two of the giant monitors, to the left of the 1870 McKillican and Mobley General Store, at the bridge among the "Clampicnic" grounds (erected by E Clampus Vitus, a fraternal organization). The trail begins across the footbridge next to yet another monitor.

The trailhead is actually the starting point for two trails: the Town Trail, which leads uphill—you'll be returning via this trail—and the Church Trail, which leads to the cemetery. Walk 0.2 mile up to the cemetery, with the fence to your right. The church and schoolhouse are off to the left, and a trail sign at the corner of the fence indicates that your trail goes onto Diggins Loop Trail. Five hundred feet down the trail is your marker to turn left on Diggins Loop. Your trail winds downhill under foothill pine, white fir, and Douglas fir. A set of large steps cut into the trail will help you down toward the floor of the diggings.

As you pass some large piles of cobble and gravel, the trail is very distinct. This is not always the case. You are entering what is essentially a giant bathtub, with a drain at the far west end. After every rain, the sand-and-gravel trail can get washed and shifted around. The trail is mostly distinguishable because it is made of compacted gravel that often looks like a sidewalk, but it can become rather indistinct at times. The park has done a good job of placing trail signs at just about every point at which a hiker would wonder where the trail goes.

At the obvious crossing, continue to walk straight across the road. A trail sign will help you, but it isn't visible until you cross. Another sign, just ahead, will direct hikers onto either the north or south portion of the trail. The described hike takes the south fork and proceeds clockwise around the basin.

Pass some old discarded mining gear, nozzles, and pipes as you walk to a vista point on the right. While you're still a bit above the floor, this vantage point affords a breathtaking view of the basin and surrounding hills. As you hike west along the gravel path, watch for rattlesnakes—they seem to be plentiful in the diggings.

Trail signs will keep you going in the right direction as you continue west past a side trail to the monument honoring the North Bloomfield Gravel and Mining Company, the "creators" of the Malakoff Diggins site. After a junction with another spur trail coming from the overlook parking, you again pass discarded and rusting pipes, monitor stands, and other mining gear surrounded by the encroaching manzanita.

After you've walked 2 miles, notice the sign on the right of this packed-dirt trail, which points out the entrance to the Hiller Tunnel. Water that entered the diggings was drained through here. Just downhill to the right, in a shaded, grassy area, is the opening to the small tunnel; during dry times, you can walk its entire length. Insufficient for the amount of water that needed to be drained, the Hiller Tunnel was replaced in 1874 by the 8,000-foot-long North Bloomfield Tunnel, an engineering feat at the time.

Another trail sign at the west end of the loop marks the intersection with the West Point Trail. Leave the loop for a few hundred feet to see another monitor, which appears to have been left in the position it was on the day operations ceased. The water-supply pipe, which runs downhill, is still connected to the monitor. (Contemporary photos of the diggings match closely to the facts on the ground today.) Continue north along the stark white "hillsides." These are excellent displays of the alluvial sands and gravels that contained gold.

Your walk along the north side of the loop is less well defined and requires a bit more route-finding than does the trek along the south side. The local map and a compass will help, though they're not a necessity. Trail markers have been placed quite frequently, but only a few are visible from one marker to the next. Generally, you will follow the base of the cliffs as you walk across wet, sandy stretches of trail. When the trail turns away from the cliffs, it follows a gravel stream (or the trail merely becomes a gravel stream) for several hundred feet. Four-inch-square posts topped with yellow paint serve as markers to help guide you. The thick willows here are fringed with bush lupine; both often conceal the markers. Keep your eyes open and anticipate the path's course, and you won't have any real difficulty. Waterproof footwear is a real bonus on the north side.

When you can see a large white needle of sandstone, you'll have hiked about 3.5 miles. The trail along here is quite indistinct (especially so the day after a rain), so you will need to mind the markers to stay on course. Take a look at the small metal tab on the side of each post. The tabs are labeled N-15, N-16, N-17, and so on. When you reach N-18, turn south-southeast to stay on track.

Another pipe graveyard follows the trail's uphill turn to the east. The pipes, made from riveted steel, are 1–2 feet in diameter. Follow some trail signs up a stony wash and a stairway set into the hill. When you reach the next intersection, you'll recognize it as the north–south split you crossed earlier. Take the big steps uphill to the junction with the Slaughterhouse Trail. You can return to the trailhead via the Church Trail by retracing your steps, or you can hike up the Slaughterhouse Trail to get an excellent view of the diggings from the rim.

Turn left at this junction and hike uphill for about 0.5 mile. The last few hundred feet will have you huffing a bit as you intersect the road. Turn left onto this paved road. The overlook is marked another few hundred feet up to the left. After your side trip to the overlook, turn left again when you return to the pavement, and walk past the group campground, on your left.

Your trail to return to the town site is opposite the covered assembly area next to the group campground. A trail sign past the toilets marks the head of the Town Trail and points the way to Blair Lake Trail. Turn right and head downhill, passing the amphitheater on your left. The dirt-and-duff trail is a cool and shady respite from the openly exposed trail in the diggings, but it still offers plenty to discover. Rusted scoops, buckets, pipes, and cables—some partially buried, some not—are hard evidence that the mining here was not done by individuals (as panning was) but rather undertaken on an industrial scale.

Just before you cross a small footbridge, you'll see a marker indicating your right turn onto the Town Trail. You'll descend along a creek to your left through thick cover of Douglas fir, foothill pine, and incense cedar. In about 0.5 mile, you'll emerge from the trees at the trailhead bridge, where your hike originated.

NEARBY ACTIVITIES

The Humbug Trail (see previous profile) leads inquisitive hikers down 1,000 feet over the course of 3 miles from the diggings to the South Yuba River. Historic mining relics can be seen along the way, and pleasant pools adorn the river.

APPENDIXES

APPENDIX A:
OUTDOOR SHOPS

BIG 5 SPORTING GOODS
big5sportinggoods.com
2556 Grass Valley
Auburn, CA 95603
530-887-8326

4794 Manzanita Ave., Ste. 1
Carmichael, CA 95608
916-972-1067

7833 Greenback Lane
Citrus Heights, CA 95610
916-726-5566

1301 W. Covell Blvd.
Davis, CA 95616
530-758-7731

6608 Laguna Blvd.
Elk Grove, CA 95758
916-691-9112

1902 N. Texas St.
Fairfield, CA 94533
707-426-5026

606 E. Bidwell St.
Folsom, CA 95630
916-984-7148

123 W. McKnight Way
Grass Valley, CA 95949
530-274-1562

2411 W. Kettlemen Lane
Lodi, CA 95242
209-366-1514

3637 Elkhorn Blvd.
North Highlands, CA 95660
916-332-6511

284 Placerville Road
Placerville, CA 95667
530-295-8290

10755 Folsom Blvd.
Rancho Cordova, CA 95670
916-852-0898

1909 Douglas Blvd.
Roseville, CA 95661
916-773-4773

3420 Arden Way
Sacramento, CA 95825
916-488-5060

980 Florin Road, Suite A
Sacramento, CA 95831
916-393-1831

6251 Mack Road
Sacramento, CA 95823
916-427-0978

1053 March Lane
Stockton, CA 95207
209-957-3095

2030 Harbison Drive
Vacaville, CA 95687
707-452-0168

431 Pioneer Ave.
Woodland, CA 95776
530-669-7013

1252 Colusa Ave.
Yuba City, CA 95991
530-671-3410

REI
2425 Iron Point Road
Folsom, CA 95630
916-817-8944
rei.com/stores/86

1148 Galleria Blvd.
Roseville, CA 95678
916-724-6750
rei.com/stores/74

1790 Expo Parkway
Sacramento, CA 95815
916-924-8900
rei.com/stores/21

SPORT CHALET
sportchalet.com
8511 Bond Road
Elk Grove, CA 95624
916-714-5740

10349 Fairway Drive
Roseville, CA 95678
916-773-6828

2401 Butano Drive
Sacramento, CA 95825
916-977-1730

SPORTS AUTHORITY
sportsauthority.com
8217 Laguna Blvd.
Elk Grove, CA 95758
916-691-4380

2799 E. Bidwell St.,
Building M-10
Folsom, CA 95630
916-983-5821

6740 Stanford Ranch Road
Roseville, CA 95678
916-789-8436

1700 Arden Way
Sacramento, CA 95815
916-564-3400

3631 N. Freeway Blvd.
Sacramento, CA 95834
916-419-3140

APPENDIX B:
MAP SOURCES

ALPENGLOW SPORTS
415 N. Lake Blvd.
Tahoe City, CA 96145
530-583-6917
alpenglowsports.com

BASSETT'S STATION
100 Gold Lake Road
Sierra City, CA 96125
530-862-1297
bassetts-station.com

CALIFORNIA SURVEYING AND DRAFTING SUPPLY, INC.
4733 Auburn Blvd.
Sacramento, CA 95841
916-344-0232
csdsinc.com

CHICO SPORTS LTD.
698 Mangrove Ave.
Chico, CA 95926
800-875-4583
chicosportsltd.net

EL DORADO NATIONAL FOREST
www.fs.fed.us/r5/eldorado

Headquarters
100 Forni Road
Placerville, CA 95667
530-622-5061

Amador Ranger District
26820 Silver Drive
Pioneer, CA 95666
209-295-4251

Georgetown Ranger District
7600 Wentworth Springs Road
Georgetown, CA 95634
530-333-4312

Pacific Ranger District
7887 Highway 50
Pollock Pines, CA 95726
530-644-2349

Placerville Ranger District
4260 Eight Mile Road
Camino, CA 95709
530-644-2324

FOREST STATIONERS
531 Main St.
Quincy, CA 95971
530-283-2266
foreststationers.com

GRANITE CHIEF SKI & MOUNTAIN SHOP
11368 Donner Pass Road
Truckee, CA 96161
530-587-2809
granitechief.com

JACKSON FAMILY SPORTS
275 E. Highway 88
Jackson, CA 95642
209-223-3890
jacksonfamilysports.com

KITTLE'S OUTDOOR AND SPORT CO.
888 Market St.
Colusa, CA 95932
530-458-4868
kittlesoutdoor.com

MOUNTAIN HARDWARE AND SPORTS
11320 Donner Pass Road
Truckee, CA 96161
530-587-4844
mountainhardwareandsports.com

MOUNTAIN RECREATION INC.
491 E. Main St.
Grass Valley, CA 95945
530-477-8006
mtnrec.com

O.A.R.S.
P.O. Box 67
Angels Camp, CA
209-736-4677
oars.com

PARADISE SURPLUS AND TRADING POST
7691 Skyway
Paradise, CA 95969
530-872-9307

PIONEER MINING SUPPLIES
878 High St.
Auburn, CA 95603
530-823-9000
pioneermining.com

PLACERVILLE NEWS COMPANY
409 Main St.
Placerville, CA 95667
530-622-4510
pvillenews.com

REI
(See page 306 for store locations)

SIERRA NEVADA ADVENTURE CO.
2293 Highway 4
Arnold, CA 95223
209-795-9310

SIERRA WEST LAND SURVEYING
1359 Sand Hill Court
Oakdale, CA 95361
209-845-2773
sierrawestls.com

SODA SPRINGS GENERAL STORE
21719 Donner Pass Road
Soda Springs, CA 95728
530-426-3080
sodaspringsgeneralstore.com

SOPER-WHEELER COMPANY
19855 Barton Hill Road
Strawberry Valley, CA 95981
530-675-2343
soperwheeler.com

STANISLAUS NATIONAL FOREST
fs.usda.gov/stanislaus

Calaveras Ranger District
5519 Highway 4
Hathaway Pines, CA 95233
209-795-1381

Mi-Wok Ranger District
24695 Highway 108
Mi-Wuk Village, CA 95346
209-586-3234

SURPLUS CITY
4515 Pacific Heights Road
Oroville, CA 95965
530-534-9956
surpluscity.com

TAHOE NATIONAL FOREST
fs.usda.gov/tahoe

Headquarters
631 Coyote St.
Nevada City, CA 95959
530-265-4531

American River Ranger District
22830 Foresthill Road
Foresthill, CA 95631
530-367-2224

Sierraville Ranger District
317 S. Lincoln St.
Sierraville, CA 96126
530-994-3401

Truckee Ranger District
10811 Stockrest Springs Road
Truckee, CA 96161
916-587-3558

Yuba River Ranger District
15924 Highway 49
Camptonville, CA 95922
530-288-3231 or 530-478-6253

TAHOE SPORTS LTD.
4008 Lake Tahoe Blvd.
South Lake Tahoe, CA 96150
530-542-4000

U.S. GEOLOGICAL SURVEY
store.usgs.gov

VALLEY SPORTING GOODS
901 N. Carpenter Road
Modesto, CA 95351
209-523-5681
valleysg.com

APPENDIX C:
HIKING ORGANIZATIONS

AMERICAN RIVER CONSERVANCY
348 Highway 49
P.O. Box 562
Coloma, CA 95613
530-621-1224
arconservancy.org/xoops

**AUBURN STATE RECREATION AREA
CANYON KEEPERS**
530-885-3776
canyonkeepers.org

CHICO HIKING ASSOCIATION (Facebook)
tinyurl.com/chicohiking

HIGH SIERRA HIKERS ASSOCIATION
P.O. Box 8920
South Lake Tahoe, CA 96158
highsierrahikers.org

**NORTH FORK AMERICAN RIVER
ALLIANCE**
P.O. Box 292
Gold Run, CA 95717
530-389-8344
nfara.org

PACIFIC CREST TRAIL ASSOCIATION
1331 Garden Highway
Sacramento, CA 95833
916-285-1846
pcta.org

PLACER LAND TRUST
11661 Blocker Drive, Ste. 110
Auburn, CA 95603
530-887-9222
placerlandtrust.org

**SACRAMENTO BACKPACKERS
MEETUP GROUP**
meetup.com/backpackers-121

**SACRAMENTO
HIKERS WITH KIDS GROUP**
meetup.com/Sac-Hikers-With-Kids

SACRAMENTO HIKING MEETUP GROUP
meetup.com/sachikinggroup

SIERRA CLUB MOTHER LODE CHAPTER
801 K St., Ste. 2700
Sacramento, CA 95814
916-557-1100, ext. 119
motherlode.sierraclub.org

SIERRA CLUB PLACER GROUP
P.O. Box 7167
Auburn, CA 95604
916-781-4926
motherlode.sierraclub.org

APPENDIX D:
MANAGING AGENCIES

BUREAU OF LAND MANAGEMENT

Mother Lode Field Office
5152 Hillsdale Circle
El Dorado Hills, CA 95762
916-941-3101
blm.gov/ca/st/en/fo/folsom.html

Ukiah Field Office
2550 N. State St.
Ukiah, CA 95482
07-468-4000
blm.gov/ca/st/en/fo/ukiah/cachecreek.2

**CALIFORNIA DEPARTMENT OF
FISH AND GAME**
dfg.ca.gov

Bay Delta Region Office
7329 Silverado Trail
Napa, CA 94558; 707-944-5500

Grizzly Island Wildlife Complex
2548 Grizzly Island Road
Suisun City, CA 94585
707-425-3828

Spenceville Wildlife Area
530-538-2236

**CALIFORNIA DEPARTMENT OF PARKS
AND RECREATION**
parks.ca.gov

Headquarters
1416 9th St.
Sacramento, CA 95814
916-653-6995

Auburn State Recreation Area
501 El Dorado St.
Auburn, CA 95603
30-885-4527

Calaveras Big Trees State Park
1170 E. Highway 4
Arnold, CA 95223
209-795-2334

Caswell Memorial State Park
28000 S. Austin Road
Ripon, CA 95366
209-599-3810

Empire Mine State Historic Park
10791 E. Empire St.
Grass Valley, CA 95945
530-273-8522

Folsom Lake State Recreation Area
7755 Folsom–Auburn Road
Folsom, CA 95630
916-988-0205

Indian Grinding Rock State Historic Park
14881 Pine Grove–Volcano Road
Pine Grove, CA 95665
209-296-7488

Malakoff Diggins State Historic Park
23579 North Bloomfield Road
Nevada City, CA 95959
530-265-2740
(*Note:* scheduled to close in 2012
or 2013)

**Marshall Gold Discovery State
Historic Park**
310 Back St.
Coloma, CA 95613
916-622-3470

South Yuba River State Park
17660 Pleasant Valley Road
Penn Valley, CA 95946
530-432-2546

CITY OF LODI PARKS & RECREATION
125 N. Stockton St.
Lodi, CA 95240
209-333-6742
www.lodi.gov/parks_rec

COSUMNES RIVER PRESERVE
13501 Franklin Blvd.
Galt, CA 95632
916-684-2816
cosumnes.org

EAST BAY MUNICIPAL UTILITY DISTRICT

Lake Camanche South Shore Recreation Area
11700 Wade Road
Wallace, CA 95252
209-763-5178
camancherecreation.com

Mokelumne Watershed and Recreation Division
5883 E. Camanche Parkway
Campo Seco, CA 95266
209-772-8204
ebmud.com/recreation

EFFIE YEAW NATURE CENTER
2850 San Lorenzo Way
Carmichael, CA 95608
916-489-4918
sacnaturecenter.net

ELDORADO IRRIGATION DISTRICT

Sly Park Recreation Area
P.O. Box 577
Pollock Pines, CA 95726
530-295-6824
eid.org/recreation/trails.htm

PLACER COUNTY PARKS DIVISION
11476 C Ave.
Auburn, CA 95603
916-886-4901
placer.ca.gov/Departments/Facility/Parks.aspx

SACRAMENTO COUNTY DEPARTMENT OF PARKS AND RECREATION
916-875-6961
www.msa2.saccounty.net/parks

SONOMA COUNTY PARKS
2300 County Center Drive, Suite 120
Santa Rosa, CA 95403
707-565-2041
sonoma-county.org/parks

TAHOE NATIONAL FOREST
(See page 308 for contact information)

UNIVERSITY OF CALIFORNIA, DAVIS

UC Davis Arboretum
1 Shields Drive
Davis, CA 95616
530-752-4880
arboretum.ucdavis.edu

UC Davis Natural Reserve System
nrs.ucdavis.edu

U.S. ARMY CORPS OF ENGINEERS

New Hogan Lake
2713 Hogan Dam Road
Valley Springs, CA 95252
209-772-1343
tinyurl.com/newhogan

YOLO COUNTY FLOOD CONTROL AND WATER CONSERVATION DISTRICT
34274 State Highway 16
Woodland, CA 95695-9371
530-662-0265
ycfcwcd.org/waterinfo.html

APPENDIX E:
ADDITIONAL READING

The American River. Auburn, CA: Protect American River Canyons, 2002.

Arno, Stephen F. *Discovering Sierra Trees.* Yosemite, CA: Yosemite Association, 1973.

Basey, Harold E. *Discovering Sierra Reptiles and Amphibians.* Yosemite, CA: Yosemite Association, 2004.

Halfpenny, James. *A Field Guide to Mammal Tracking in North America.* Boulder, CO: Johnson Books, 1986.

Hill, Mary. *Geology of the Sierra Nevada.* Berkeley: University of California Press, 2006.

Horn, Elizabeth L. *Sierra Nevada Wildflowers.* Missoula, Montana: Mountain Press Company, 1998.

Laws, John Muir. *The Laws Field Guide to the Sierra Nevada.* Berkeley: Heyday Books, 2007.

Miller, Millie, and Cyndi Nelson. *Talons: North American Birds of Prey.* Boulder, CO: Johnson Books, 1989.

Murie, Olaus J. *Peterson Field Guide: A Field Guide to Animal Tracks.* Boston: Houghton Mifflin Company, 1974.

Niehaus, Theodore F., and Charles L. Ripper. *Peterson Field Guide: a Field Guide to Pacific States Wildflowers.* Boston: Houghton Mifflin Company, 1976.

Russo, Ron, and Pam Olhausan. *Mammal Finder.* Berkeley, CA: Nature Study Guild, 1987.

Storer, Tracy I., Robert L. Usinger, and David Lukas. *Sierra Nevada Natural History.* Berkeley: University of California Press, 2004.

Thomas, John H., and Dennis R. Parnell. *Native Shrubs of the Sierra Nevada.* Berkeley: University of California Press, 1974.

Underhill, J. E. *Sagebrush Wildflowers.* Blaine, WA: Hancock House, Inc., 1986.

Whitman, Ann H., ed. *Audubon Society Guide: Familiar Trees of North America: Western Region.* New York: Alfred A. Knopf, 1988.

INDEX

Check out these other great titles from
── Menasha Ridge Press! ──

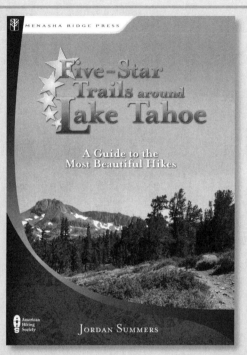

Five-Star Trails Around Lake Tahoe

By Jordan Summers
ISBN: 978-0-89732-959-0
$15.95, 1st Edition

296 pages, 5x7, paperback
maps, photographs, index

Covering the region surrounding the 22-mile-long Lake Tahoe, Jordan Summers guides hikers along 40 of the region's best trails—all within 25 miles of the lake's shoreline. Trekkers can easily find the perfect hike with the complete trail descriptions for 27 day-hike and 13 overnight destinations. An accurate map, directions to the trailhead with GPS coordinates, and an elevation profile of each trail prepare hikers with the full picture of the route ahead. Intended for outdoorspeople of all ages and abilities, *Five-Star Trails Around Lake Tahoe* describes great hikes in the Desolation, Mt. Rose, Granite Chief, and Mokelumne Wilderness areas, as well as along sections of the Pacific Crest National Scenic Trail and portions of the Tahoe Rim Trail. Ranging across forest- and granite-covered terrain to more than a dozen peaks and several dozen lakes, the hike profiles include details on natural history, geologic features, and places of historic note.

With *Five-Star Trails Around Lake Tahoe*, hikers will follow in the footsteps of pioneers such as Kit Carson and the historic Donner Party along the Pony Express Trail and the Emigrant Trail, often with stunning vistas of Lake Tahoe, Emerald Bay, Fallen Leaf Lake, or the Crystal Range.

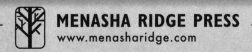

MENASHA RIDGE PRESS
www.menasharidge.com

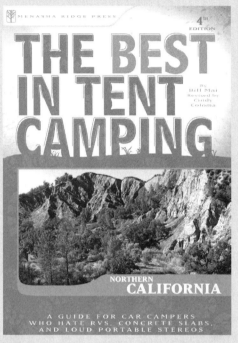

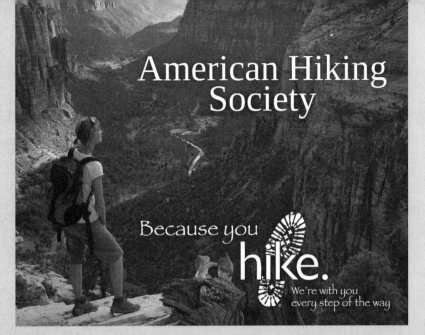

American Hiking Society

Because you hike.
We're with you every step of the way

Since its founding in 1976, **American Hiking Society** has been the only national voice for hikers—dedicated to promoting and protecting America's hiking trails, their surrounding natural areas and the hiking experience. **American Hiking Society** works every day:

- Speaking for hikers in the halls of Congress and with federal land managers
- Building and maintaining hiking trails
- Educating and supporting hikers by providing information and resources
- Supporting hiking and trail organizations nationwide

Whether you're a casual hiker or a seasoned backpacker, become a member of **American Hiking Society** and join the national hiking community! You'll not only enjoy great members-only benefits but you will help ensure the hiking trails you love will remain protected and will be waiting for you the next time you lace up your boots and hit the trail.

American Hiking Society

We invite you to join us today!

1422 Fenwick Lane · Silver Spring, MD 20910 · (800) 972-8608

DEAR CUSTOMERS AND FRIENDS,

SUPPORTING YOUR INTEREST IN OUTDOOR ADVENTURE, travel, and an active lifestyle is central to our operations, from the authors we choose to the locations we detail to the way we design our books. Menasha Ridge Press was incorporated in 1982 by a group of veteran outdoorsmen and professional outfitters. For 25 years now, we've specialized in creating books that benefit the outdoors enthusiast.

Almost immediately, Menasha Ridge Press earned a reputation for revolutionizing outdoors- and travel-guidebook publishing. For such activities as canoeing, kayaking, hiking, backpacking, and mountain biking, we established new standards of quality that transformed the whole genre, resulting in outdoor-recreation guides of great sophistication and solid content. Menasha Ridge continues to be outdoor publishing's greatest innovator.

The folks at Menasha Ridge Press are as at home on a white-water river or mountain trail as they are editing a manuscript. The books we build for you are the best they can be, because we're responding to your needs. Plus, we use and depend on them ourselves.

We look forward to seeing you on the river or the trail. If you'd like to contact us directly, join in at www.trekalong.com or visit us at www.menasharidge.com. We thank you for your interest in our books and the natural world around us all.

SAFE TRAVELS,

BOB SEHLINGER
PUBLISHER